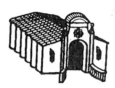

HACIENDA PUBLISHING, INC.

Presents for Review

Vandals at the Gates of Medicine—Historic Perspectives on the Battle over Health Care Reform

Publication Date: November 24, 1994 (Thanksgiving Day; but shipping now).

Edition: First edition.

Specifications: 403 pages, 6 x 9 trim with four-color process dust jacket.

CIP/LC: 94-077392

ISBN: 0-9641077-0-8, book alone, $41.95.

A copy of your review to the address below would be appreciated.

Hacienda Publishing, Inc., P.O. Box 13648, Macon, Georgia, 31208-3648
Telephone: (800)757-9873, Fax: (912)757-9725

REVIEW COPY
NOT FOR SALE

VANDALS AT THE GATES OF MEDICINE

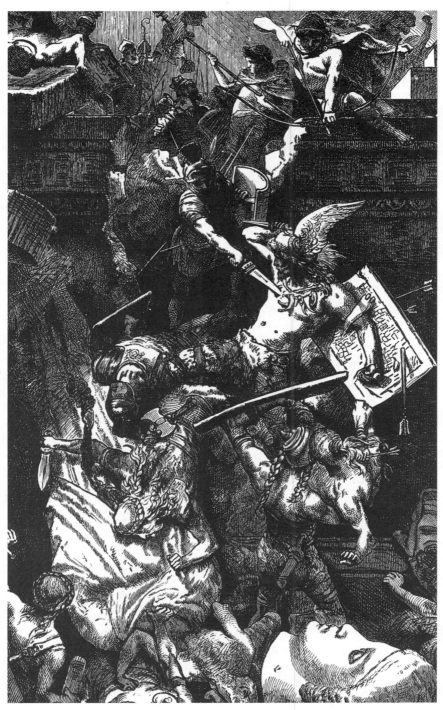

The Attack on Rome by the Vandals. Mansell Collection, London, England.

VANDALS AT THE GATES OF MEDICINE

Historic Perspectives
On The Battle Over Health Care Reform

BY MIGUEL A. FARIA, JR., M.D.

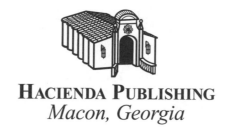

HACIENDA PUBLISHING
Macon, Georgia

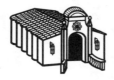

HACIENDA PUBLISHING
Macon, Georgia

Copyright © 1994 by Miguel A. Faria, Jr., M.D.

First edition.

All rights reserved.

No part of this publication may be reproduced, stored in a retrieval system, or transmitted in any form or by any means, electronic, mechanical, photocopying, recording, or otherwise, without prior written permission of the publisher, except in the
case of brief quotations embodied in critical articles and reviews. Inquiries should
be addressed to Hacienda Publishing, Inc., P.O. Box 13648, Macon, Georgia 31208-
3648, 912-757-9873. FAX: 912-757-9725.

1 3 5 7 9 10 8 6 4 2

Library of Congress Catalog Card Number: 94-77392
ISBN: 0-9641077-0-8

Printed and bound in the United States of America on acid-free paper.

DEDICATION

This book is dedicated to my father, Miguel A. Faria, Sr., M.D., whose ultimate decision to embark upon that hazardous but fateful three-month odyssey that began in February, 1966, ended in freedom – and changed my life.

ACKNOWLEDGEMENTS

I would like to acknowledge the two individuals who made the writing of this book possible. My eternal gratitude goes to my devoted and loving wife Helen, and my former secretary and friend, Mrs. Regina Kirkland.

CONTENTS

PART SIX: MIDDLE AGES

PART SEVEN: THE RENAISSANCE

ILLUSTRATIONS

PREFACE

There is a historical precedent in medical history and medical ethics for the reintroduction and reimplementation of truly free-market, ethical, patient-oriented medical care in both the academic and private setting. In fact, it is the only system which has ever been in existence that can provide the proper incentives for the patient, for the doctor and even for society at large, in our effort to promote equitable access to health care for all citizens whilst controlling costs. It is the only proven system that has the proper built-in structural and mechanical incentives to reduce cost because it places the informed patient in the driver's seat in controlling his/her health care.

No health care delivery system will succeed unless the two parties who have the most at stake in the system – the patients and the doctors – cooperate, without coercion from the state. Therefore, for the patient, we should rekindle the consumer-based incentives (based on self-interest) to contain costs; this point is particularly important as our population ages, technologic advances proliferate, and expenses mount as further demands are placed on our overburdened health care system.

Interestingly, as the public and the medical profession both clamor for change and as sociopolitical and economic issues inevitably attain global dimensions, it behooves us to ponder about how to solve the present problems in health care and implement the best health care for our citizens.

In this book we will ratiocinate history, for I am deeply convinced that many of the answers to today's perplexing questions regarding health care reform and the allocation and use of medical resources, not to mention the direction that health care should take, can be found in the wisdom recorded on the pages of history. If we know history, at the very least, we can avoid the mistakes of the past. And this fact is what this book will try to establish, not so much from an economic basis, as from a socio-political and cultural perspective.

Moreover, the economic basis for the modern free-market capitalist system has already been well established by such economic giants as Milton Friedman (b.1912), Ludwig von Mises (1881-1973), Friedrich von Hayek (1899-1992), Henry Hazlitt (1894-1993), and others.

I hope to build my case and rely on the political, philosophic, and historic insights provided to us from the lessons of history, as well as on the unique role of venerable and commendable physicians from antiquity up to the Renaissance. Perhaps, so enlightened by the physicians of yore, we can contribute something tangible to the present health care debate. Perhaps, so endowed, we can contribute time-honored and proven answers as solutions to the quandary in which we are all embroiled today.

This book will attempt to unravel the interconnections amongst medical science, philosophy, political history, keeping in mind that many books have been published about these topics individually. Few until now, however, have been published in which the interrelationship of all of these disciplines has been discussed seriously using history as a reflective background.

Physicians, an essential component in any health care system, have been given very little opportunity to participate in the recent pivotal discussions regarding health care delivery. Why is it that private practitioners, the backbone of the health care delivery system, have been essentially excluded from the policy debate process and discussions of health care initiatives by the government policy-makers? The American Medical Association (AMA), that once wielded great power, has been seemingly emasculated and beaten into submission by the ever-growing power of the federal government. Then, who is really pulling the strings behind the scene of health care reform, and what is their agenda?

Our discussion will touch on the origin, development, and implications of the ethics of the medical profession as a whole – both as a matter of principle and as a matter of practical importance – no trivial matter to be sure; on the contrary, a matter of utmost importance for the survival of the practice of medicine and the autonomy of American physicians. The basis of medical ethics also concerns not just practicing physicians but patients, the consumers of health care, who will be most affected by changes in health care delivery.

We will not discuss specific ethical issues seen in medical practice such as abortion, self-referral, end-of-life directives, or euthanasia, except perhaps tangentially, as these issues are well covered by present-day ethicists, not to mention the mainstream media which has joined the ever-growing crowd of self-proclaimed judges of medical ethics. Suffice it to say that we deal with the overall picture: the origins and sources of philanthropy, humanitarianism, and charity.

But physicians have their work cut out for them. Now that the doctors are finally willing to participate in the health care debate, the medical profession has been given only scant opportunity to participate in the gladiatorial arena of the health care reform contest. The AMA has been scoffed by the Clinton Administration. Why is this? Is it fear of the once great and mighty profession, or a hidden agenda much more sinister? We will try to answer these questions in our search for truth. I believe that despite the perilous waters in which physicians find themselves navigating, there is hope for the future. The consciousness of the new Renaissance physicians, like an undying ember, will be rekindled and the new healer, like a knight armed with resourcefulness and courage, will lead us out of the present morass in which we are mired. We are concerned, therefore, with the path that we have taken in the past and the direction that we will be taking as we embark on change in the health care delivery system. Yes, we are today standing at the crossroads of change in medical care, and physicians have a moral obligation to render advice to the public and to health care planners. In fact, a recent (1993) national survey revealed that more than 75% of American citizens wanted to know and expected to be advised by their physicians about what they [the physicians] think of health care reform and their [the physicians] opinions regarding the direction that health care reform should take. Physicians must lead the way out of the morass in which the profession finds itself mired, trapped, and seemingly unable to gain its freedom. But before the House of Medicine marches forward, it must first look back to see what lessons can be learned from past mistakes, as well as from past accomplishments and achievements.

In this book, we retrace historic steps as far back as prehistoric times, antiquity – aeons ago, to those archaic times when the line between historic facts and myths become blurred. We delve into the history of Western civilization because, before we can comprehend the history of medicine and explore the minds and hearts of physicians, we must first learn about the psyche and soul of man. And for this, we must search and find the earliest facts, the earliest hints, the earliest sentiments that led the first humans to build a civilization and their motives behind rendering aid to their fellowmen, the first instance of one man helping another.

Our saga begins in the haze of prehistory and the mist of myth as we begin our search for historic precedents in those obscure and uncertain times and follow the course of civilization. We will travel the historic path through ancient Mesopotamia and Egypt, splendorous Greece, mighty Rome, and resurgent Europe living through the barbarism of the Dark Ages and the somnolence of the Medieval period to emerge resplendent in the glittering light of the Renaissance. We shall relate the splendor of Greek and the grandeur of Roman civilization, the problems plaguing Greek democracy and the virtues of the Roman Republic; the rise and fall of empires, all the while, recounting (when we can) the trials and tribulations of the physicians and their patients during those tumultuous periods in history.

We will deal with the plight of the perplexed and hapless masses during the apocalyptic visitations of the great plagues of antiquity, recounting the survival instinct of populations held hostage to disease, pestilence, and death. All of these calamities lashing at humanity whilst two dedicated professions, the medical profession and the clergy, attempted in vain to stamp out the menace. The clergy, armed with religion and faith, and physicians, possessed of rudimentary medical knowledge and reason, both impotent to protect a hapless and hopeless population held ransom, not only by disease and pestilence but also by their ignorance and superstition.

For its part, the ecclesiastical power became a force to be reckoned with as a result of a series of events: the conversion of Constantine and his forged Donation, the legitimate donation of Pepin, and the writings of St. Augustine and St. Thomas Aquinas. Yet the Church would lose some of its luster and prestige because of its failure to heal the ailing massses and stop the plague of the 14th Century.

Yes, in this book, we are concerned with the overall picture (and direction) that the profession has taken in the past, is taking at the present time, and must take in the future if it is to survive the present crisis and remain a caring and compassionate profession. As we teeter at the brink of major health care reform, what will be the guiding light leading us safely out of this morass in which we are mired? How can we make sure that in the ongoing battle over health care reform we proceed in the right direction and for the good of the nation? I believe that the answers to today's perplexing questions regarding the direction health care reform should take can be found in the wisdom recorded on the pages of history.

With that said, let us now proceed with our discussion of antiquity, the origins of civilization, and the birth of medicine.

Miguel A. Faria, Jr., M.D.

Macon, Georgia
April, 1994

PART ONE: ANTIQUITY

CHAPTER 1

PRIMITIVE MEDICINE

Any sufficiently advanced technology is indistinguishable from magic.
Arthur C. Clarke
Scholar, historian

In the beginning...following the ebb of the glacier and the recession of the last major Ice Age 40,000 years ago, Cro-Magnon man (modern man) migrated from the African interior to North Africa, across the Middle East, and eventually made his way to the European continent. By 30,000 B.C., Cro-Magnon man was flourishing in Europe, whilst the slower-witted Paleolithic Age Neanderthal man had, by now, become extinct. Remains of Cro-Magnon men found in the caves of the Dordogne River valley in southwestern France, northern Spain, and other parts of Europe revealed the first traces of early modern man and with him, the first doctors, the medicine men of 20,000 to 30,000 years ago. Incidentally, along with evidence of the presence of the earliest medicine men, we also find tangible evidence of paleolithic art – splendid cave paintings, including enigmatic images of animals and female (fertility) figures, as well as small sculpted figurines – remnants of the period commencing immediately after the interlude of the last great Ice Age.

We can speculate that organized medical care was needed from the beginning....We can, for example, hypothesize that from the first blunt head injury due to the fierce clubbing by a paleolithic enemy to being trampled upon in a futile attempt to escape from a wounded and furious Mastodon, or the first penetrating head trauma from man's unexpected encounter with a saber-toothed North American tiger – man recognized the need for tending to the wounded in his clan. Also, when he became ill from imbibing the stagnant water of a polluted pond, he also recognized the need to be provided with aid and comfort during sickness...and to be nurtured back to health.

A bit later in the Neolithic period (8000-3000 B.C.), we begin to find paleontologic and archaeologic evidence for medical care associated with the earliest healing rites and rituals. Circumstantial evidence points towards a tendency to care for the wounded and the sick in the depths of the near-impenetrable caves of Europe. Medical ethics likely began the day that the earliest Siberian shaman, American medicine man, African witch doctor, or Scythian priestess took responsibility for the care provided to the injured members of his/her tribe during this Stone Age period. It may have been pure and true *altruism*, the instinctive need to help others in need; or *idealism*, the need to do what is right, ennobling, and courageous; or camouflaged self-interested *individualism*, the opportunity to gain favor with the other members of the tribe and gain prestige and power; or ultimately, *pragmatism*, the recognition that at the time, it was the thing to do after weighing and balancing the options.

I personally doubt the latter scenario, since pragmatism seems to be the product of a much more recent vintage – and, I may venture, the seemingly prevailing philosophy of today. For we must remember that we were dealing with *Homo sapiens,* with brains similar to ours and with the same needs for self-preservation and sur-vival. Moreover, it would appear that since the dawn of history, circumstantial evi-dence suggests that human nature has remained unchanged. We can speculate motives, and we can pretend to know the thoughts and secrets of the human heart, but it is just that, speculation. In the end, only man's outward acts and objective actions can truly be judged. Motives may be hidden so that subjective intention is only a matter of conjecture.

If there is a way to judge intent and the contents of the human heart other than by the expressed word, it remains objective action based on known facts, or lacking that, judgmental action based on prevailing views and beliefs as to known facts. And that is the way in which the work of physicians should be judged throughout the ages.

It is highly probable that ritualistic medical care began with the fertility cults of high-priestesses in the Neolithic period who worshipped primal Earth-Mother goddesses and nature – prior to the Aryan (Indo-European) invasions of the epoch circa 2500-1500 B.C., invasions that took place from northeastern Europe to the southeastern regions of Europe, Asia Minor, the Middle East, and areas of southwestern Asia; and by warring nomadic Semitic peoples of the Arabian penin-sula from the south. As waves of invaders converged on the Middle East, especially Mesopotamia, the period of indigenous matriarchal cultures that heretofore existed suddenly came to an abrupt end.

The invaders brought with them war chariots, an agricultural economy, and a new age – the Bronze Age. Although primal matriarchal cultures had ended, many rituals of the high-priestesses continued. Evidence suggests that in many areas where the invaders settled, primal Earth-Mother goddesses continued to be worshipped, locally or by sects, in cults and rituals presided over by high-priestesses or a sacerdotal class of male priests.

So, at the dawn of history, patriarchal cultures had been established by both Aryans from the north and Semitic peoples from the south. And the land between the rivers, Mesopotamia, was the hub of civilization. In the worship of the supreme Aegean Earth goddess, Gaea – daughter of chaos and mother and wife, respectively, of the sky god, Uranus, and sea god, Pontus – the Oracle at Delphi originated. It was only later, after the Aryan invasions had swept upon the Aegean and Minoan cultures, that the shrine became the principle temple and the supreme Oracle of Apollo. As late as the 6th Century B.C., the oracles were still spoken by high-priestesses in a state of frenzied possession and spiritual wisdom, to then be interpreted by male priests who spoke or wrote the oracle in enigmatic or prophetic verse to the awed and profoundly affected supplicants.

The great Mother-goddesses in the ancient Middle East symbolized the Earth's fertility, and as the primal fertility symbols in nature, they were worshipped syncretistically under many names: Ishtar in Babylon; Isis in Egypt; Cybele in Asia Minor; and in ancient Greece and Rome, Demeter and Ceres, respectively.

SHAMANISM AND THE MEDICINE MAN

With the advent of the medicine man, we see man's first attempt to treat injuries and exorcise disease. Primitive man could now find solace in the thought that if and when he was wounded whilst hunting or warring, he would no longer be left to die unattended. It was a simple but comforting thought, that if ever in need, he would be cared for and treated by the medicine man of his tribe. Rudimentary care, and perhaps even more importantly, attention and sympathy were now given to the injured man.(1)

From the earliest beginnings in the most primitive societies, the medicine man occupied an important place and fulfilled a unique role in the tribe. Moreover, because his role called for authority, he was given power and vested with a special status that reflected the authority which was required for fulfilling his role and shouldering his responsibilities. We can surmise that the labor of attending the ill and ministering to the wounded required economic sacrifices from the rest of the cave dwellers which could have only been enforced by the chieftain or his perennial second-in-command, the medicine man, the witch doctor, or the Shaman – later this would be a member of the sacerdotal class, the priest or priestess. Since power was necessary to enforce his decrees for the proper care of the sick and wounded, the status of the medicine man would later evolve to that of the caste of physician-priest, a position which carried not only immense responsibility but also unprecedented prestige and power within the tribe. Likewise, in the matriarchal societies, the high-priestess assumed ultimate authority and presided over the fertility and healing rituals of her tribe.

Prestige, respect, and responsibility went with the territory, whilst power, both in the form of spiritual guidance and tribal authority, was an indispensable necessity of his office. As a result of his moral burden and hierarchical obligations, he was responsible not only for interpreting omens and making predictions but also advising on planting and cultivating the soil before the growing season. Most relevant to our story, he was in charge of the health and well-being of the members of the tribe – and for that, the medicine man was rewarded with material possessions. He was second-in-command and thereby, he had second best in everything. He occupied the second best place in the cave or in the village, for he was second in the position of the tribal hierarchy.

The chieftain would often consult with him on important matters before the tribe, for the medicine man possessed cryptic and forbidden knowledge that separated him from the rest of the clan. But these attributes, power, respect, material possessions, and relative wealth, were not a given, they were associated with proven benefits for the tribe. The privilege to wear elaborate ceremonial costumes emblematic of his office and symbolic of his power (not necessarily preordained) were contingent upon fulfilling properly his responsibilities to the tribe. However, failure to deliver the expected beneficial results – either by dereliction of duty or simply bad luck – endangered his status and his power. And power was essential and necessary to frighten wicked spirits and protect the tribe. Loss of power and loss of his magic could bring evil, sickness, and disease upon the tribe – and lead to defeat in war with enemies of his clan. Proper decorum and propriety were necessary to command respect from his fellow tribesmen, who in turn, needed him for maintenance of health and well-being, not to mention, recovery from sickness or injuries. As a result he was respected...and the survival of the tribe depended on it.(1)

Overindulgence could result in bad fortune and, even possibly, divine retribution from the myriads of fiends that roamed the land, especially at night, and evil spirits that inhabited the forests, fields, and streams. Overindulgence or dereliction of duty could also result in earthly punishment, such as dismissal from office, banishment from the tribe, corporal punishment, or even death. In time, simple rites, such as offerings, supplications, imbibition of magical potions, drinking of herbal remedies, simple magic and exorcisms, etc., evolved to more complex rituals involving incantations, prayers, libations, and even animal sacrifices which entailed more complex ceremonies. For these acts, as we have mentioned, a new caste was required, a new sacerdotal class, the priesthood. Simple treatment with herbs and potions may have been incorporated into rites of passage and fertility rituals by the priesthood. So, to primitive generic man, we surmise that we owe the origin of the primeval doctor.

In those primordial times, disease was attributed to supernatural causes. The early medicine man, the primeval physician-priest – whether an African witch doctor or a Siberian shaman – used magic,[1] the power of suggestion, and trance states to cure the sick. The medicine man would also use his magic and power of divination in an attempt to manipulate and control earthly and heavenly events that would benefit and impress the tribe.

Disease was ascribed to the acts that offended or neglected previously friendly or utterly unfriendly spirits, and/or the deliberate casting of spells by spirits or demons, or the invocation of curses from enemies of the tribe.(1-5)

The belief in the power of the supernatural or the supernatural origin of disease is universal with primitive cultures, from the Blackfoot Indians of the United States to the Taiga tribesmen of Siberia (from which the word *Shaman* itself originates), from the Stone Age cavemen of 20,000 to 50,000 years ago to the presumed matriarchal cultures in the Neolithic period, the warring and conquering patriarchal cultures of the Bronze[2] and Iron Ages.[3] And this belief in the supernatural origin of disease remained entrenched in man's collective mind up to the time of the zenith of Greek civilization c.600 B.C.

Ascribing pestilences, illnesses, and natural calamities to a supernatural causation provided, at least, a needed explanation for unknown phenomena; indeed, it provided a remarkable explanation that attributed not just diseases but also every calamity and every misfortune, even plagues and famine, to the deeds of whimsical evil spirits and demons. The noted medical historian, Dr. H.W. Haggard, in *The Doctor in History* puts it very clearly and succinctly: "Egotism makes us believe that what we accomplish successfully is due to our own fine qualities, and that what we do poorly is owing to no fault of our own but to some outside influence. Like the savage, we all wish to take credit for our success and to blame our failures on someone else."(1)

On the tendency of members of primitive cultures to blame the bogeyman for misfortune and unfavorable acts, Haggard further states: "Confronted by disease, they blamed their misfortunes on something other than their own ignorance, on something outside themselves....The spirits were the invisible agents of misfortune...misfortunes could be blamed on the spirits. It was a very satisfying belief indeed."(1)

---

[1] Magic within this text is the purported ability to exert extraordinary power or influence either by knowledge of nature's secrets or by manipulation of supernatural forces or powers.(2)

[2] The Bronze Age was the technologic period when metals were used to make tools and weapons. Casting of copper and bronze began in the Near East by 3500 B.C. and in the New World as late as 1100 B.C. The Bronze Age revolution may be said to have brought about the first nation states.(2)

[3] The Iron Age began with the Egyptians or the Hittites between 1350 B.C. and 1200 B.C. However, iron technology was not exported to other areas of the Middle East and the rest of Europe until c.800-500 B.C. (2)

It was important that the medicine man maintain decorum in the tribe to elicit the proper respect and deference needed for performing his work and to set an example for the other members of the tribe. Yet, he also needed to impress his audience for his spells and magic potions to work. Haggard writes: "The medicine man built his treatment into a ceremony....His efforts were always intended to remove the evil spirit that he imagined caused the illnesses. He dressed to impress the spirits and carried charms to make them obey him; he danced, he shouted, he shook his rattle...to frighten demons away. But more importantly, his antics made an impression on the patient and on those who watched him."(1)

Furthermore, Haggard is likely correct when he posits that comfort and relief of worries and responsibilities had a beneficial effect on the mind of sick or injured tribesmen. He believed that the medicine man encouraged the sick man, "comforted him, removed his fears; he took over responsibility for the disease and so relieved the patient's mind of responsibility. In consequence the sick man might feel better, and suffer less...because he believed in the medicine man."(1)

As we have seen, the origin of medicine is intricately related to magic and the origin of primitive religion. One wonders how against such odds, primitive man managed to survive. He had to contend with predatory animals stronger than he, live with a scarce and uncertain food supply, and lastly, endure disease. He invented weapons not only to defend against predators but also to hunt for food.(1-5) In time, though, he insured his food supply with the development of farming and the domestication of animals such as sheep and cattle, but these developments did not come until approximately 8000 B.C.

The third hazard, however, the most elusive and dangerous to human existence, disease, remained beyond his control. To conquer disease man needed knowledge, medical knowledge, the most priceless of his possessions. "Knowledge is man's greatest triumph in his struggle for existence, the struggle for safety, food and health."(1)

ANIMISM

History are fables agreed upon.
> *Voltaire (1694-1778)*

One of the theories proposed for the origin of religion was Animism, the belief that everything in nature – trees, brooks, wind, mountains – has a soul.(3) In fact, animism is a word derived from the Latin *animus* which means "soul or spirit." In the book, *Primitive Culture* (1871), Sir Edward B. Tylor (1832-1917), Professor of Anthropology at Oxford, argued that animism was the origin of religion and that primitive man presumed everything in nature had a spiritual as well as a corporeal existence.(3) This idea was further expounded by the Scottish anthropologist, Sir James G. Frazer (1854-1941). In his book, *The Golden Bough*, Frazer wrote:

> *After men had peopled with a multitude of individual spirits every rock and hill, every tree and flower, every brook and river, every breeze that blew, and every cloud that flecked with silvery white the blue expanse of heaven, they began, in virtue of what we may call the economy of thought, to limit the number of the*

spiritual beings of whom their imagination at first had been so prodigal.
Instead of a separate spirit for every individual tree, they came to conceive of a
god of the woods in general, a Sylvanus or what not;...To put it otherwise, the
innumerable multitude of spirits and demons were generalized and reduced to a
comparatively small number of deities, animism was replaced by polytheism.(4)

Polytheism was in time supplanted by monotheism, sequentially by Jews, Christians, and Moslems, but the theory of animism did not go unchallenged. The late R. R. Marett, Professor of Anthropology at Oxford, pointed out that "supernaturalism, the attitude of the mind dictated by awe of the mysterious, which provided religion with its raw material, could exist apart from animism and might be the basis on which animism was founded."(5)

The most recent archaeologic and anthropologic data indicate that the earliest form of deity was that of the Earth-Mother goddess, which reflected primitive man's desire for fertility and renewal. Furthermore, Tylor's and Frazer's dualistic conception of the soul – inner self and outer body – did not appear in Western history until Greece c.600 B.C.; evidence extracted from ancient Egyptian and Mesopotamian texts points to a melding of the physical and spiritual, rather than a stark separation of body and soul.(5)

Interestingly, this cultural tradition, namely, that of the medicine man, persists to this day, not only in such faraway peoples and places as the cultures of the Bushmen of Central Africa, the Guarani Indians of the Amazon river basin, the Maori of New Zealand, or the Aborigines of the Great Australian deserts, but even in the United States. The presence of the medicine man is felt today in the U.S. in the form of "root doctors," practitioners who derive their origins from the slave cultures of Africa and the antebellum South. Adherence to "rootwork medicine" combines supernatural causation of illnesses, such as by magical spells,[4] with cures by sorcery; amazingly, it also embodies the more recent empirical tradition that emphasizes natural causation of illnesses and believes in mundane treatment and the attainment of cures with the use of old remedies and the ingestion of medicinal herbs.(6)

Another example of the medicine man is found in American Indian culture where he still uses a wide repertoire of medical treatments derived both from the natural (herbalism) and the supernatural (magic). Through the centuries, many methods that rely on empiricism[5] were utilized to effect treatment, and at the head of this list, is the process of casual inference. Included in these methods of casual inference were the doctrine of signatures, the "trial and error" method, and serendipity.(7)

Supernatural methods of treatment include such disparate practices as the Aleutians' practice of piercing of the skin to let out "bad air," and natural treatments such as bleeding to let out "bad blood" and relieve headaches. Furthermore, Drs. J.H. McWhorter and S.D. Ward write, "the Aleuts wash wounds and suture with bone needles and sinew thread....And, the Upiks treated fractures of a limb by realignment and the encasing of the limb in tough hardened animal skins as a splint."(7)

Botanical medicine included remedies utilized as cathartics, emetics, and astringents. Cathartics and emetics cleanse the body as well as rid it of evil spirits.

---

[4] Whilst black magic is said to be intended to harm, white magic is believed to be conducted for the benefit of the community, as in fertility rituals or to heal an individual suffering from the effects of black magic.(2)

[5] Empiricism is the philosophic doctrine that maintains that knowledge is gained by human experience, whether derived from the mind or the senses, and denies rationalism as a method of obtaining knowledge.

Amongst such medicines we find cascara, podophyllum, and senna which have been used for centuries and are still used today in modern medicine. And the list of astringents included such medicaments as wild geraniums, hemlock, oaks, persimmon, and witch hazel; febrifuges (antipyretics) included dogwood and wild cherry.(7)

The similarities of parallel development in cultures is inescapable and may be discerned in present-day societies in which individuals are prone to seek both spiritual as well as physical healing for problems presumed to be caused by both natural and supernatural causes. Thus, according to McWhorter and Ward as well as Dr. H.F. Mathews, a pluralistic approach to medical care maybe sometimes necessary to treat such individuals and members of certain cultural minorities.(6,7) For treatment and successful therapy, patients with these cultural and ethno-medical backgrounds and beliefs may require evaluation by sundry health personnel such as physicians, herbalists, ministers, or faith healers; and, if all is still not well, ultimately, a medicine man or root doctor.(6,7)

MAGIC AND MEDICINE

If the reader would permit, I would like to digress for just a moment to say a word about magic and medicine, I think such an indulgence would be of interest to the reader.

Dr. Pasquale Accardo writes that the physician and cleric, Michael Scot of Balwearie (1175-1235), was put by Dante in the Eighth Circle of Hell (the circle of the fraudulent) in part because "his accurate but ultimately ineffective prediction relating to his own and Emperor Frederick II's death lent support to the medieval tendency to equate excessive learning with black magic."(8) He also quotes Dorothy Sayers who wrote about the many forms magic can take, "ranging from actual Satanism to attempts at 'conditioning' other people by manipulating their psyches; but even when it used the legitimate techniques of the scientist or the psychiatrist, it is distinguished from true science by the 'twisted sight,' which looks to self instead of to God for the source and direction of its power."(9)

THE DAWN OF CIVILIZATION

Without culture, and the relative freedom it presumes, society, even when perfect, is no more than a jungle. This is why every authentic creation is a gift to the future.
Albert Camus (1913-1960)
French existentialist and Nobel Prize winner
in Literature in 1957

In the wake of the last glacial era 10,000 years ago and the end of the Mesolithic period, which witnessed both the gradual domestication of plants and animals and the formation of very early communal living,[6] we begin our story of

---

[6] Again, it must be noted that the earliest evidence for communal living – e.g. man-made shelters, communal gathering, hunting, and belief systems based on magic and the supernatural as evidenced in rock carvings, paintings, sculpted figurines, and other artifacts – dates to the end of the Paleolithic era (Upper Paleolithic) of Cro-Magnon man.(2)

civilization. With the dawn of the Neolithic Age (7000-3200 B.C.), the Earth-Mother goddesses, perhaps the earliest and most primal form of deities, were venerated as the source of life, fertility, and renewal. Medicine, still inextricably linked to religion and ritual, was first organized as healing cults of the supernatural and reflected man's primordial desire for survival, security, and the renewal of life. It was during this time, according to the noted historian Joseph Campbell, that two major developments occurred, almost simultaneously: agriculture and animal domestication. We have already intimated the importance of these developments to civilization. The area where these developments occurred included the Middle East region (Mesopotamia, "the land between the rivers," Sumer, Ur, and Jericho, 5000-2340 B.C.), Southwest Asia and the Indus Valley (Mohenjo-Daro and Harappa, c.2500-c.1500 B.C.), Asia Minor and Southeastern Europe (Çatal Hüyük), and Mesoamerica (Mexico) and South America (Peru).

In all of these ancient regions, archaeologic remains such as those found in the biblical city of Jericho and in the temples of Çatal Hüyük, where archaeologists have unearthed large pueblo-like constructions as well as small stone figurines Mother-goddess motifs feature prominently. Moreover, Mother-goddesses were birth-giving goddesses and performed health and life rituals as well as sacrificial ceremonies. Ceramic vases discovered at these archaeologic sites show figurines with motifs depicting the various representations of the Mother-goddesses, i.e., lion goddesses, serpent madonnas, and mythologic figures reminiscent of the Garden of Eden.(10)

By the end of the Neolithic period (at approximately 3200 B.C.), two developments took place in Mesopotamia which heralded a new age. These landmark developments in civilization included the invention of writing (near Sumer) and the invasion of the fertile crescent region of the Middle East by two different groups. The first group of invaders, the Aryans (Indo-Europeans), migrated from the Trans-Caucasus region of the north. They herded cattle, domesticated the horse, and introduced the then invincible war-chariots to the area. The other invaders were the Semites who came from the Arabian peninsula from the south and who herded sheep and goats. These arriving patriarchal cultures are believed to have overthrown and supplanted the cult of the Earth-Mother goddesses in southwestern Asia and southeastern Europe, ending the matriarchal cultures.

We should pause to note that the city of Sumer in 4,000 B.C. Mesopotamia may have been not only the first city to emerge, but also "the cradle of (the first) civilization." It is here that the invention and development of cuneiform writing took place at approximately 3200 B.C. With the fall of the Earth-goddess cultures throughout Europe and Asia and the close of the Neolithic period, a new order was established. Between 1500 and 1350 B.C., the Indo-Europeans, still on the march, invaded northern India, and the Indus Valley civilization was transformed, with complete assimilation of the indigenous culture and blending of the races and languages. The invasions established the Brahmin (or Brahman) class, felt to be the direct descendants of the Indo-Europeans and who wrote in Sanskrit, as the highest Hindu caste – the priesthood – in the Indian peninsula.(10) Although the concept of the invading Aryans (or the Indo-Europeans) as a distinct race has been discredited in anthropology, because of the extensive mixing of the races during this period and throughout history, the distinction is still valid within the context of the Indo-European linguistic group.

Likewise, in the Western Hemisphere, in Middle and South America, ancient Pre-Columbian civilizations developed Neolithic cultures by 1500 B.C. For example, the ancient Peruvians apparently performed trephination (skull surgery) successfully, as great numbers of trephined skulls with healing edges have been found in South America. Moreover, the Olmecs of Veracruz performed human sacrifices and carried out elaborate jaguar rites and fertility rituals, in their, as of yet, poorly understood cults. The Mayans devised a distinct system of writing, the Mayan glyphs, composed of phonetic writing intermixed with pictorial representations (ideograms). Also deeply preoccupied with time and endless calculations and representations of the latter, they invented a calendar as accurate as our own. The Mayans built complex cities amidst dense jungles, erected steep majestic pyramids crowned with temples for worshipping closer to their gods, and constructed extensive irrigation systems to water their fields and sustain their ever-growing population.

Between 3200 and 1500 B.C., the next stage was set for the establishment of the powerful sacerdotal class of physician-priests in Mesoamerica, in southeastern Europe and Asia Minor, southwestern Asia, the Middle East, and the northeastern corner of North Africa.

PRIMITIVE SURGERY

The earliest evidence for surgery is found in the skulls of primitive peoples of the Neolithic period in Europe, North Africa, Japan, and South America. Trephining – the surgical opening and/or removal of sections of the skull – was done in accordance with the belief system of supernatural causation of disease previously discussed, and we believe, for cases of epilepsy, insanity, and recalcitrant headaches; but there is no concrete evidence, as of yet, for these educated guesses. In other cases, segments of the skull may have been removed from already deceased persons and used as charms and amulets to guard against evil spirits.(11) We do know that the Peruvians, at least, had medical instruments designed for trephining, such as the Tumi, which was a definitely effective surgical instrument designed for this specific purpose.

In fact, hundreds of trephined skulls with partially healed edges and regenerated bone have been found, at the very least proving that some of the patients miraculously survived the operation-ordeal. Cranial surgery in Peru has captured the imagination of many investigators and has been extensively studied and written about by such eminent physicians as the anthropologist-neurosurgeon Paul Broca (1824-1880), and many others.(12-14)

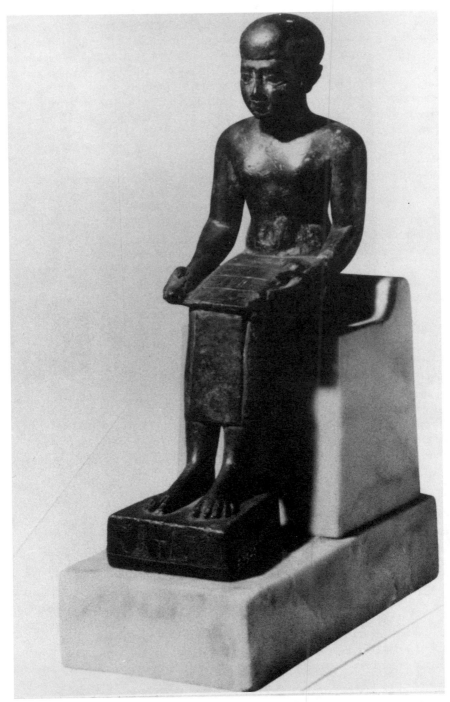

Plate 1 – Seated figure of Imhotep, vizier, scribe, architect, and the first physician to step out of the mist of history. Bronze statue c.2600 B.C. Musée du Louvre, Paris.

CHAPTER 2

THE DAZZLING EGYPTIAN CIVILIZATION

A race preserves its vigour so long as it harbours a real contrast between what has been and what may be, and so long as it is served by the vigour to adventure beyond the safeties of the past. Without adventure, civilization is in full decay.
Alfred North Whitehead (1861-1947)
English mathematician and philosopher

PHARAONIC RULE AND THEOCRACY IN EGYPT

In Egypt, Mesopotamia, and almost uniformly in other pockets of civilization, the nascent states were administered by a sacerdotal class, a primeval bureaucracy headed by a priest-king or a physician-priest. High tributes were levied, arduous labor was exacted, and strict discipline was demanded from the people to sustain the livelihood of the ruling classes as well as the splendor of their burgeoning civilizations. Feats of engineering and empire-building, such as pyramid and complex temple constructions, were attained in antiquity with limited technology but at great human cost.

In Egypt, pharaonic rule was based on the incarnation of the god Osiris and protected by the falcon-god, Horus, the son of Osiris and Isis. The first pyramids were established at approximately 2300 B.C. The celebrated Grand Vizier, a deified physician and illustrious architect – Imhotep, himself – may have designed the imposing Step Pyramid at Saqqara, near Memphis, as early as 2600 B.C. for the pharaoh, Dzoser, a ruler of the III Dynasty of the Old Kingdom (3110-2258 B.C.). Imhotep was the first physician of whom we have a written record, and from the Ebers Papyrus (c.1750 B.C.) we know that he was also a magician, a sorcerer, and a priest.

It was during the Middle Kingdom of Egypt (2000-1786 B.C.), beginning with the VIIth Dynasty, that the biblical Abraham migrated from the kingdom of Ur in Mesopotamia to southern Israel. Abraham (c.2000 B.C.), you remember, was the first Hebrew patriarch, "the father of a multitude of nations." In Israel, he founded the lineage that, according to biblical tradition, produced the Twelve Tribes of Israel. Also, it was during the period of the Middle Kingdom that the Hyksos, a Semitic nomadic people, conquered Egypt and founded the foreign XVth Dynasty; the latter, after just over 200 years, were driven out by the resurgence and reassertion of the native aggressive Egyptian rulers of the New Kingdom.

In 1420 B.C., Amenhotep III (14th Century B.C.) of the XVIII Dynasty began a Golden Age in Egypt. He was an able and adept ruler who exerted and maintained peace in his realm. He built the splendorous temples at Luxor and the Great Temple of Amon-Ra, the latter to the supreme Egyptian deity. Unfortunately, the thriving kingdom that he had so carefully nurtured quickly came to an end after the accession and rule of Amenhotep IV (pharaoh, c.1372-1354 B.C.).[7]

Egypt was not ready for this new king. Soon after taking the reigns of power, Amenhotep IV changed his name to Akhenaton – after Aton, the new sun-god. Akhenaton made Aton the sole god of Egypt and introduced the cult of Aton, an elaborate sun-worshipping ceremony, which offended the ruling theocracy. The priests were suppressed and forced to abolish the worship of the other Egyptian deities including Amon-Ra.(15) Akhenaton even moved the capital from ancient religious Thebes to his new capital at Amarna. Obsessed with his solar, monotheistic religion, Akhenaton neglected the secular affairs of state and the actual ruling of the empire, with devastating consequences for Egypt and its dominion.

The boy-King Tutankhamen (fl.c.1350 B.C.) succeeded Akhenaton, and with his ascension, the old priesthood, with its worship of Amon-Ra and the other gods, was restored to its former glory in the Egyptian pantheon. Evidence of the new religion which had been inaugurated by Akhenaton (including monotheism) was erased throughout the empire, so that only traces of its existence remained for posterity. And of the empire over which he ruled, only Egypt and the Upper Valley of the Nile remained; all other provinces were lost.

Interestingly, a recent author who is both a pediatrician and medical historian, Dr. Harry Bloch, has implicated Akhenaton's solar theology not only as a possible source for the impetus of monotheism in nearby cultures, particularly the Israelites – but also as the possible inaugurator of the use of solar energy as a source of healing and health, (i.e., heliotherapy and phototherapy) in more recent centuries.(16)

The XIX Dynasty was a power house of rulers: the founders, Horemheb (c.14th Century B.C.) and Ramses I (d.c.1314 B.C.), were followed by the energetic rulers, Seti I (fl.1313-1301 B.C.) who reconquered Palestine and Syria, and whose daughter pulled Moses from the bulrushes, and Seti's son, Ramses II, "the Great" (pharaoh, 1292-1225 B.C.). Ramses II built huge public monuments, thus keeping the Egyptian masses occupied in national projects. Abu Simbel and other major constructions were built at his direction. Under his rule, Egypt expanded its frontiers to southern Syria and to the 4th Cataract of the Nile (modern Sudan). Egypt reached another age of splendor.

Ramses II was not only a stern ruler but apparently also an able diplomat. In 1298 B.C. at the Battle of Qadesh, Ramses II and Mutawallis, King of the Hittites, clashed in what must have been a spectacular battle, and when the dust had settled, both leaders had adeptly retreated, each claiming victory in their respective nations. Ramses II later concluded a peace treaty with the Hittites and married a Hittite princess to consolidate the gains of his empire. He also left such majestic temples as are found at Karnak, Luxor, and Thebes. The Hittites, for their part, left a mark in history following this encounter in which one or both armies may have used iron weapons for the first time.

It was probably during Ramses the Great's rule that the Israelite Exodus, led by Moses, took place in the 13th Century B.C. (the date heretofore given as

---

[7] Amenhotep IV (Akhenaton)'s wife, Nefertiti (fl.c.1372-1350 B.C.) was queen of Egypt. A splendid limestone bust of her can be seen in the Egyptian collection of the Berlin Museum. She was also aunt to Tutankhamen.

1250 B.C., as we shall see, has been questioned by more recent research). It is of interest that the biblical parting of the Red Sea described during the Exodus and recorded in the Old Testament has been studied and explained by some scholars as a natural phenomenon, and therefore, not inconsistent with holy scripture. In fact, a special project conducted by an international corps of engineers actually constructed a model in which the nature and intensity of the winds in that area, coupled with the fact that there is a large sand bar across the bottom of the Red Sea, were carefully studied in an attempt to examine the possibility that the biblical event was indeed explainable as a natural phenomenon. To the satisfaction of biblical scholars, the modern experts found that the sand bar – which, interestingly, had been discovered and noted by Napoleon's engineers during their excursions against the Mamelukes of Egypt in 1798 – made the event physically plausible. Indeed, it was their conclusion that the parting of the Red Sea could have taken place as described in the Bible.(17)

Egyptian history abounds with interesting twists and unexpected turns. Recent paleontologic and forensic medical research, supported by historic accounts from holy scriptures, points to Menerptah, Ramses II's son, as the pharaoh of the Exodus. Forensic studies and x-rays performed on Ramses II's mummy suggests that this energetic, resourceful, and powerful pharaoh most likely died at the ripe old age of 85 – and without evidence of acute trauma or death by injuries. Moreover, at that age, it would have been unlikely for an old ruler to have acted so brazenly, mentally or physically, especially given the profoundly aggressive and tempestuous attitude as was displayed historically and biblically by the bold and irascible ruler (and almost of necessity, young) pharaoh of the Exodus. Moreover, a recent author, M. Bucaille, argues, Menerptah was young, and his mummy, unlike that of his father, was found to show forensic evidence of cranio-cerebral trauma: a wound in the right parietal region capable of causing rapid traumatic death.(18)

Regardless of which pharaoh presided over the Egyptian debacle, Moses was able to lead the Israelite Exodus across the Red Sea and through the desert to Canaan, the Promised Land. At Mt. Sinai, Moses received the summary of divine law (the Mosaic law) directly from God, and the Ten Commandments; this sacred decalogue, was then delivered to the Israelites (Exodus 20:2-17 and Deuteronomy 5:6-21). These divine precepts formed the basic tenets of the ethical foundations of Judaism, Christianity, and Islam.

THE LEGEND OF OSIRIS

If there is a sin against life, it consists perhaps not so much in despairing of life as in hoping for another, and in eluding the implacable grandeur of this life.
        Albert Camus

The Egyptian pantheon of gods and their fascinating mythology can be best discussed by referring to the legend of Osiris.

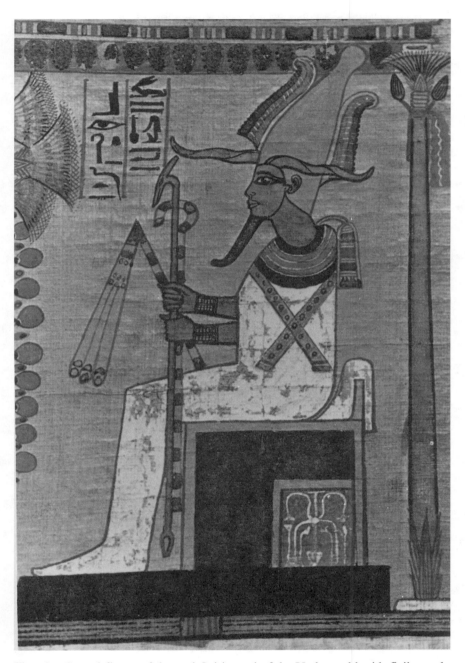

Plate 2 – Seated figure of the god Osiris, god of the Underworld with flail, crook, and scepter. From the opening scene of the papyrus of the *Book of the Dead* (c.1400-1350 B.C.). Courtesy of Museo Egizio, Torino.

GENEALOGY AND MYTH OF OSIRIS

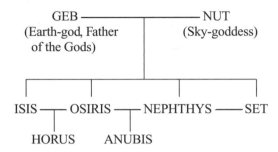

Though Amon-Ra, the supreme Egyptian god, occupied the highest place in the pantheon of Egyptian deities, other gods came close to being just as powerful. Some gods and goddesses were even more familiar to the Egyptian laity and common folk – especially those living outside the large cities, for example, the deities representing health, life, death, and the underworld. In this context, we can discuss the major deities, Isis and Osiris, who are of singular concern to us for reasons that will become self-evident.

Osiris was the personification of the Nile, as well as the Lord of the Dead and Judge of the Underworld. His sister-wife, Isis, was the primeval Earth-Mother goddess (perhaps the only one whose cult persisted and survived with vigor in the form of the cult of Isis-Hygeia during Hellenistic and Roman times). In fact, as we will find in our narrative, her cult actually grew in popularity in those later days and even competed with the charming astral temples of Æsculapius (also Asklepios) in the Græco-Roman World.(19) Isis was the embodiment of the ruling house and the throne of Egypt itself, whilst still being worshipped as a healing goddess by the upper and lower classes. Horus was the falcon-god, the god of health and healing, and light and the noon-day sun. He was also the personification of the pharaoh.

The importance that the Egyptians paid to health and medical treatment is corroborated by the pantheon of gods dealing with health matters, diseases, cures...and death, as well as the numerous extant inscriptions and hieroglyphics dealing with these subjects.

The Osirian legend of the birth of Horus has been recorded by the Greek biographer and priest at the Delphic Oracle, Plutarch (A.D.46-119) and is worth recounting.(20) The legend is concisely and well told by Dr. Morad Tavallali from a compendium of sources and follows:

> *Geb, the supreme deity, transferred his powers to his son Osiris, god of the dead, who with his sister/wife, Isis, began to govern the world. This aroused the jealousy of their brother, Set, who set out to destroy Osiris. At a fateful feast, Set abducted Osiris, bundled him into a chest, and drowned him. Isis, however, began a search and finally returned the body of Osiris to Egypt. Undaunted, Set stole the corpse and dissected it into fourteen pieces which he scattered about the world. Once more, Isis searched for her husband's remains and was able to recover all of the parts except for the phallus; she then proceeded to create the first mummy from the remains of Osiris, and after his reanimation bore him a son named Horus.*

Under protection of his mother, Horus grew to be a warrior and set out to reclaim his inheritance from Set and avenge his father's murder. A series of battles followed between the two; finally, in hand-to-hand combat, Horus was justly able to emasculate his uncle, at which time Horus suffered the loss of an eye. (In a later adaptation of the legend, Set buried the eye of Horus in a mountain, where it grew to form the lotus flower.) The other deities intervened and at a tribunal, restored Horus to his inheritance as Lord of Egypt and ancestor to the Pharaohs, while Set was consoled by being allowed to howl in the sky as the god of storms. Thoth, the god of medicine and physicians, was instructed to heal both parties. Horus had his eyes restored after Thoth spat into the orbit. As a gesture to the spirit of his father, Horus presented his new eye (the Udjat) to him, and replaced it in his own head with the divine serpent, the Uraeus, which thenceforth became the symbol of royalty.

This dramatic saga set the stage for the rise in popularity of this heavenly family, and the Eye of Horus or Udjat became known as a symbol of restored health by divine intervention.(21)

Horus lost one eye in his struggle with Set – his ceremonial penance for the resurrection of Osiris. Set, for his part, lost his testicle. Tavallali adds another interesting bit of information which was that: "Horus also was known as the god of the noonday sun, flying across the sky in the shape of a hawk, and the Udjat was worn in the design of an amulet to confer the strength of the sun and the security of health on its bearer."

Tavallali goes on to explain the origin of the Rx symbol used in prescribing medication; he argues convincingly that the Rx sign which physicians use today in their medical prescriptions has its basis in the Udjat, the eye of Horus.(21)

Thoth, the physician of the gods and source of all knowledge, as we have seen, healed the eye of Horus and became the patron god of both physicians, the source of medical knowledge, and scribes, the legendary inventors of Egyptian writing.

Many of the lesser figures within the Egyptian pantheon are known as healers of the sick; amongst them are Serapis, a local divinity who later rivaled Æsculapius as god of healing amongst the common folk of Alexandria.

By the 6th Century B.C., Thoth, himself, the physician to the gods, had been replaced by our colleague Imhotep, whom Sir William Osler (1849-1919) called, "the first figure of a physician to stand out clearly from the mist of antiquity."(19)

Moreover, during his deification process and heavenly ascension, Imhotep was even given a divine father, the god Ptah, to further establish his legitimacy in the Egyptian pantheon.

As an interesting aside, allow me to mention a ruler who was thought to have medical knowledge and magical power. Her name was Queen Hatshepsut (d.1468 B.C.), who assumed the powers of government after the death of her husband and half-brother, Thutmose II (pharaoh, c.1495-1490 B.C.), whilst becoming the regent to her young son, Thutmose III (d.1436 B.C.; pharaoh, 1468-1436 B.C.).(19) Thutmose III would become a great conqueror [8] and would build many magnificent temples and impressive obelisk

---

[8] The Thutmose rulers were great conquerors. Thutmose I (pharaoh, c.1525-1495 B.C.) conquered lands up to the Third Cataract of the Nile, and advancing through Syrian territory, reached the Euphrates. His son, Thutmose II, ruled ably guided by Queen Hatshepsut (who held the real power). Thutmose III was not only sole ruler of Egypt but also embarked on expeditions that consolidated his rule over Syria, the Aegean islands, and all the powers north of the Euphrates except Phoenicia. He enriched Egypt with the wealth of foreign lands and their much needed manpower – both were used to build magnificent temples along the Nile.(2)

including many of the misnamed "Cleopatra's Needles," still standing in such Western cities as London and New York. Under his rule the Egyptian empire would reach its farthest extent and a pinnacle of glory.

THE EGYPTIAN AFTERLIFE AND THE BOOK OF THE DEAD

Death will smite with its wings whoever disturbs the peace of the Pharaoh.
Inscription found over the tomb of
King Tutankhamen,1921.

The combination of a dry climate and the sandy soil of Egypt preserved records as well as the bodies of persons who had been buried for centuries. *The Book of the Dead* is a guide to prepare royalty and ordinary Egyptian citizens for the afterlife. Because Egyptians believed that after death the spirit of a man survived and lived in another world, the priests prepared the body by mummification in elaborate rituals. The mysterious and sometimes inscrutable *Book of the Dead* also described Egyptian medicine and the treatment of diseases by specific rites or elaborate rituals, the muttering of prayers, the recitation of incantations, the imbibition of magical potions, the wearing of amulets, the use of divinations, the act of sacrificial libations, the utterance aloud of supplications, and the singing of praising songs and chantings. Curiously, I have recently discovered that no two books of the dead contained all of the same incantations and supplications, thence, no two of the *Book of the Dead* papyri were ever alike!

Because of Egyptian preoccupation with death and the afterlife, the Egyptian *Book of the Dead* not only had rituals, incantations, and supplications for the dearly departed but also clear instructions for burial practices and elaborate rituals to prepare the physical body for receiving the life force necessary for resurrection.(22)

It was ancient Egyptian belief that the living human body was the abode of the divine spirit or soul, *Ka,* a spiritual double which remained with the properly embalmed body after death to make sure that proper ritual was instituted, that the priests followed the precise rites of the "opening of the mouth" ceremony depicted and discussed in the *Book of the Dead*. For example, embalming rituals called for placement of each of the deceased's organs (the liver, lungs, stomach, and intestines) into four stone canopy jars to preserve them and ensure that they would function for eternity. The intracranial contents, however, were removed through the nostrils and discarded! The body cavities, skull, chest, and abdomen were washed with exotic herbs and aromatic spices, and the body was soaked in a mixture of clay and salts, carbonate sulfates.(19) For embalming, the body was prepared with gums and resins and then wrapped in long strips of linen.

Of interest to us is the fact that despite their knowledge of embalming procedures, Egyptian anatomy, physiology, and pathology remained rudimentary and inadequate.(19) Nevertheless, the Egyptian physician-priest, despite his medical shortcomings and meager knowledge of anatomy and physiology, was aware, by keen observations, of certain facts of nature. For instance, "to the Egyptian physician," writes Woodward, "the heart and the circulatory system simulated the Nile River and its system of canals used for irrigation."(23) So that they seemed to possess an inkling of the relationship of the heart to the circulatory system but had no knowledge of its purpose. And Woodward reminds us that even to this day, the minister consoles us with comforting words: "Let not your heart be troubled." And, he adds, "on February 14th, the symbol of St. Valentine's Day is the heart, not the liver or brain" that we celebrate.(23)

The Egyptian priests ministered to the living as well as to the recently departed and did everything within their power to promote a smooth transition from this life to the afterlife.

To this end, the Egyptian physician-priests were obliged to perform precise rituals and recite ancient incantations to the gods, especially to Osiris and Anubis. Osiris, as we have said, was the Lord of the Dead and Judge of the Underworld, and Anubis, the jackal-god, the god of mummification.

According to Egyptian mythology, Anubis, the son of Osiris and Nephthys (Set's wife), was conceived as a result of what today, I suppose, would be considered a case of mistaken identity. This is apparently what happened: in the darkness of a hot passionate Egyptian night, the fervidly impassioned Osiris mistook the goddess Nephthys for Isis. According to the late historian Joseph Campbell, this was a case of "inattention to detail," so to speak, and it was this act that sparked Set's revenge against Osiris that led to the saga of the resurrected Osiris that we have already described.

It suffices to say that the jackal-god, Anubis, presided over the "opening of the mouth" ceremony and was the god of embalming. As the jackal-god, we see him frequently depicted in the marvelous paintings on the walls of the awe-inspiring Egyptian tombs of antiquity. Osiris is usually portrayed as the elderly, yet imposing, seated figure with a distinct goatee and a grayish-green morbid (ashen) complexion, who solemnly presides over the ceremony of death from his regal throne in the realm of the Underworld. He often carries the symbol of power, the Egyptian *flail* in one hand, signifying discipline and justice; just as the flail was used to beat the wheat to separate the chaff from the grain, so Osiris fed his people with discipline and justice. In his other hand, he holds the *crook* of royalty which signifies statesmanship and leadership and the emblem of a god of mercy who is charged with leading his flock through the proper path.(10) In these characteristic Egyptian paintings with frontal torsos and facial profiles, the departing pharaoh is depicted carrying the *ankh*, the symbol of life and everlasting peace.

Thus the pharaohs ruled by divine authority, as they were considered living gods, living personifications of Osiris, and sons of Amon-Ra; their throne, their source of power, was the emblem of the primeval Mother-goddess, Isis.(24) The sacred asp which projected from their headdress, the *Uraeus,* symbolized their magical power as well as life and wisdom.(25)

These religious beliefs endured and survived for centuries, and ironically, it was a sacred asp that ended pharaonic rule in Egypt. It was the striking of a queen's bosom by an asp in 30 B.C. that ended Ptolemaic pharaonic rule after the disastrous defeat of the combined fleets of two lovers: the Roman Mark Antony and the astute Egyptian queen Cleopatra at Actium in 31 B.C.

EGYPTIAN SURGERY

In 1862, American archaeologist and Egyptologist, Edwin Smith (1822-1906) made a fortuitous discovery, a discovery that was to become a notable contribution to the history of civilization and particularly medical history. He came across a collection of old papyri which described the diagnosis and treatment of 48 case-histories of traumatic injuries, starting with head trauma and proceeding down the body to include injuries of the spine. The hieroglyphics contained in the Edwin Smith Papyrus, after whom the scrolls (truly papyri) were appropriately named, provide us with the earliest written record of the practice of surgery and the first written medical book in history.(1,11,13,19,26)

The papyri together were 15 feet long and described in detail both natural means of treatment, such as immobilization of the injured and the setting of broken bones, as well as instructions as to supernatural treatment in the form of magical formulae and incantations.

Amazingly, some of the natural treatments outlined in the text could effectively be used today. For example, the positioning for proper reduction and immobilization of clavicular fractures was accurately described. Even the prognosis of spinal injuries was described, and the ancient Egyptian physicians recognized, for example, the grave prognosis associated with flaccid quadriplegia (limp paralysis of all four limbs) and priapism (spontaneous pathologic erection) following a severe cervical spine injury.

The rest of the hieroglyphics, which presumably included sections on the chest and abdomen, unfortunately were (and remain) missing. The manuscript itself is believed to be a copy of an earlier manuscript dating back to 3000 B.C., and thus, the original text is as old, if not older, than the great pyramids of Giza. Curiously, and of great historic significance, the eminent American Egyptologist, James Henry Breasted (1865-1935), who studied and translated the precious document in 1930, believed that the earliest known physician, the Grand Vizier Imhotep, had written this papyrus 5,000 years ago!(11)

The medical and surgical instruments that have been found near Thebes are characteristic of the Bronze Age and reflect the expected needs of the ancient Egyptian surgeons. The gods Amon-Ra (also Ra), Isis, Thoth, and Horus were all called upon to preside over invocations, prayers, and magical incantations preceding the use of medical prescriptions and natural remedies. Regarding surgical judgment and treatment, the noted medical historian M. Neuburger quotes from the Ebers Papyrus:

> When thou findest a purulent swelling with the apex elevated, sharply defined and of a rounded form, then sayest thou, 'It is a purulent tumor which is growing in the flesh. I must treat the disease with a knife.'
> When thou findest a growth upon the throat of a patient containing matter...and thou findest its top raised like a wart, know that the matter moves within it.
>
> When thou findest a fatty growth in the neck, and findest it like an abscess of the flesh and soft to the fingers, then sayest thou, 'He has a fatty growth on his neck. I will treat the disease with the knife, paying heed to the vessels.'
>
> When thou findest a tumor of the flesh in a particular part of a person's body, and findest it like skin upon his flesh, it being moist, moving with the fingers except they be still, the movement being thus due to the fingers, it is a tumor of the flesh; then sayest thou, 'I shall treat the disease by trying to cure it with fire.'(27)

In addition, we also know from the Ebers Papyrus that the Egyptian physician-priests had instructions for the proper dressing and treatment of wounds and the care of the wounded.

Circumcision and castration were old customs in the ancient world, especially in Egypt and Mesopotamia. The prominent physician and medical historian, Richard A. Leonardo, states that for centuries Egypt was the world's leading contributor of eunuchs.(11) Lithotomy was an important procedure in Egypt, and Egyptian lithotomists were the first to keep the art of urology a secret for centuries. In fact, at the time of the Hippocratic Oath, skilled itinerant Egyptian lithotomists practiced urology, and the reference to: "I will not cut a person who is suffering with a stone, but will leave this to be done by practitioners of this work"...(28) is a reference to these itinerant lithotomists. Moreover, in my opinion, this clause was not a condemnation of lithotomy as a surgical procedure *per se*, but a plea to physicians, many of whom were not familiar with this surgical procedure, to refer those patients afflicted to the qualified practitioners who were more experienced and adept in this surgical specialty. It was to be many centuries, perhaps not until the time of the great surgeon, William Cheseldon (1688-1752), before lithotomy became a recognized and legitimate part of medicine and surgery.

EGYPTIAN MEDICINE

The Ebers Papyrus was named for the German scholar, George Ebers (1837-1898), who studied the hieroglyphic scrolls he had discovered in Luxor in 1872. The papyrus dates from approximately 1750 B.C. Largely a collection of medical recipes, the Ebers Papyrus contains over 800 medical prescriptions and remedies as well as herbal ingredients used for concocting medicinal drugs. Ebers believed this papyrus to be one of the most sacred books of the moon god, Thoth.

Thoth, as we have seen, was also an important and powerful deity, closely identified with medicine and healing. He was incarnated in the Ibis, and because the latter with their long beaks instinctively injected sea water into their rectum, Thoth, by association, was credited with the invention and use of enemas.(29)

Egyptian physicians, in general, believed that internal afflictions were caused by supernatural causes, whereas, external injuries were caused by natural events. The former, therefore, were treated with magic and religion; the latter, with salves, bandages, and wound care, as well as surgery. The best known Egyptian goddess, Isis, according to ancient Egyptian myth, taught the Egyptians the art of hygiene and sanitation. Perhaps it is because of her association with cleanliness and good health that Egyptian priests bathed four times daily and abstained from foods known to produce bad breath and flatulence, such as pork, beans, and onions.(29)

As mankind took his first steps and ascended the ladder of civilization, he no longer believed that spirits inhabited inanimate objects, e.g., rivers, streams, or trees. Instead, in the minds of men, omnipotent, omniscient, and not always benevolent supernatural denizens of other worlds, gods and goddesses, ruled mightily with the power of incarnation over living things and with the awesome power to direct and control the ordinary events of ordinary human beings. Amon-Ra was worshipped throughout Upper and Lower Egypt as the sun god, a powerful god who each morning fought and won the struggle to rise as the sun, the source of life and fertility in Egypt. As we have seen, Egyptians were polytheistic, worshipping many deities, some of whom are even more central to our story. The solemn god, Osiris, quarreled, and through his wife, Isis, and son, Horus, defeated his evil brother, Set, the god of Upper Egypt, who now along with his many minion demons constantly created evil and spread disease amongst the earthly dwellers of the kingdom of the Nile.(1)

The Egyptian upper class of physician-priests were conversant with the ways and cognizant of the secrets of the merciful gods as well as evil demons. And thus, they followed the instructions of the *Book of the Dead* to the letter, chanting sacred hymns, reciting incantations, concocting magic potions, and performing rituals – all to drive away the evil spirits, to brake wicked spells and curses, and stamp out sickness and disease. The priests of Egypt, then, were the descendants of the earlier medicine men (or witch doctors), and supreme amongst them, as we have mentioned, was the physician, Imhotep. So much so did his reputation grow after his death, that by the time of the Persian conquest of Egypt by the Achaemenid King of Persia, Cambyses II,[9] Imhotep had become an important god of Egypt.

Amongst the incantations that have come down to us from Egyptian hieroglyphics recorded on the pages of history is the introduction to the Ebers Papyrus, which was intended to be recited when applying external remedies and so reads:

> *Words to be said with exactitude and repeated as many times as possible when one applies remedies over a member of some one who is ill, in order to destroy all cause of disturbance residing within him.*

> *Isis has delivered Osiris, has delivered Horus from evil things which his brother Set had done him by killing his father Osiris. O Isis, great goddess of incantations, deliver me, free me from all bad, evil and cruel things, deliver me from the god of pain, from the goddess of pain, from a death, from the penetrating which penetrates me, in the same way as thy son Horus was delivered and freed. For I have entered into fire, I have come out of water, I have not fallen into the snare of today. I have said that I have been a child, that I have been small. O Sun, speak with your tongue! O Osiris, intercede by your intervention. Now thou hast delivered me from every bad, evil and cruel thing, from the god of pain, from the goddess of pain, from death.(30)*

We also have incantations to be recited by Egyptian physician-priests when internal remedies are to be administered: "Come remedies, come and expel the things of my heart, of my limbs. Incantations are good for remedies and remedies are good for incantations. Do you not remember that Horus and Set were brought within the great temple of Heliopolis when the question of their legitimacy was being discussed? He is now prospering as he was when on earth, he does everything that he desires, like the gods among whom he now resides."(30)

The late medical historian Dr. Charles G. Cumston reminds us that these

---

[9] There was a major Persian incursion into Egyptian territory during this time. The veritable invasion was led by Cambyses II (King of Persia, 530-522 B.C.) in 525 B.C., who continued the wars of conquest commenced by his father, Cyrus the Great. Cambyses II succeeded in conquering Egypt and capturing the religious and cultural centers of Thebes and Memphis. However, in the midst of his conquests, the conqueror suddenly and mysteriously died in North Africa (poisoning has been speculated) whilst planning further campaigns and expeditions to Ethiopia and Carthage.

incantations were to be recited "as exactly as possible and as many times as possible whenever the patient drank a potion."(30)

Another example was in the treatment of tapeworms which appeared to have been a common infestation in pharaonic Egypt; in these cases the remedies administered were associated with the incantation: "May these words expel the painful creeping progression traced in my belly by him who winds within! It is a god that has created this enemy! May he charm it and expel the affection that he has produced in my belly!"(30)

And when all else failed, magic formulae gave way to execrations in conjunction with emetics in an attempt to exorcise the malevolent spirit: "O demon who art within the abdomen of So-and-so, son of So-and-so, O thou whose father is surnamed He who causes heads to fall, whose name is death, whose name is the male of death, whose name is accursed to Eternity."(30)

ANCIENT MEDICAL JURISPRUDENCE:
HAMMURABI'S LEGACY AND THE EDWIN SMITH PAPYRUS

Most of us spend too much time on the last twenty-four hours and too little time on the last six thousand years.
>> *Will Durant*

At the time of his travels, the great historian, Herodotus (c.484-424 B.C.), the Father of History, was meticulously collecting information about different peoples, their cultures, and their faraway lands. It was from his accounts about Egypt that we get a glimpse as to the status of Egyptian physicians in the 5th Century B.C. "The art of medicine is thus divided among them: Each physician applies himself to one disease only, and no more. All places abound in physicians; some physicians are for the eyes, others for the head, others for the teeth, others for intestines, and others for internal disorders."(11)

Moreover, the influence of the celebrated Babylonian king, Hammurabi (fl.1792-1750 B.C.) – of whom we will have more to say about later – was more widespread than was heretofore believed, not only in Mesopotamia but also in Egypt, especially in the incipient field of medical jurisprudence and its effect on ancient medical practices.

According to the ancient Greek historian, Diodorus Siculus (fl.20 B.C.), Egyptian physicians were regulated by the state:

> *In expeditions and journeys from the country all are treated free of charge, for the physicians receive a salary by the state, and they provide their services according to a written law compiled by many famous physicians of ancient times...and if after following the laws read from this sacred book they are not able to save the patient, they are safe from any accusation, but if they act contrary to the written law, they may expect capital punishment, as the legislator considers that only few men would have knowledge better than the method of treatment observed for many years and prescribed by the best masters.(11)*

There is no doubt that the message conveyed in the above paragraph gives a boost to the present-day proponents of practice parameters, which in the same or similar fashion are seen not only as educational materials for physicians but also as a method to reduce medical liability amongst those doctors who followed the guidelines. By the same token, opponents of practice parameters call it "cookbook medicine," decry the fact that in today's litigious climate, parameters will not deter litigation, and contemplate the possibility that practice parameters could actually reduce innovation and even lead to mediocrity in a stagnant medical environment.

Although we will discuss Mesopotamia in the next chapter, I would like to mention the Code of Hammurabi at this point, as it appears to have profoundly affected medical practice in ancient Egypt – far more than had ever been imagined.

The Code of Hammurabi strictly and harshly dealt with an "eye for an eye" justice, as well as general medical jurisprudence in Akkadian Babylonia, c.1750 B.C. For example, regarding surgical fees and operations, the code promulgated:

> If a physician shall cause on anyone a severe operation wound with a bronze operating-knife and cure him, or if he shall open a tumor (abscess or cavity) with a bronze operating-knife and save the eye of the patient, he shall have ten shekels of silver; if it is a slave, his owner shall pay two shekels of silver to the physician.

> If a physician shall make a severe wound with the bronze operating-knife and kill him, or shall open a growth with a bronze operating-knife and destroy the eye, his hands shall be cut off.

> If a physician shall make a severe wound with a bronze operating-knife on the slave of a freed man and kill him, he shall replace the slave with another slave. If he shall open an abscess (growth, tumor, cavity) with a bronze operating-knife and destroy the eye, he shall pay the half of the value of the slave.

> If a physician shall heal a broken bone or cure diseased bowels, he shall receive five shekels of silver; if it is a matter of a freed slave, he shall pay three shekels of silver; but if a slave, then the master of the slave shall give to the physician two shekels of silver.(11)

Lower class Egyptian physicians (apparently no members of the priesthood) were in fact subject to many strict rules and regulations that affected medical practice.

A thoroughly fascinating study by Dr. James Salander of the Edwin Smith Papyrus should be of great interest to the readers. Salander studied what is considered the world's oldest surgical textbook and after years of researching a translation of the papyri (provided by the University of Chicago), Salander was able to elucidate very interesting details regarding medical practice in Egypt c.1500 B.C. His copy of the Edwin Smith Papyrus was translated and annotated by the renowned scholar, James Henry Breasted. Salander confirmed that the papyri were a collection of 48 cases, 45 of which were trauma cases, a fact which suggests that these scrolls may have been an ancient military textbook.(26)

Case stories were presented "in anatomical sequence, beginning with injuries of the head and onward down the body." In the papyri, he continues, "each case is assigned a prognosis...." Then a very important ethical statement follows: "In cases in which injury was so severe that a favorable outcome seemed unlikely, the practitioner declined to treat the patient. Fifteen of the 45 trauma cases received unfavorable verdicts." The report went on to say, "not all patients denied care suffered devastating injuries." Dr. Salander reports that closed fractures of the mandible and open-rib and nasal fractures were all considered "untreatable." The student of history will agree with Salander's explanation for the unfavorable prognoses rendered in these cases, and that is that the strong influence of the Code of Hammurabi which dates from the same era and "holds strict accountability to the physician with uncomfortably severe penalties..." made Egyptian physicians wary of treating those injuries which carried a high degree of failure or deformity.(26)

Like Moses, who received the Ten Commandments from God, Hammurabi claimed to have received his laws from the Babylonian sun-god, Shamash, god of justice. The laws are inscribed in 4000 lines of Akkadian cuneiform writing containing 300 legal provisions covering not only an oppressive code of medical "ethics" imposing heavy penalties for physicians who injured patients or obtained a bad result with their treatment but also voluminous rules covering businesses, criminal laws, agricultural provisions, and rules of conduct in all ways of life, public and private. The polished black diorite stele is an impressive $7\frac{1}{2}$ feet tall and bears a bas-relief of a standing Hammurabi receiving the laws from a seated Shamash.

Nevertheless, its jurisdiction was pronounced by the King in the presence of his advisors and established, "an eye for an eye" justice, in which the state was supreme. It was oppressive to medical practitioners. Medical progress would have to flourish elsewhere.

A college textbook further explains, "the Code of Hammurabi was based on a caste society: injuries to men of the upper classes are fined more heavily than injuries to a 'freeman' and injuries to a freeman came higher than injuries to a slave."(31)

The implications, of course, are tremendous and are relevant to the present-day adversarial litigious climate that permeates our society. What we have found here is that knowledgeable Egyptian physicians, the most knowledgeable physicians in the civilized world at the time, were advising that medical knowledge not be used to treat patients as a self-protective measure – *defensive medicine* – against potential government reprisals in case of treatment failure or in the case of nasal fractures, patient dissatisfaction. The practice of medicine, then or now, cannot thrive in a milieu of government oppression, coercion, and intimidation, and as we have just found, this is true whether we are speaking of an era 4,000 years ago or the environment of today.(32)

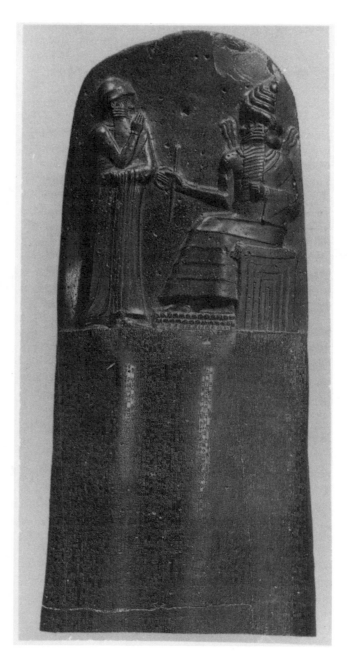

Plate 3 – King Hammurabi receiving his code of laws from the sun-god, Shamash, as depicted on the famous polished black diorite stele c.1750 B.C. Musée du Louvre, Paris.

CHAPTER 3

MESOPOTAMIA AND THE EMPIRES OF THE NEAR EAST

We are in the first age since the dawn of civilization in which people have dared to think it practicable to make the benefits of civilization available to the human race.
Arnold J. Toynbee (1889-1975)
English historian and internationalist

THE CRADLE OF CIVILIZATION

As Mesopotamia, the cradle of civilization, and surrounding territories circling the fertile crescent have an entwined political, economic (trade), and military history, it is appropriate that we recount important historic events of Western civilization that occurred in this region in order to gain a better understanding of the tenor of our story. Mesopotamia, "the land between the rivers," the Tigris and Euphrates, is now the setting of the next scene in our drama. This ancient region was indeed one of the earliest community settlements where the first nomadic hunters settled to become gatherers of seed and grain and develop a new way of life. For the first time in history, the land was tilled to produce enough crops to support the establishment of new societal classes including merchants, traders, craftsmen, as well as the sustenance of a sacerdotal or priestly class whose members served as religious leaders, political administrators, scriveners, and physicians.

The Sumerians were the first people to settle in Mesopotamia in approximately 5,000 B.C. and to develop a true civilization with an agricultural economy, division of labor, and commercial interdependence between the various city states in the region (i.e., Ur and Lagash). More importantly, the Sumerians devised the first system of writing, the cuneiform method ("wedge-shaped") which was done on clay tablets and was well established as a form of writing by 3200 or 3100 B.C.. Fortunately, clay tablets have been relatively well preserved for scholars and for posterity.

Along with the invention of writing, a powerful sacerdotal priesthood developed to serve local deities and build temples of worship for the Sumerian pantheon of gods. By 2300 B.C., the Sumerians would be subdued by the Akkadian invaders, as we shall see, led by King Sargon I who created the first Mesopotamian empire.

Interestingly, many old Sumerian stories are purported to be the source of inspiration for some biblical stories. For instance, the story of Noah [10] and the Flood, which is now believed to have occurred sometime before the Sumerian settlement, is a good example. A gigantic flood reminiscent of the biblical flood of Noah is recorded and described in the Sumerian epic of Gilgamesh, the King of Uruk (Ur), which details the extraordinary saga of the legendary Babylonian hero.

Another biblical story, the Tower of Babel, has also been studied by biblical scholars and has been offered as a plausible explanation for the almost sudden explosive

---

[10] The biblical story of Noah in which he built a great ark under divine guidance and saved the human race and species of animal life during the great deluge is told in the Old Testament (Genesis 6-10).

development of various Semitic languages in the region.(17) Historically, the Tower of Babel was probably a Sumerian *ziggurat*, one of the many great towers built with sun-baked bricks in the region during this time. The most impressive ziggurats, such as the Tower of Babel and the Ziggurat of Ur (Sumer), were architectural culminations of centuries of improvement in mound-building engineering. These pyramidal structures with receding tiers of construction were elaborate edifices which served the Sumerians (and later the Babylonians and Assyrians) as temples of worship for their many deities.(2)

Ur was then the historic capital of Sumeria in the delta of the Euphrates and Tigris rivers, and the birthplace of Abraham, the father of Judeo-Christian monotheism 4000 years ago. The Ziggurat of Ur is perhaps the best preserved model of the biblical Tower of Babel.(33)

The achievements of the Sumerians and early Babylonians were indeed monumental in the history of civilization. In addition to the invention of cuneiform writing on clay tablets, the first method of writing and the prerequisite for any truly blossoming civilization, they developed the wheel and put it to proper use. They also conceived of and used the 60-minute hour as a unit of time, the 360-degree circle as a unit of angular measurement in engineering, and the first written code of laws. The alphabet, of course, was a gift to civilization by the nearby entrepreneurial maritime Phoenicians.

The legendary biblical paradise of the Garden of Eden is believed to be located near the ancient city of Ur in Sumeria in lower Mesopotamia, which was also near the region where the ancient Sumerian cities of Erech and Lagash were located.

THE FIRST INVASIONS AND THE BABYLONIAN KINGDOM

Territorial aggression on a grand scale commenced with the conquests of the Akkadian King Sargon I (c.2334-2279 B.C.). After subduing and conquering the native population of Sumer, he founded the first Semitic empire in Mesopotamia, c. 2300 B.C. His empire extended from Sumer "to the Cedars of Babylon, silver rich Anatolia and the stone-rich Elam"(Iran)(1) – and thus, he controlled much of southwestern Asia and its prize, much of the fertile crescent extending from Mesopotamia to Palestine (but not Egypt). A few centuries later, the aggressive Hittites conquered Babylonia in 1925 B.C. and ruled for nearly a century until they were repulsed and replaced with the first Babylonian dynasty, established in 1830 B.C. This dynasty (the Amorites) reached its zenith with the ascension of King Hammurabi, whom we have already discussed. Semitic Babylonian peoples of Akkadian and Amorite stock continued to rule Babylon until approximately 710 B.C. After a millennium of relative peace, the war machine of the Assyrians arrived on the scene and overpowered the old Babylonian kingdom. Hammurabi's empire was destroyed, but his legendary code of laws inscribed on the column of Susa survived as one of the marvels of antiquity.

THE ASSYRIANS

The war-like Assyrians were led by King Sennacherib (705-681 B.C.). By 689 B.C., Sennacherib and his mighty Assyrians had conquered and destroyed Babylon and with slave labor built their imperial capital and royal palace at Nineveh

(701 B.C.). The old and more modest capital city of Kalah was abandoned and eventually fell prey to the detritus of time. Yet, the black obelisk of Kalah resides today in the British Museum in London, and its inscriptions detail the conquests of the war machine of the Assyrians. Bas-relief sculptures depict the vanquished and hapless prisoners held captive by the Assyrians. Amongst the depicted prisoners are the Israelites marching under the yoke of their captors. Literally, tell-tale cuneiform clay tablets have been excavated both from Kalah and Nineveh.

The mighty armies of the Assyrians captured Samaria and squelched both the kingdoms of Israel (722 B.C.) and Judea (682 B.C.).[11](34) Under Ashurbanipal II (King of Assyria, 669-633 B.C.), Assyrian conquests reached a pinnacle of power. Ashurbanipal II ruled Mesopotamia, Palestine, and most of the fertile crescent.(31) He even had the audacity to invade and sack the Egyptian city of Thebes in 663 B.C.

The Assyrian war machine consisted of heavily armed warriors mounted in light-weight, two-wheeled chariots. They used swords, spears of iron, and siege warfare, both standing and besieging armies, and psychologic warfare against their encircled enemies. It is of interest to note that the light two-wheeled chariots dominated the area in warfare – from the 9th to the 7th Century B.C.

For all his fame as a warrior and military genius, Ashurbanipal II was also a scholar who built a magnificent and opulent library at Nineveh and who enjoyed sumptuous living when not involved in warfare. His library, which was rediscovered by Layard in the year 1845 to 1847, was reputed to have contained 22,000 clay tablets inscribed in various Semitic languages. Under his rule, the arts, especially sculpturing and architecture, flourished. His capital was decorated with ornate gates and his palaces with sculptured figures of colossal winged-bulls, walls decorated with imposing bas-reliefs of fierce lion hunts, and heroic scenes of battles and sieges. Yet, the Assyrians were cruel and ruthless to their enemies, and it shows on these extant bas-reliefs. They are frequently portrayed decimating, with swords or with bow and arrows, their retreating or falling enemies. In addition, their use of battering rams during sieges, smoldering and demolished cities, impalement of captives, and massacres of prisoners are all scenes vividly depicted in Assyrian bas-reliefs.(35)

The Assyrians controlled an empire for the period between 883 and 612 B.C. which stretched from the Persian Gulf, through Mesopotamia and Palestine, all the way to Egypt. Ashurbanipal II was their last great king; his empire collapsed a few years after his rule.

The Assyrian empire had been founded on a single pillar and that was military power (and raw terror) and not on any lasting formula of philosophic, religious, or economic foundation. Their empire established by the sword was destined to fall by the sword. In 612 B.C., the mighty Assyrian empire, these once seemingly invincible conquerors, were overran by a combination of enemies that included Babylonians, Medes, and Persian tribes. Nineveh, as predicted in biblical scripture of the Old Testament – was destroyed by fire, flood, and war – but unlike the phoenix, it never rose again from its ashes.(36)

---

[11] King Sargon II, who founded the last Assyrian dynasty, completed the conquest of Samaria and dispersed the Israelites so widely throughout his kingdom that they became "the lost tribes of Israel."(2)

THE SECOND BABYLONIAN EMPIRE

The next power to rise and leave its mark on the land of Mesopotamia was the Chaldean empire whose greatest ruler was the king Nebuchadnezzar II, "the great" (ruler, 605-561 B.C.). Nebuchadnezzar ruled his empire from his capital at Babylon. Once in power, Nebuchadnezzar II, the undisputed ruler of Babylonia, built an architectural masterpiece, Babylon's celebrated Hanging Gardens. Babylon was the greatest city of antiquity in her time and the Hanging Gardens, without a doubt, were considered a marvel and a great feat of engineering. Later, the Hanging Gardens of Babylon would be recognized as one of the ancient Wonders of the World.(37) A beautiful description of Babylon written by John A. Halford and Keith Stump is found in *Babylon – Past, Present and Future,* Copyright ©1991 Worldwide Church of God. This is their description based on biblical scholarship, historic records, and ancient archaeologic evidence:

Under Nebuchadnezzar, Babylon grew to become the most impressive city of its time – the largest city on earth. The Greek historian, Herodotus, declared that it surpassed in splendor any city in the known world. Its population may have exceeded 200,000. Nebuchadnezzar's vast city included immense fortifications. It had two walls, inner and outer, impossible to scale or breach. A hundred gates of bronze were set in an impregnable wall, which was buttressed at regular intervals by defensive towers.

The city's central feature was the great Temple of Marduk, chief of the Babylonian gods. Just to the north was its associated ziggurat or temple tower known as Etemenanki, the house that is the foundation of heaven and earth. The seven-storied tower was topped by a temple in magnificent blue glaze.

From the Temple, the paved Processional Way lead northward to the spectacular Ishtar Gate, decorated with magical bulls and dragons molded in relief in the colorful glazed brickwork. The avenue – its wall decorated with enameled lions – continued through the Ishtar Gate and northward to a temple outside the city walls. Nebuchadnezzar's immense royal palace...lay between the Processional Way on the east and thickly walled citadel to the west. The palace contained five great courtyards. Nebuchadnezzar's throne room – probably also the site of Belshazzar's feast and Alexander the Great's death - lay directly to the south of the central courtyard. Greek tradition refers to the palace's magnificent Hanging Gardens, regarded as one of the Seven Wonders of the Ancient World.(38)

Nebuchadnezzar quickly invaded and conquered the surrounding territories, including the kingdom of Judea which was annexed to the Babylonian empire. The Chaldeans occupied and sacked Jerusalem in 586 B.C. taking the Israelites with them to Babylon in the famed Babylonian Captivity, a historic chapter also described in holy scripture.

THE FALL OF BABYLON

But the great city of Babylon would not last long after the reign of Nebuchadnezzar. Like the Assyrians before them, the Babylonians failed to build a moral or economic foundation for their empire, thus making themselves vulnerable to external attack from their besieging enemies as well as from subjugated peoples within.

Both Herodotus and Seneca have recounted the events leading to the fall of Babylon. The Medes and Persians under Cyrus the Great, as portended by the prophet Daniel (36,38), diverted the Euphrates river to a dried out lake, allowing the level of the main river flowing through Babylon to fall. Using this opportunity, they sneaked into Babylon under cover of darkness, marching under Babylon's defenses over shallow water with the assistance of spies already placed within the gates of Babylon. All this whilst Belshazzar, the indulgent grandson of Nebuchadnezzar and king of Babylon, refusing to heed the advice of the prophet Daniel and unable to decipher the warning, *Mene, Mene, Tekel Upharsin,* which portended the overthrow of the Babylonian kingdom and the rise of Cyrus the Great and the Persian empire, reveled and feasted in his palace, believing that the city's defenses were impregnable to its enemies.

In 539 B.C., the wondrous Babylonian capital with its Hanging Gardens was overrun by a combination of Medes and Persians. The Persians would capitalize from this gain by establishing themselves in the premier position as empire builders. From their capital at Persepolis, the Persians went on to found the successor empire, an impressive empire that would dominate the geopolitical scene of the inchoate Western world for the next 200 years.

THE HITTITES

Three other groups deserve mention in our story because of specific contributions they made which are relevant to our narrative. One of these is the Hittites of Anatolia (c.1200-1500 B.C.) who were of European origin and spoke an Aryan (in Sanskrit "chosen or noble ones") tongue which has now been deciphered. They introduced iron to the area and almost inconspicuously moved civilization from the Bronze Age to the Iron Age. It is with this important development (the use of iron in weaponry) that we mentioned them earlier in reference to the Battle of Qadesh.

THE PHOENICIANS

Another distinct group that should be mentioned, as they also influenced important world events, was the Phoenicians. Most importantly, they invented the alphabet (c.1300 B.C.) and founded faraway colonies in the Mediterranean including Carthage in 814 B.C.(31) They were exemplary seafarers who circumnavigated Africa by sailing from the Red Sea around the Cape of Good Hope and then northward up the Atlantic, finally returning to Egypt via the Mediterranean. They had sailed under the aegis of the Egyptian pharaoh Necho in their maiden voyage.

THE ISRAELITES

The Israelites founded two kingdoms: Israel, with its capital at Samaria which fell to the Assyrians in 721 B.C., and Judea, with its capital at Jerusalem which fell to the Chaldeans (Babylonians) under Nebuchadnezzar in 601 B.C.

It was also during this period that the Jews were persecuted and forced to disperse. First, there was the Assyrian capture and destruction of the Kingdom of Israel (c.745-625 B.C.), and then the Babylonian invasion of Judea and the fall of Jerusalem with the destruction of the Temple of Solomon (the First Temple) in 587 B.C.(34) Hebrew leaders were taken prisoner in the Babylonian Captivity previously mentioned, but under the more tolerant Persians, the Jewish captives were allowed by Cyrus the Great to return to Jerusalem, the biblical capital of their homeland. Nevertheless, the sack of Jerusalem by the Babylonians would not be the last time Jerusalem would be captured, burned, destroyed, and then rebuilt. As we shall see in a later section on Jewish Revolts within the Roman Empire, the Second Temple would again be destroyed in A.D. 70.

Suffice it to say that their struggles have continued to the present age, and only recently – with the peace treaty consummated in October 1993 between Yasir Arafat, Chairman of the Palestine Liberation Organization (PLO) and Israeli Prime Minister, Yitzhak Rabin (head of the Labor Party of Israel) – does a lasting peace seem within reach. To this author, however, despite the peace overtures, the survival of Israel as the homeland of the Jewish people appears uncertain. The Middle East remains an insecure region, a perpetual tinder box, within a shrinking smaller modern world – a serious situation if history is a guide. Moreover, today, ancient powers (although referred to generally by different names) are possessed of modern weapons of mass destruction – i.e., Iraq (Babylonians), Iran (Persians), Syria (Assyrians), Turkey (Hittites), and Lebanon (Phoenicians). The area remains restless and inherently unstable, a historic reminder of an ancient and endless struggle in a land plagued by antediluvian conflicts and ancestral rivalries.

THE PERSIANS

The Persians came into the limelight of the historic scene around 559 B.C. when Cyrus the Great (King of Persia, 559-530 B.C.) unified the various warring Persian tribes. Once unified, the Persians led by their intrepid king set out to topple their Babylonian overlords. With victory after victory, the Persians overran Asia Minor, Mesopotamia, and finally conquered Babylonia in 539 B.C. Judea and Phoenicia, "both proud and independent kingdoms," became Persian provinces.(34) Despite his war successes and his indefatigable spirit, Cyrus was a tolerant ruler who, as we have mentioned, allowed the Jewish exiles to return to Judea. Cyrus' son, Cambyses (ruler, 530-521 B.C.), as we have noted, continued the conquests of his father, extending his dominion to North Africa and briefly conquering Egypt in 525 B.C. His successor, King Darius I (ruler of Persia, 521-486 B.C.) put down Greek revolts in Ionia during the first Persian expedition. It was at this time that the Achaemenid Dynasty (c.550-330 B.C.) and ancient Persian rule reached their zenith of power and their pinnacle of glory.

Yet, it was at their zenith in 490 B.C. that King Darius suffered a major setback in his aspiration of known-world domination during his second Persian expedition in Ionia. He was decisively defeated by the combined power of the independent-minded Greek city-states (but mostly Athenian forces) at the decisive Battle of Marathon.(39) King Darius died before he could proceed with the plan of his next expedition and complete his dream of Persian world hegemony. Nevertheless, his dream and his plans of conquest were undertaken by his son, Xerses I (ruler of Persia, 486-465 B.C.).

In 480 B.C., Xerses raised a grand army of 180,000 men, very likely the largest army ever assembled in history up until that time. He also built and manned a huge and powerful fleet, before embarking on a third expedition against the unruly and contumacious Greeks. The Spartans led the Greek city-states. At the Battle of the Pass of Thermopylae, 300 legendary Spartans under the leadership of King Leonidas were poised to defend the critical and strategic pass against the huge and mighty Persian army. Heroically, the 300 Spartans and a handful of Theban reinforcements held their post and, for a considerable and crucial time, halted the march and onslaught of the huge Persian army, allowing the Greek army to save their most powerful asset, the Athenian fleet, and prepare it for the yet to come decisive maritime battle. The Spartans, however, were betrayed by a Greek traitor who led the Persians behind their lines. The brave Spartans were annihilated as they defended the strategic path to the last man. Nevertheless, the massacre of the heroic Spartans was not in vain, for the Persian fleet was destroyed by the Athenians led by Themistocles (c.525-c.460 B.C.) at the naval Battle of Salamis that same year. Moreover, at the Battle of Plataea, the Persian army was decisively defeated by the combined armies of the Greek city-states. Persian hegemony in Ionia and the threat to the Greeks had ended.

MESOPOTAMIAN MEDICINE

The earliest civilization, as we have seen, developed along the banks of the Tigris and Euphrates river and fertile Mesopotamia, a civilization which developed almost in parallel with the Egyptian civilization along the fertile banks of the Nile. It is from Mesopotamian cuneiform writings that we know that medical and surgical practice was regulated in the cultures of Babylonia and Assyria.

Mesopotamian medicine consisted of divination, an offshoot of the pseudo-science of astrology (which was born here and would later contribute in part to the true science of astronomy taught in the medieval universities), magic, rituals, incantations as well as treatment with charms, herbs, and minor surgery. The liver was regarded as the seat of the soul and the center of life. Therefore, divination and hepatoscopy were to Mesopotamian medicine what incantations and supplications were to Egyptian medicine; both relied on magic and elaborate ritual for treatment of disease as well as healing and preservation of health. Other courses of treatment in Mesopotamian medicine consisted of medicinal baths, anal suppositories, catheterization and the blowing of medications directly into the urethra, and phlebotomy. Dr. Theodore Woodward describes hepatoscopy and Mesopotamian medicine as follows:

> The technique of hepatoscopy, performed by divination, was a ritual performed before the statue of a god. Usually an animal was sacrificed and the liver of the animal was examined and compared with a clay model of the liver. Various changes, colors, and prominences of the fresh liver were then used to

gauge diagnosis and prognosis for the patient. Illnesses were treated with drugs, fumigation, medicated baths, and hot and cold water baths. At times, drugs were given in anal suppositories and even by blowing medications into the urethra..."(23)

Prevalent diseases of Mesopotamia included: rheumatism, tumors, heart disease, abscesses, jaundice, respiratory problems, venereal diseases, diseases of the ear, eyes, and skin as well as pestilential diseases such as malaria, dysentery, typhoid fever, and leprosy.(23) Popular drugs used during this time were Hellebore (*Colchicine*, still used today in the treatment of gout), *opium* (morphine and derivatives, still our mainstay for the control of severe or acute pain), and hemp.

In Mesopotamia, the god of the moon, Sin, was also identified with medicine, and under his aegis, medical men gathered medicinal plants by moonlight to concoct their medical preparations.(11)

The long-standing but no longer acceptable ethics of not treating hopeless cases, embraced by philanthropic Greek physicians in later times, began here in Mesopotamia. Babylonian p hysicians felt that the practice was sound and protected the sick and vulnerable from charlatans and mountebanks who would take economic advantage of seriously-ill patients who were beyond medical help.

Codified laws were for the first time formulated to regulate public health and enumerate the duties and responsibilities of physician-priests.(11,23,29) Along with these duties went stiff legal penalties that we have already discussed. Thus, under King Hammurabi, the first code of "ethics" was imposed on the medical profession. Woodward explains: "If an operation caused loss of an eye, the physician might have his hand amputated; if a high-born person died as a result of treatment, the physician lost his life."(23)

Unearthed, deciphered cuneiform texts revealed that ancient Mesopotamians also believed in demonology, and thus, many diseases were thought to be caused by evil spirits or by spells cast upon unwary victims. Cure was sought by physician-priests who were versed in astrology and in divination. In his travels in Babylonia, Herodotus noted:

They bring out their sick to the market-place, for they have no physicians; then those who pass by the sick person confer with him about the disease, to discover whether they have themselves been afflicted with the same disease as the sick person, or have seen others so afflicted; thus the passers-by confer with him, and advise him to have recourse to the same treatment as that by which they escaped a similar disease, or as they have known to cure others. And they are not allowed to pass by a sick person in silence, without inquiring into the nature of his distemper.(11)

MESOPOTAMIAN SURGERY

We have just alluded to regression to a more primitive state of affairs in Babylonian medicine. We also learn from the writings of Herodotus that at least on occasions, when physicians were scarce or non-existent, the whole community seemed to have acted as a collective of physicians utilizing a communal, empirical approach.

Yet, in Egypt, as the Edwin Smith Papyrus illustrates, the physician-priests emerged as having definite knowledge about the diagnosis, treatment, and even prognosis of specific traumatic injuries. The Egyptian physicians' ingenuity was only impeded, it seems, by the necessity to follow written guidelines ("cookbook medicine") and to protect themselves from the harsh "eye for an eye" Akkadian justice (defensive medicine) to fend off lawful reprisals from possible bad outcomes (medical liability).

We can surmise that Mesopotamian surgery was even more restricted and may have been impeded even further in innovations and techniques by the natal and closer legacy of the harsh code of laws of Hammurabi. Unfortunately, given the ravages of time, these lessons have been forgotten. Despite all that we now know about the extensive regulations and impositions of the Code of Hammurabi, we know very little about actual Babylonian operative techniques or surgical practice.(1,11,13,19,30)

We have already referred to the subject of medical jurisprudence and Hammurabi's legacy under the topic of Egyptian surgery, and the point establishing the detrimental effect on society of oppressive laws on medical practice has clearly been made. Let us now discuss what we know about the surgical knowledge of other groups that resided in this area.

We do know that the Medes and the Persians practiced surgery at a level, perhaps, above that practiced by the Babylonians and the Assyrians. For instance, we know that Persian physicians were divided into three classes: those who practiced with herbs; those who practiced with words (counselling); and those who practiced with the knife. Nevertheless, Persian physicians and surgeons were considered second rate to their Egyptian counterparts, and Persian rulers, such as Cyrus the Great and Darius I, were known to seek medical care from Egyptian physicians.(11)

Ancient Israelites did not practice medicine as a separate profession. Their priests considered medicine and healing as part of their priestly duties and believed in disease as a result of divine retribution or punishment inflicted by God for worldly sins. So it may well be said that the earliest Hebrew priests practiced medicine and their *sine qua non* was the belief in the power of prayer to heal.

The medical historian, Dr. Richard A. Leonardo, believed that in later biblical times, physicians evolved as distinct healers, true medicine men. He maintained:

> *In the Bible a physician is always called a physician and not a priest and for this professional physician the expression "rophe" was used. These physicians seem to have been handicapped in their struggle for recognition because of the religious beliefs and superstitions of the people as well as because of the antagonism of the priests. An often quoted instance of this is the sarcastic story about the illness and death of King Asa who "in his disease sought not to the Lord, but to the physicians," with the result that he "slept with his fathers" (II Chronicles, xv1,12,13).(11)*

Yet, physicians came to be respected by the Israelites for their work, their dedication, and their compassion. This is perhaps best expressed in the words of Jesus, the son of Sirach, who declared in 180 B.C. (Ecclesiasticus (R.V.) Chapter xxxviii) his profound respect for physicians in the following statement: "Honor a physician according to thy need of him with the honors due unto him: For verily the Lord hath created him."(11)

The beginning of Jewish medicine and surgery dates from the time of the Old Testament and the Five Books of Moses (the *Pentateuch*) collected at the time of King Solomon (d.922 B.C.). There are several mentions of surgical procedures in the Old Testament. For example, the ear lobe perforation with the awl as the surgical instrument (Deuteronomy 15:17) and circumcision. Circumcision was also practiced by Egyptian surgeons, but in the case of the Hebrew surgeons, it was practiced as a religious rite.

According to Hebrew scriptures, Abraham in 1897 B.C., at the ripe old age of 99, was the first man to undergo the procedure. In those days, stone knives were used, and even when bronze became available, the traditional stone knives continued to be used for the ceremony. The first written record of the operation c.800 B.C. was recorded in Genesis 17 as follows:

And God said unto Abraham, 'Thou shalt keep my covenant therefore, thou, and thy seed after thee in their generations. This is my covenant, which ye shall keep, between me and you and thy seed after thee; every man child among you shall be circumcised. And ye shall circumcise the flesh of your foreskin; and it shall be a token of the covenant betwixt me and you. And he that is eight days old shall be circumcised among you, every man child in your generations, he that is born in the house, or bought with money of any stranger, which is not of thy seed. He that is born in thy house, and he that is bought with thy money, must needs be circumcised; and my covenant shall be in your flesh for an everlasting covenant. And the uncircumcised man child whose flesh of his foreskin is not circumcised, that soul shall be cut off from his people; he has broken my covenant.'

The Talmud – a compilation of Hebrew law in association with rabbinical commentaries and the authoritative body of Jewish tradition (written between 586 and 538 B.C.) – records Jewish medicine and surgery from the time of the Babylonian Captivity up to A.D.500. And from this body of knowledge we know that Hebrew priests in their role as physicians were capable of suturing wounds, repairing imperforate anus, distinguishing uterine from vaginal bleeding; they also knew of mild anesthetics that could be used to decrease pain, of dental prosthesis that could be used as artificial teeth (made of hard wood and gold), of techniques of amputations and the fitting with wooden legs, etc.(11)

Despite all of these surgical advances, the greatest achievement of Hebrew medicine during this time was its emphasis on public health, sanitation, and personal hygiene.(11,27,40)

CHAPTER 4

THE EASTERN RELIGIONS AND PHILOSOPHIC INFLUENCES

Books are the treasured wealth of the world and the fit inheritance of generations and nations....Their authors are a natural and irresistible aristocracy in every society, and, more than kings or emperors, exert an influence on mankind.

Henry David Thoreau (1817-1862)

THE 6TH CENTURY B.C.

There is no question that immeasurable influence was exerted on the development of Western thought and values by the ethics of Judeo-Christian religion and philosophy. Likewise, Judeo-Christian ethics were paramount in the development of Western medical ethics and the making of medical history. In fact, it may be said with little exaggeration that the raison d'être for the Western intellectual tradition may be found in the twin pillars of the Judeo-Christian heritage and the Græco-Roman legacy. In this regard, before we proceed further with the main thread of our discussion, let us discuss those Eastern religions and philosophic influences that in the crucible of time became seasoning ingredients in the forging of Western medical history and ethics.

Eastern thought reached its peak of emanating influence in antiquity in the wake of the 6th Century B.C., with the advent of some of the most influential theophilosophies of the ancient world. This influence was neither as intense nor as lasting as the influence that Judaism exerted throughout this time and Christianity exerted a millennium later during the Dark Ages and the Medieval period.

Curiously, it was also during the 6th Century B.C. that Greek philosophy and by extension the incipient ethics of secular Greek medicine were being constituted. We will, therefore, address those emergent theologies and philosophies of the East that were born during that remarkable century which not only paved the way for other Eastern religions but also influenced directly or indirectly the evolving tenets and mores of Greek secular philosophy, scholarship, and medicine.

The remarkable 6th Century B.C. gave birth to, or rise to, three of the world's major religions and/or moral philosophies. Their teachings influenced the course of history, moral philosophy, and personal ethics within the East, and not unexpectedly they also influenced Western thought even up to the present age. This century also influenced the course of medical ethics – first indirectly, via the ancient Greeks, and later, circuitously via the contributions of the Islamic physicians and other Middle Eastern scholars during the Middle Ages.

CONFUCIANISM

Confucius (551-479 B.C.) was a Chinese secular philosopher, not a religious leader. In fact, he did not consider himself a prophet but only a gifted man who could disseminate the wisdom of the sages of ages past. His philosophy was based on enlightened personal morality and uncorrupted political conduct. His main precept was that a ruler should not only serve his people well, but also rule by moral example.(41) Moreover, a ruler should not exempt himself from the rules he imposes on others. This noble idea, which most likely originated with Solon in Greece in the early 6th Century, was to substantially influence millions of people for centuries. It would have the biggest impact in ancient Greece and Rome and later in enlightened Western countries, most notably England. Confucius preached a variant of the golden rule: "What you do not want done to yourself, do not do to others." Note the similarity to the Christian golden rule: "Do to others as you would have them do to you." (Luke 6:31).

Confucius' political outlook was conservative, espousing obedience to elders and the integrity of the family; likewise he predicated obedience and allegiance of vassals to their overlords, but he did not condone tyranny.(41) It is not surprising then that Confucian philosophy was suppressed in 3rd Century B.C. China by the powerful emperor, Ch'in Shi Huang Ti (259-210 B.C.; emperor, 238-210 B.C.) who wrought to subdue vassals, end the Chinese feudal system, and unify China. It is understandable that such a mighty ruler obsessed with centralization of the country would suppress Confucian philosophy, which amongst other things, stressed moral obligations, decentralization, and individual responsibility.

Ch'in Shi Huang Ti was the most powerful ruler of ancient China. As emperor, he unified China with his sheer military prowess and the force of arms. He established the framework of cultural unity that has preserved China for centuries. Historically, he sought to make "a clean break with the past," in much the same fashion as the communist Chinese under Mao-Tse-Tung (1893-1976) and his successors, notably his widow Jiang Qing, head of "the Gang of Four," attempted to do. On the other hand, the present (still communist) leader, Deng Xiaoping (b.1904), appears to have come to terms with the past with at least partial liberalization of economic policies, but myopically, political repression persists as of this writing. As the Chinese communism riddle unravels, it is not difficult to discern why the modern Chinese communists also attempted to eradicate Confucius' teachings, whilst resurrecting the spirit of Ch'in Shi Huang Ti as a national hero: They wanted to justify totalitarianism and authoritarianism in the guise of nationalism and patriotism.

The iron-fisted Ch'in Shi Huang Ti is also the national leader from which China takes her name, though he presided over one of the shortest ruling dynasties in Chinese history. Ch'in's young son and immediate successor ruled for only a few years.

Toward the end of his rule, Ch'in became increasingly paranoic, fearing assassination and trusting no one but his closest minister. Aware of the advancing years and the workings of time, he incessantly searched for the mythical fountain of youth and the key to unlock the secret to immortality. He built great monuments such as the Great Wall of China to keep "barbarians" out of his kingdom, and he also built an astonishingly impressive tomb for himself. In it, we find an impressive army of ceramic soldiers, imperial horses, carriages, ships, and even his royal retainers who were poised in full military regalia to guard his afterlife. Soldiers and retainers were life-size, and each preserved their own likeness in their terra-cotta representation. These amazing and monumental archaeologic finds have been recently excavated and featured in popular magazines including *National Geographic*.(42) Spectacular display pieces from the royal tomb have also been exhibited in museums throughout the world.

The importance of Confucianism is that its teachings stress ideals and eternal truths such as the supremacy of merit and competence over birthright and lineage as the basis for employment and career advancement in government posts and civil administration, and by extension, the right of the individual to be accepted for his own accomplishments, and to pursue happiness, and be rewarded with the fruits of one's labors. Despite Ch'in Shi Huang Ti's efforts to eradicate Confucianism, the philosophy – based upon justice, fairness, obedience (especially to elders), economic freedom, individual responsibility, and accountability – survived, making it possible for Chinese society to build a solid philosophic underpinning and historic foundation that was planted on firm ground and remained stable from 100 B.C. to A.D. 1900 – two millennia in which China was, perhaps, one of the best ruled and most stable nations in the world.

TAOISM

Although Taoism was not a philosophy or religion of the 6th Century B.C. it is worth discussing at this time. Taoism, together with Confucianism and Buddhism, formed part of the predominant theology and moral philosophy of the Chinese people, the most populous nation on Earth.

The enigmatic Lao Tzu (4th Century B.C.), believed to have been a royal librarian, lived two centuries after Confucius, yet he remains an even more puzzling historic figure.(2,41) The book of this Chinese philosopher written in 320 B.C. sets down the tenets of Taoism. It should be noted that, of all the thousands of Chinese texts, the most widely circulated, not only in China but throughout the world, is the *Tao Te Ching*, the relatively slender tome in which the philosophy on Taoism is promulgated.

The central theme of Taoism is that the individual should not struggle against the *Tao*, "the way" or the "natural order," but should cooperate and conform with the spirit of Tao. For one thing, according to Taoist philosophy, it is not only immoral but also futile to exercise power against nature. Violence and greed are to be avoided as are fame and prestige.(41)

Lao Tzu believed that to lead the people, leaders should "walk behind them." Moreover, "as for the best leaders, the people do not notice their existence. The next best, the people honor and praise. The next, the people fear, and the next, the people hate. When the best leader's work is done, the people say, 'we did it ourselves.'"(43)

Perhaps most relevant to today's political climate and globally projected dimensions of government are Taoism's insistence on a government that is decentralized, deliberately weak, and overtly benevolent. It stresses the avoidance of war, warns against the implementation of ambitious government projects, and encourages non-enforcement or outright popular rejection of bad laws. According to Lao Tzu, one should not have the audacity to unravel and reform the intricacies of the world, but rather, respect it. Intended as a secular philosophy, Taoism has been used by many sects, including college groups in the U.S. during the 1960s who militated to develop the secular precepts into a religious movement, perhaps to fill the spiritual void created by the relentless attack on conventional religion and social institutions that occurred during those turbulent years of U.S. government growth and involvement in the Vietnam War.

It is of interest that whilst in our 20th Century United States, the *Bible* and Ayn Rand's *Atlas Shrugged* have been the most widely read and supposedly most influential books,(44) it has been the *Bible* and the *Tao Te Ching* that have been the books with the greatest number of English language translations (for the *Tao Te Ching* at least 40 translations).(41) Taoism has not only had a direct influence on Western pacifist philosophy, but as we shall see shortly, also a substantial influence on traditional Buddhist philosophy.

BUDDHISM

Buddhism, the religion founded by Gautama Buddha (in Sanskrit, "the Enlightened One"; 563-483 B.C.), originated in India in the prophetic 6th Century B.C. and remains influential in certain parts of Asia, notably Nepal and Tibet. Buddhism lost influence in Southeast Asia with the advent of communism in that region, in spite of the outright sympathy by many of its priests and followers for the communist Vietcong and totalitarian North Vietnamese regime. One need only recall the ghastly drama widely seen on television of the self-immolation of the Buddhist priest protesting the war, or rather U.S. involvement which was the only impediment to the communist takeover of South Vietnam. The image of the serene monk in a busy street of Saigon putting himself aflame whilst posing in front of U.S. cameramen is an image not easily forgotten and its pacifist intention not easily discounted or swept aside.

The barbarous Khmer Rouge and communist Vietcong, who carried brutal totalitarian Marxist policy to an extreme, abhorred religion and also proceeded to systematically kill hundreds, if not thousands, of Buddhist monks and desecrate their holy shrines and temples during their communist conquests of Cambodia and South Vietnam.

But let us now return to Buddha, whose original name was Prince Siddhartha Gautama. He was born in a small kingdom of India near the Nepalese border. A soothsayer is said to have presaged the birth of a great teacher, a *swami,* just as he was being born to the warrior caste, the son of a Hindu king. As a young man he decided that "there must be more to life than transitory pleasure, chronic suffering and death."(41) He therefore abandoned his luxuriant life and worldly possessions and pledged himself to the search for truth – grappling with these mundane problems as well as the meaning of human existence. It has even been said that Buddhism arose as a revolt against the rigidity and stratification of the caste system in India.(19)

After years of wandering, meditating, and attaining physical and spiritual discipline, Buddha, at the tender age of 35, is believed to have achieved supreme enlightenment. The story goes that one day beneath a giant fig tree, Buddha solved the puzzle of the meaning of life and human existence, and thus, so immersed in spiritual wisdom he became "the enlightened one."(2,31,41) He preached the "Four Noble Truths": First, life is unhappy. Second, unhappiness is caused by selfishness and desire. Third, attainment of *Nirvana* is possible by abandoning those desires and passions. And fourth, follow the "Enlightened Path": right views, right thoughts, right speech, right actions, right livelihood, right effort, right mindfulness, and meditation.(41)

Buddhism grew as a major religion, sweeping through India, fanning out into China and Southeast Asia, and then streaming across the Sea of Japan to influence Samurai society. The sect of the Zen-Buddhists was, in fact, adopted to Japanese stoicism, and thereby, immensely influenced Japanese feudal society. Zen-Buddhism established a moral basis for the iron-willed Japanese Samurai code, which called for self discipline, meditation, stoicism, and the attainment of enlightenment through intuitive insight. Nevertheless, we must recognize the fact that for the most part, as exemplified in the more recent histories of China and Vietnam as well as elsewhere, mainstream Buddhism *per se* has had a strong pacifist non-violent tradition, especially when viewed in comparison with Christianity or Islam.(31,45)

Ultimately, eternal bliss is possible through the teachings of Buddhism, despite its admittance of the concept of the existence of evil of the flesh as embodied in the concept of original sin. In Buddhism, one can find eternal peace in *Nirvana*, the peaceful release from earthly existence and the attainment of salvation, made possible by leading an ascetic life, a life of charity and good works.

ZOROASTRIANISM

The Iranian prophet Zoroaster (c.628-c.551 B.C.) was successful in preaching and making converts to his religion in the Persian empire, after proselytizing King Vishtaspa himself, the ruler of northern Persia. Zoroaster became his friend, and the king in return became his fervent protector. Zoroaster, himself, wrote part of the *Avesta*, the sacred scriptures of Zoroastrianism. His theology was a mixture of monotheism and dualism. The latter concept represented a cosmic, constant, and perpetual struggle between the forces of the "true God" and Evil incarnate.[12] In Zoroastrianism, there is philosophic room for free will, free will for man to be able to choose between these forces. Zoroastrianism also professes a belief in the afterlife. Good ethical principles include righteousness and truthfulness. There is no asceticism or celibacy, and, curiously, various rituals are centered on the purity and sanctity of fire.(45) The three moral precepts of Zoroastrianism are "good deeds, good works and good thoughts."(41)

Since individuals have the ability to choose via free will, they are responsible for their actions, and they are judged by their actions for an afterlife of earned salvation in heaven or damnation in hell.(46) But even though punishment in hell is made to fit the crime, damnation is not eternal. The punishment is to reform "so that on the day of resurrection all may be raised by the Savior to face the final judgment." (45)

Zoroaster died about the time that Cyrus the Great (c.600-529 B.C.)

---

[12] Goodness is supported by good spirits or *ahuras*, led by Ahura Mazdah, and they are countered by evil and wicked spirits, the *daevas*, led by Ahriman.(2)

conquered Persia. Zoroastrianism was adopted by the Persian rulers at the height of the Achaemenid empire, but it declined rapidly after the advent of Alexander the Great's Macedonian conquests.

Zoroastrianism, to Westerners initially exposed to it, is an abstruse and arcane religion that calls for elaborate ceremonies, including the preservation of the sacred fire in the temples of the faithful, as well as the disposition of the Zoroastrian decedents by placing the corpses on towers to be eaten by vultures. This funerary custom, incidently, is still practiced by the Parsees (or Parsis) in India. The Parsees build circular towers, which they call Towers of Silence, where they dispose of their dead by this ancient religious ceremony.(45) Since they revere fire as one of the manifestations of Ahura Mazdah, their central divinity, and also highly respect water and earth, their religion precludes cremation, internment, or disposal by water, since all of these elements would then become contaminated by the "impurities" of the dead. "Death is the work of the devil, so a corpse is the abode of demons."(45) Instead, the deceased are placed on the parapets surrounding the aforementioned towers, and travelers report that the vultures waiting around these parapets can pick a corpse clean in less than one hour. The bones, after being cleaned by the vultures, are allowed to bleach and dry in the sun and air. The remains of the skeleton are then allowed to crumble to dust in the special wells where they are deposited.

During the resurgence of the Persian empire by the Sassanid Dynasty (c.A.D.226-651), Zoroastrianism was resurrected and formerly readopted by the empire, only to be abandoned after the conquest of the Persians by the Arabs in the late 7th Century A.D. when the population converted *en masse* to Islam. The remaining Zoroastrians fled to the island of Hormuz, a name easily recognizable today because of the recent Gulf wars and the geopolitical significance ascribed to the Strait of Hormuz in the Persian Gulf for the important continuance of the flow of Middle Eastern oil to the West.

From this tiny island, the faithful fled to India, where they are known as Parsees (because of their Persian ancestry) and where they comprise a prosperous community of over 600,000 followers. The largest community is in Bombay. Moreover, there are still an estimated 10,000 to 20,000 Zoroastrians in Iran today.(41,45,46)

ZOROASTRIAN MEDICINE

Unfortunately, not much is known about Zoroastrian (Persian) medicine. The Medes and Persians, both considered Aryan tribes, succeeded the Chaldeans in Babylonia and ascended to a zenith of power in the region. The Persians believed in the sacred scriptures of the *Zend Avesta* (or *Avesta*) which were supposedly written by Zoroaster himself.(2,11,45) This sacred book is imbued with both religious themes, the duality of the supreme deity and the struggle between the forces of darkness and the forces of light, and with the workings of nature with health rituals and the rudiments of medicine.(11) Nevertheless, as we have already related, Persian rulers, even during the golden age of the Achaemenid Dynasty and the first period of Zoroastrianism, despite the availability of Persian (Zoroastrian) physicians, initially sought the services of Egyptian physician-priests – and later, the advice and treatment of secular Greek physicians. Therefore, not much is known about natural treatments and surgery performed by Zoroastrian physicians. We do know that rules governing medical practice in ancient Persia at the time of Darius I, "the Great" (c.558-486 B.C.), were set down in writing in the Persian *Vendidad*, one of the two main liturgical texts of the *Avesta*.(19)

MANICHAEISM

Zoroastrianism had a great influence on Judaism and Christianity, as well as on Manichaeism, the religion founded by Mani (A.D.216-276), another important Persian prophet, who also believed in the concept of duality and the struggle between good and evil.(41)

Manichaeism is a religion of the 3rd Century A.D. but, like Taoism, deserves to be mentioned at this time, for not only did it borrow elements of the prophet Zoroaster, but it also synthesized elements from earlier religions, gnosticism and Christianity.(2)

In Manichaeism, the dual forces are equal in power; God, the Father of Greatness, is opposed by Evil, the Prince of Darkness. In Zoroastrianism, as we have intimated, the forces of good are believed ultimately to prevail.

Manichaeans believe that man's soul is the good principle and his body the evil principle. Yet there is ample room to allow for salvation and the transmigration of the soul.(45)

Manichaeans believed that "the elect" of the church, not the ordinary members, were prohibited from engaging in sex, ingesting meat, or drinking wine. It was also "the elect" whose souls went straight to paradise after death. Mani, working in 3rd Century A.D. Persia, at first was allowed to preach his religion (at the outset of the Sassanid empire), but conflicts arose with the highly-placed priests of the Zoroastrian religion, the Persian state religion of the time, and the conflict ended with Mani's imprisonment and his death in captivity in A.D.276.(41)

Manichaeism, at its height, spread across three continents from Spain to China, and in the 4th Century A.D., became a rival to Christianity. St. Augustine (of Hippo, A.D.354-430) was a Manichaen for 9 years before he was proselytized to the Christian faith and became a Christian leader. I suppose St. Augustine was practicing Manichaeism when he allegedly wrote: "Lord, make me chaste – but not yet."(43)

Manichaeism was outlawed in the Roman Empire after Christianity became the state religion and by A.D. 600, it had been virtually eliminated from the West. Manichaeism continued to decline and ultimately became extinct with the advent of the teachings of the prophet Mohammed (A.D.570-632), the expansion of the warring Arab empire, and the ushering of the new crusading age of Islam in the 7th Century A.D.

It is interesting to note that the Albigensians of southern France (12th-13th Century A.D.), who considered themselves Christians, were an offshoot of Manichaeism. They were considered heretics of Christian dogma and were persecuted by the powerful Pope Innocent III (pope, 1198-1216). They were inevitably crushed by the crusade called against them by the popes between 1209 and 1244, ending their revolt in southern France and their heresy in Europe.[13]

HINDUISM

I will not discuss the ancient Hindu religion or its caste system at length. But I would like to ascertain a few facts. First, Hinduism, the religion of the invading Aryans or Indo-Europeans (c.1500 B.C.), was intermixed with the belief system and practices of the indigenous peoples and established a rigid caste system on the Indian subcontinent – in which the highest caste was the sacerdotal class occupied by the priests (Brahmins or Brahmans). The next highest caste was that comprised of the kingly-warrior class (*kshatriya*); next came the merchant class (*vaishya*), followed by the serfs (*shudra*). The lowest estate was occupied by the "untouchables."(45)

Second, intrinsic to Hinduism is the strict doctrine of *transmigration of souls*, whereby saintly life leads "to ultimate freedom from flesh and reunion with the perfect," whereas sinful life leads to reincarnation in a lower caste or animal life and perpetual suffering.(45) Salvation is attained by ascetic denial and virtuous life. This precept of ascetic denial leading to salvation is inherent in the Eastern concept (or law) of *Karma*, which, not surprisingly, is best exemplified by the Hindu religion. The concept of karma holds that one's station in life and corporeal existence is the result of past moral behavior or spiritual incarnations and that one's destiny (future incarnations) is determined by present moral action, spiritual conduct, and behavior.(45) Exempted are "only those who have attained *Nirvana*" and "have transcended karma."(2) Deliberate human action and behavior have their own consequences; therefore, corporeal existence during transmigration of souls is the result of one's own volitional acts. Morally upright individuals assume "heavenly or human bodies" and evil ones, "infernal or animal ones."(45) In its essence, however, Hinduism is characterized by the caste system and the belief in their most sacred scriptures, the *Vedas*. [14]

HINDU MYTHOLOGY AND MEDICINE

Ancient Hindu scriptures refer to medicine and surgery as recorded in the sacred writings of the *Vedas* (meaning "knowledge" and comprising the oldest scriptures of Hinduism) written in Sanskrit, the language of the Indo-European (Aryan) invaders of 1750-1500 B.C.

[13] The Albigensian Crusade of 1233 triggered the Inquisition which, although organized by the Roman Catholic church and Pope Gregory IX (pope, 1227-1241) to suppress heresies such as Albigensianism, was later used by the church and the Spanish monarchy to establish religious uniformity as well as to stamp out political enemies. The later church-led Inquisition of the Renaissance, reintroduced to suppress Protestantism, ebbed over the centuries and was replaced in 1965 by the Congregation of the Doctrines of the Faith. The secular Spanish Inquisition, led by the Spanish monarchs and independent of the church, came to a close when it was formally abolished in 1834.(2)

[14] The *Vedas* comprise the liturgy and exposition of rituals of the Hindu religion, including sacrificial rites, and the mystic literature of the *Upanishads* that contain the doctrine of the Brahman and absolute reality contained in the self and the objective of Hinduism, "liberation from the cycle of rebirth and the suffering brought about by one's own actions," one's karma.(2)

The *Vedas* consist of four types of Hindu literature compiled between 1000 to 500 B.C. Of these sacred writings, two are particularly relevant to us because they contain ancient knowledge (traced to the Aryan invaders) used for medical purposes such as healing rites and rituals: The *Rig-Veda* contains invocations to the gods and hymns, the *Atharva-Veda* contains magic formulae, incantations, and spells.

Additional medical texts were later written by the two Hindu physicians, Charaka, (1st Century A.D.) who compiled the *Charaka Samhita*, and Susruta, (4th Century A.D.) who authored the *Susruta-Samhita*. Both claimed to have received their knowledge through divine intervention from the Hindu gods themselves.(11)

The Hindu godhead is composed of a trinity: Brahman, the creator; Shiva, the fierce deity of destruction, regeneration, and conqueror of death; and Vishnu, the preserver of the world who is as powerful but better disposed than Shiva. A remnant of matriarchy, the Hindu Earth-Mother goddess, Shakti, became spouse to Shiva. She has a dual personality. As Parvati, she was Shiva's beautiful consort and immensely gentler than her alter-ego deity, the malevolent and blood-thirsty Kali.(45)

It is of interest to note that recent archaeologic evidence from excavations at Mohenjo-Daro and Harappa, chief cities of the Indus Valley civilization, reveal that these cities had a fairly advanced system of sanitation prior to the Aryan invasions. Hindu medicine – despite the remarkable advances in the use of medicinal herbs (pharmacopoeia) and the innovations in surgical techniques that came about from the forging of the knowledge of the Aryans and the native inhabitants of the old Indus Valley civilization – was deeply immersed in magic, mythology, and religion. Invocations to a myriad of deities, mystical recitals of magical incantations (referred to in the Sanskrit as *Mantras*), oblations, libations, and other forms of ceremonial offerings to the Hindu trinity were as, or more important, than natural therapies in treating the sick and afflicted.

It also appears that treating spiritual ailments by supernatural means was given as much emphasis as the use of herbal remedies or home recipes in treatment. Surgery was definitely used for treatment of external ailments or physical injuries. Nevertheless, medicine was immersed in the supernatural. For example, the Hindu goddess Kali was associated with disease, death, and destruction, whereas Agni, the god of fire, was invoked in cases of febrile illnesses. Moreover, the Hindu deities were sometimes identifiable in some aspects with some of the Western gods; for instance, Shiva, the omnipotent god of the Hindu trinity, sometimes shot arrows to inflict pain and suffering as did the Greek god, Apollo, and his twin sister, the goddess Artemis (Diana).(19)

The *Susruta* not only contains detailed descriptions of various surgical procedures and treatments but also contains references to the use of anesthesia. For example, the *Susruta* says, "wine should be used before operation to induce insensibility to pain."(11) Moreover, there is an account of two brother surgeons in A.D.927 who performed what might have been the first successful brain operation recorded. According to the account, the King of Bhoja of Dhar was afflicted with a brain tumor and underwent a craniotomy (opening of the skull) whilst anesthetized by a drug called *Samohini*. The operation was successful, according to the narration. The tumor was removed, and the wound was closed by stitching. The King was revived from the soporific anesthetic with the administration of another drug named *Sanjivani*.(11,16)

Comments: Moral Conduct, Past and Present

Now let us return for a moment to the present. And, this brings to mind a beautifully written issue of *Iatrofon* [15] by its late editor, Robert S. Jaggard, M.D. In this particular issue, Dr. Jaggard pointed out how four of the major religions, Judaism, Buddhism, Christianity, and Islam, all have a similar central theme, that is, that "individuals should recognize the basic rights of others and have an acceptance (if not actual love) for his neighbor and fellowman."(47) He went on to discuss that philosophers differ amongst themselves about what they believe is the individual's responsibility to help others in society, *altruism*, or to help himself, *individualism*, with the recognition that by working for his or her own enlightened self-interest, ultimately one can be of benefit to others in the exchange of goods and services in a free society without intimidation or coercion by government.

Furthermore, Dr. Jaggard bemoaned that charity, which should be voluntary, has been coercively extracted from one individual and given to another by government in the name of the welfare state and that it has been legislated, creating envy and jealousy where there should have been love and charity. Forgotten are the ancient Hebrew admonition that one should not covet his neighbor's goods and St. Paul's Christian teachings that charity comes from the individual. Instead, a leviathan government has been created that does not follow the wise teachings of antiquity nor any moral code except the force of majority legislation supported by activist judicial decrees – all at the expense of individual liberties.

If one lesson can be learned from these religions and moral philosophies, it is just as Dr. Jaggard correctly contended, that government is not the instrument to enforce religion, ethics, or morality, even if it claims to enforce the provision of "the greatest good for the greatest number."(47) Religion and philosophy are the proper vehicles to achieve the incarnation of the spirit of charity and rekindle the fire of voluntary philanthropy that is present within the individual. Charity must come from the heart, nurtured by tradition, family values, and societal institutions, because when it is forced upon the individual, it is no longer charity, it becomes tyranny.

These theo-philosophies, despite their differences and the passage of centuries, have much to say to us about what is right and what is wrong in our present society; this is true even though they differ in what they expect of us as individuals. However, one common thread runs through them regarding government and morality, that whatever impositions are placed on moral conduct, it is the individual who has free will and who is accountable for his/her deeds. Yet it was not until the advent of Marxist theory in the 19th Century and democratic socialism and communism in the 20th Century that these religions and moral philosophies were used to provide a moral basis for threatening the individual with force and economic destruction to implement charity and coercive compassion in the name of the common good. [16]

---

[15] The now defunct newsletter was the official bulletin of an international organization of private (independent) physicians who follow the traditional Hippocratic ethics of medicine.

[16] Dr. Robert S. Jaggard was recognized, prior to his untimely demise on March 4, 1993, for his indomitable spirit and his indefatigable efforts in the defense of freedom and the preservation of the private practice of medicine. He was awarded the first Medal of Freedom by the Association of American Physicians and Surgeons (AAPS). R.I.P., Dr. Jag.

PART TWO: GREECE

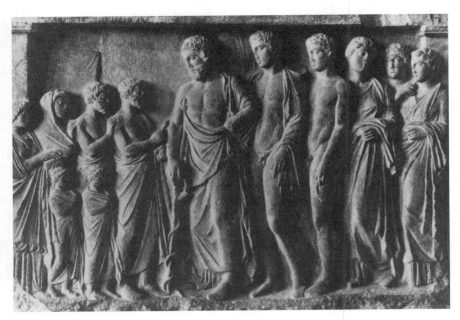

Plate 4 - Mythic Æsculapius and his family including his sons, Machaon and Podalirios, and his daughters, Hygeia and Panacea. Depiction on votive tablet c.370-270 B.C. National Archaeological Museum, Athens.

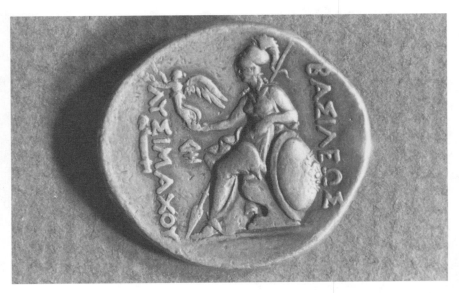

Plate 5 – The goddess Athena enthroned holding the insignia of victory. Silver tetradrachm, Kingdom of Thrace (297-281 B.C.). Author's private collection.

CHAPTER 5

GODS, ASKLEPIADS AND SYMBOLISM IN MEDICINE

A civilized society is one that exhibits the five qualities of truth, beauty, adventure, art and peace.

Alfred North Whitehead

Similarly, as had happened with the Indo-European invasions of northern India, waves of Aryan invaders descended from the Trans-Caucasus sweeping through southeastern Europe. These newcomers descended and established themselves on the mountainous and arid terrain of the Grecian peninsula. The Neolithic inhabitants – purportedly worshippers of Earth-Mother goddesses as the indigenous Minoans (considered matriarchal) as well as the Myceneans (likely patriarchal) peoples – were overrun by the aggressive invaders armed with superior weapons. Thus, by 1000 B.C., Achaeans, Ionians, and Dorians and other Greek-speaking peoples had settled in the region that today encompasses modern Greece. [17] The fusion of these cultures, and later their reemergence as a network of independent city-states resulted in time in the formation of Greek civilization.(1,2)

Much of Greece's ancient history comes from the great epics, *The Iliad* and *The Odyssey*. In these epics, formulated in the oral tradition of the 11th or 10th Century B.C. and composed into epic poetry by the blind minstrel Homer in the 8th Century B.C., we get a panoramic and comprehensive view of Greek religion, history, philosophy, and even medicine. It may be said that these epic poems provide more than a bird's eye view of Greek mores and customs in everyday life, although inextricably entwined with the heroic actions and unpredictable deeds of the humanized gods and goddesses. Thus, we learn in the pages of these epics that the gods were anthropomorphic with all the emotions, desires, and frailties of the human heart; yet they were also possessed of the cleverness and resourcefulness of the human brain. In short, they were separated from men and women and their human attributes only by their immortality. The gods were venerated, though they lived apart from mankind, leading sumptuous lives, drinking and feasting heartily, and enjoying all the amenities of their elysian paradise at their empyrean abode on Mount Olympus.

Paradoxically, although at times they seemed totally oblivious to man's suffering on earth, at other times, they interfered constantly in man's affairs, as is well testified in the many volumes of Greek mythology and literature. Time and again, they came to the rescue and succor of mythologic heroes who were frequently their offspring from sexual escapades with mortals of the opposite sex and who then, with their godly assistance, were able to escape from seemingly inescapable dangers or perform laborious, time-consuming, and formidable tasks. The male Olympians were often stricken with insatiable lust, as in the case of Zeus, the supreme god, and when this became the case, no mortal female could escape his

[17] By the 8th Century B.C., colonies had also been established from Asia Minor to Spain (Magna Graecia).(1)

concupiscence. Zeus's philandering conquered all, whether by charm, subterfuge, or brutal force.

From time to time, the gods and goddesses would descend from Mount Olympus to reward a lucky soul or to castigate an offender for an impious or sacrilegious transgression. With all their human follies, the amazing point is that the Greeks not only believed, but venerated their gods and goddesses "who seem to spend timeless, deathless lives in feasting, lovemaking, and often meddling in Earthly affairs."(3) Although, the rule was definitely patriarchal, Zeus and Hera ruled, at least theoretically, jointly and almost supremely, on Mount Olympus.

On the next Olympian tier, we find the mighty god Apollo and the wise goddess Athena. Apollo was the primary god of healing in the Greek pantheon as well as physician to the gods. Athena was the goddess of wisdom, and the patron goddess of Athens – to whom the Parthenon, the magnificent structure still standing on the Acropolis in Athens, was consecrated. Athena holds a special place in the Greek pantheon. She was given birth by Zeus, from his own body without the cooperation of either mortal woman or statuesque goddess, and thus, we have the origin of the word *parthenogenesis* – "virgin birth" – scientifically speaking, the birth and development of a whole individual from a single unfertilized egg.

But most relevant to our discussion is the god Æsculapius (or Asklepios) and his daughters, the goddesses Hygeia and Panacea. As the reader will remember, Hygeia was the goddess of health, and Panacea, the goddess of remedies. In Greek mythology, Æsculapius was the son of Apollo and a young Thessalian maiden named Coronis who was later killed by an arrow shot by the goddess Artemis, twin sister of Apollo, because of the maiden's infidelity to Apollo. In an act of godly grace, the infant Æsculapius was saved and given to the wise centaur Chiron to be reared. Chiron was knowledgeable in medicine, having been taught the sacred art by Apollo himself. Because of his wisdom, Chiron had also previously been entrusted with the upbringing of other superheroes such as Jason (*Jason and the Argonauts*), Hercules (the executor of the toilsome "Twelve Labors"), and Achilles (the hero of *The Iliad*). Under his tutelage, Chiron conferred upon Æsculapius "the art of healing by using herbs, potions, and incantations."(4)

According to legend, Æsculapius soon surpassed his teacher's font of knowledge and medical skills, becoming exceedingly proficient in healing the sick and the injured. He even had the audacity to resurrect a dead man from what should have been his eternal repose in Hades. This deed was an impious act in the face of the gods and a direct affront to the Olympian immortals. Æsculapius was accused by Pluto, the Lord of the Underworld, of diminishing the number of souls in Hades. Zeus was particularly incensed: He would not allow a mortal to have "power over the dead and slew Æsculapius with a thunderbolt."(4) As a result of the legend of Æsculapius and the honors bestowed upon him by the Greek populace, great temples called *Asklepia* (or Asclepia) were erected, first in Thessaly, then throughout Greece, and his cult spread throughout the Greek (and later Roman) world.

According to the medical writer, Dr. Theodore E. Woodward, two great systems of medical philosophy and healing developed during this time. The first method was *temple medicine* which was practiced at Epidarus (the largest of the Asklepia temples) and in many other smaller temples scattered throughout the Grecian countryside. These temples were usually built near idyllic locations – such as natural springs, gymnasia, and gardens, where the tall ivory-white marble columns could be discerned from a distance by the traveling, ailing patients and those seeking medical cures and treatments.(3) Once in the temples, patients were treated with diet, exercise, baths, religious suggestions, and intuitive psychotherapy.(3-5)

Dr. W. Steven Metzer has also described temple medicine as practiced by the Æsculapian physicians (Asklepiads) within those institutions. In his estimation, miracles were alleged to have been performed as follows: "Afflicted persons who sought a cure at the temples completed a process referred to as incubation. First they were purified with prayer, mineral baths, massage, and inunctions....In early times, the priest appeared in the mask of the god and performed medical treatments. Later, medical advice came to the patient in the form of a dream that was interpreted by the priest, who then prescribed medical remedies."(4)

Woodward describes the methodology further, "often healing...consisted of contemplative dreams and temple sleep. The person seeking help studied the temple writings...and was massaged. He slept at the foot of Æsculapius and dreamed about him, often with the help of a little opium. Æsculapius or his daughters...frequently appeared in the patients dreams." Woodward continues, "in a day or two, the cured patient departed but was expected to leave a little remembrance, anything affordable, such as gold, silver, ivory, songs, prayers, sheep or payment of various kinds."(3)

The cult of Æsculapius spread to Rome and its surroundings around 290 B.C. when the aid of the healing cult was requested by the Romans as the answer from the Oracle of Delphi to the question of how to combat and end an epidemic that was ravaging Rome. As we shall see, this visitation by the mythologic Æsculapius to Rome (probably an Asklepiad priest) inspired the foundation of one of the first rudimentary indigent hospital.

The cult of Æsculapius in the temples of the Asklepiads spread all over Greece from Thessaly, and later temples were erected throughout the Græco-Roman empire. By 200 B.C., these temples numbered over two hundred and were supervised by the Asklepiads who functioned as physician-priests. The Asklepias could be considered the first walk-in clinics where practitioners of the art of medicine first practiced in a setting halfway between an office and a hospital-based practice. It also becomes evident that not all Greek physicians were followers of Hippocrates and the School of Cos, and at least in the setting of the Asklepia, early Greek medicine and Greek religion were greatly entwined.

Moreover, it was not until the 5th Century B.C. that Hippocrates (who is said to have claimed to be an 18th generation descendant of Æsculapius via Podalirios) and the School of Cos and their successors began in earnest the separation of secular medicine from magic and religion, along with the development of a lofty code of medical ethics.

In fact, during the declivity of the Roman Empire and the rise of the early Christian church, there may have been more practicing Asklepiads than Hippocratic physicians – a point which we will return to in our discussion of the Roman cults.

The second method of Greek medicine was the *empiric approach* based on rational thought, observation, and experimentation – the method of the natural sciences as established by Hippocrates (460-370 B.C.) and his follower-members of the Island (school) of Cos. Empiricists, for once, denied the heretofore nearly universal idea that illness afflicted and injuries occurred as the result of divine retribution from deities offended by the actions and sins of ordinary human beings. Instead, these early physicians believed that just as injuries were the result of natural acts, illnesses were the result of natural phenomena. Consequently, they denied that illness and sickness were punishment willed by the divinities themselves. Hence, other causes of illnesses were sought, and natural remedies were prescribed.

The empiric school that later revolutionized Greek medicine was in large part the product of the Greek Island of Cos, home of Hippocrates, the Father of Medicine. Hippocrates was born near a small village on this scenic island known for its shady olive trees. Years later, as an early Asklepiad, as followers of Æsculapius were then called, the Father of Medicine taught the art and philosophy of medicine under a large and shady plane tree in the center of his village.

From a historic perspective, the greatest contribution to medicine by Hippocrates and his followers is, without a doubt, the attribution of all diseases, including epilepsy and fever, to natural causes rather than to divine punishment and supernatural events.[18] Hippocrates, his Island of Cos followers, and his later successors' should all be credited not only with the creation of a transcendental code of medical ethics still practiced 2500 years later but also with the revolutionary concept which separated illnesses from supernatural phenomena. Diseases were the result of natural causes and could, therefore, be treated by natural means rather than by magic or invocation of the gods. This revolutionary concept was indeed a giant step forward in the history of medicine. And for these and other advances that we have yet to discuss, the classical Greeks, like the Hebrews of biblical times, honored their physicians. We will come back to Hippocrates and Hippocratic medicine later in the section on Græco-Roman Medicine.

EPIC MEDICINE

In the sacred art of medicine, legendary Æsculapius was assisted by his daughters, Hygeia and Panacea. And as most of us know, these health goddesses are quite conspicuous in the opening words of the Hippocratic Oath. Less well known to us are Æsculapius' sons, Podalirios and Machaon, both of whom were trained physicians who participated valiantly in the Trojan War, perhaps as the first medics in history. As "physician-warriors" during the heroic resistance of Troy, they actively tended the sick and wounded on the fierce battlefield (c.1800 B.C.).

The Iliad of Homer is indeed a repository of medical information in legendary military history. So much so that military historians have come forth with a curious tally of all the wounds mentioned or discussed in *The Iliad*. The tally has shown a total of 147 war casualties. As recorded in the epic poem itself, the mythical catalogue of injuries includes: 106 spear-penetrating wounds, 17 sword-chops, 12 arrow-shots, and 12 sling-shots. Even the mortality statistics are ascertainable from the poetic lines and are as follows: of those wounded by spear-thrusts, the

---

[18] The pursuit of science – that is, the search for scientific facts by the use of data to corroborate or disprove the validity of theories – may be said to have begun in approximately 600 B.C. with the Ionian philosophers, such as Thales of Miletus (c.636-c.546 B.C.), "who were stimulated by their acquaintance with Egyptian scientific lore"(2) and who explained the world not from mythologic creation but from an underlying physical substance which Thales believed to be water.(1) Both the philosophers Anaxagoras (c.500-428 B.C.) and Anaximander (c.611-c.547 B.C.) were disciples of Thales.

death rate was 80 percent; for sling-shot victims, it was 2 out of 3; for the sword-chop wounded, it was 100 percent; and for the arrow victims, it was nearly 50 percent. Menelaus, the King of Sparta and husband to the most beautiful of mortal women of antiquity (Helen, the prize of the Trojan War) was one of the seven who survived an arrow wound.(14)

SYMBOLISM IN MEDICINE

The long standing controversy that started in antiquity and has continued well into the closing decades of this century regarding the true symbol of medicine is of great interest to medical historians.(4-13)

Although both the American Medical Association (AMA) in 1919 and the World Medical Association in 1956 adopted the Æsculapian staff as the world's medical emblem, the recalcitrant controversy persists. The controversy takes us back to the myths and legends of the Græco-Roman gods and to even earlier antediluvian times. Given the interest in this subject, I would like at this time to review and summarize the salient points of the disputed matter and, if possible, present it somewhat differently from the usual historic perspective.

In addition – given what we have learned about the role of dreams in the Asklepias and the interest in the meaning of dreams in modern medical practice – it is relevant and appropriate that we also say a few words about the significance ascribed to dreams by ancient medical sages and contrast it to the symbolism that was assigned to them by a turn of the century physician.

THE SNAKE SYMBOL – THE CADUCEUS

Though there is ample evidence that both the caduceus and the staff of Æsculapius can be traced to ancient Babylonia and even to Moses and the Exodus, the connection of these ancient symbols to the practice of medicine is arguably more tenuous. Much more evidence is traceable to the more familiar Græco-Roman gods, particularly those in ancient Greek mythology. For one thing, both symbols are definitely linked to Apollo. The youthful Phoebus (brilliant) Apollo, who in Greek mythology personified virile beauty, was the brightest and the best liked of the Olympian gods. He was interchangeably and simultaneously the god of music, archery, and prophecy. And of paramount importance to us here, as previously stated, is the fact that he was also the primary god of healing and the physician to the other Greek gods on Mount Olympus.

We know that at least since the Renaissance with the rediscovery and resurgence of the Greek and Roman classics, the two symbols – the caduceus and the staff of Æsculapius – have been confused, and this confusion has been carried over to the present age. Let us discuss this issue by entering the mystifying realm of legend, where history and myth merge imperceptibly. In these stories, mythology prevails grandly.

The caduceus is the wand of Hermes (or the Roman Mercury) surmounted by a pair of wings, with two serpents facing each other intertwined around the wand. Hermes, the messenger of the gods, was given the wand by Apollo as a reward for his invention of the lyre. The story relates that Hermes threw the wand between two fighting serpents and they instinctively coiled around it in a friendly gesture (or as some scholars have intimated, sexual passion). In any case, the staff was said to have the power to unite all things divided by hate.(4) The wings were later added to the staff (c.250 B.C.) making the caduceus more identifiable with the messenger god Hermes.

Finally, another significance for the snake symbol is found in remote antiquity. In Egyptian mythology, as we have seen, the *Uraeus,* the sacred asp which stood as if poised to strike from the forehead of the pharaoh, has been said to symbolize "wisdom and life as well as to communicate magic virtues to their crowns."(4)

THE STAFF OF ÆSCULAPIUS

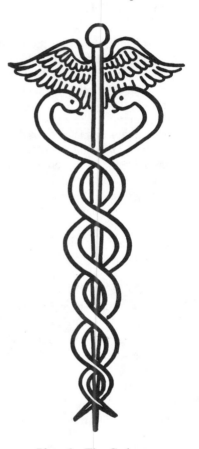

Let us briefly recapitulate the story of Æsculapius before we recount the myth of his staff that came to be emblematic of medicine.

Æsculapius, the god, was the son of Apollo who was reared and educated by the wise centaur, Chiron. Chiron taught Æsculapius the art of healing, and mythology tells us that in due time, the student surpassed his teacher. Æsculapius put his knowledge to good use, healing the sick and comforting the suffering.

Then Æsculapius, apparently becoming vainglorious from the triumphant success of his medical deeds, perpetrated an affront to the gods, a mortal sin. With his medical knowledge and skills, he resurrected a man from the dead. Zeus would not allow a mere mortal to have power over the dead. Acting as judge and executioner, Zeus slew Æsculapius with a deadly thunderbolt.(4) Another variation of the story says that Apollo himself struck down

Plate 6 – The Caduceus

Æsculapius with an arrow, "because of a successful cardiopulmonary resuscitation which incurred the gods jealousy. The arrow of Apollo then became a synonym for sudden death in Greek medical literature."(8,13)

But let us now return to the symbol...the story goes on to say that whilst Æsculapius was visiting a patient, a snake coiled itself around his staff. Instinctively, Æsculapius killed the snake, but another one appeared holding a magical herb-leaf in its mouth which restored life to the dead man.(5) The story reinforced an old Greek belief that people restored to health during illness were actually being resurrected from the dead. It also explains the reason why snakes were allowed to roam freely in the temples of the Asklepiads and were thought to even participate in healing rites in those mystifying temples.(7)

The staff of Æsculapius is a simple emblem, a short, crude, and knotty staff with a single serpent coiled around it. Æsculapius , the man, like Imhotep, was likely a mere mortal but as great physicians, both were later deified. It is possible that Æsculapius was only a myth transformed by time into a legendary man through the magical concoction of the ages.

In conclusion, I would agree with the medical writer Lou Carver who points out the similitude between the two symbols and the reasons for confusion in the past. Carver correctly asserts, in my opinion, that both the caduceus and the staff of Æsculapius had direct connections to Apollo and symbolized healing.(5) Yet given Hermes' later Roman impersonation as the god Mercury – the patron of merchants, travelers, thieves, as well as god of games and luck – the controversy today should lead to resolution with the inescapable conclusion arrived at by Dr. Walter Friedlander and others.(4,6,7,10-13) And that is, that despite medicine's woes (e.g., stifling government regulations, insufferable medical litigation, bureaucratic strangulation, spiraling health care costs, consumerism, conflict of interest issues, etc.), the staff of Æsculapius is still, and will remain in the foreseeable future, the most appropriate symbol for the medical profession. The two most serious threats to the simple wooden staff of Æsculapius presently are the strangulation of American medicine with the tangled and redundant red tape of government regulation and bureaucracy and the ever-growing devastation of the all-consuming fire of the litigation juggernaut.(15,16)

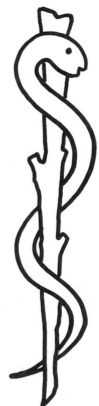

Plate 7 – The staff of Æsculapius

DREAMS AND MEDICINE

In the age-old argument between the relationship of the natural and the supernatural as a basis for the practice of medicine, the study of dreams and their significance provides an excellent medium for discussion. In this regard, and with the noted similitude between sleep (dream) and death (repose), I would like to quote an interesting passage by the neurologist writer, Dr. Francis Schiller, which is particularly symbolic of this duality between the natural and the supernatural, and the ambivalence between sleep and death:

Two major analogies regarding sleep and dreams seem to be as old as recorded human thought, one is that sleep resembles death like a twin brother...from these views follows the second analogy: dreams are an expression of the soul's survival. Proof of the paradox that dreaming, i.e., the life of the soul continues when all major evidence of the body's activity has ceased, is furnished by the fact that sensory activity, sight mainly, persists and is remembered through a period when the person was disengaged from the real world.(17)

The Greek rationalists including the philosophers Socrates, Plato, and Aristotle – all rejected a supernatural theory of dreams, as well as a divine or prophetic nature of the latter. Instead, they subscribed to a natural, physiologic explanation for sleep and dreams. Aristotle,(18) Hippocrates,(19) and Galen,(20) whilst denying the supernatural basis of dreams and in many ways "side stepping" the debate of any supernatural basis for the phenomenon, did maintain the medical significance of dreams by enabling physicians "to predict or uncover disease."(17)

The Stoic philosophers proclaimed dreams as "god-sent to enlighten or deceive you." Hippocrates, himself, asserted that "sleep is the time when the soul truly comes into its own, free from the demands of the body"(19); but he also believed, like Galen, that dreams had self-fulfillment functions. Quoting Herophilus, Galen writes, "what we wish we experience as happens to lovers when they see themselves hugging their girlfriends in their dreams."(20) And as pointed out by Schiller, in his enlightening essay, Hippocrates referred to nocturnal seminal emissions as "loves mockery."(19)

In the 20th century, Sigmund Freud (1856-1939), the Austrian psychiatrist and founder of psychoanalysis, asserted in his *The Interpretation of Dreams*, published in 1900, that the importance of dreams in medical practice was in its wish-fulfillment, ego mechanism. Moreover, he affirmed his theory of the interpretation of dreams as wish-fulfillment to be associated with confirmatory physical attributes, such as "overt sexual arousal and the penile tumescence observed in the wet dreams."(17,21) The issue of dreams and their significance has not been settled even to this day, but it is important to note here that the interpretation of the meaning of dreams and their use in medical diagnosis and treatment commenced in earnest in the temple of the Asklepiads 2500 years ago – if not earlier in Egypt or Babylonia.

Presently, there has been a resurgence in the study of sleep physiology, and the significance of dreams continues to be debated in medical circles as well as in the lay press. Sleep physiology medical laboratories for the investigation of functional and pathologic sleep disorders, as well as the study of seizures, sleep-apnea, insomnia, and other ailments plaguing us today are on the cutting edge of medical research in this closing decade of the 20th Century.

But for now, let us continue with our discussion of the other aspects of Greek culture which allowed the art and science of medicine to flourish during the Golden Age of Greece.

CHAPTER 6

THE GOLDEN AGE OF GREECE

Art not only imitates nature but also completes its deficiencies.
Aristotle (384-322 B.C.)

The Golden Age of Greece may be said to encompass the period from approximately 600 to 400 B.C. and coincides with the time when Greek democracy flourished. During this period, the arts and theoretical sciences were tenderly nourished, resulting in a veritable intellectual revolution in which Greek philosophy reached unprecedented heights. In turn, this nurturing philosophic climate made it possible for other disciplines such as politics, history, drama, literature, law, and medicine to blossom.

THE BIRTH OF DEMOCRACY

It was during this intellectual upsurge that Solon (c.638-558 B.C.), the celebrated lawgiver, statesman, and adept politician, sowed the seeds of democracy in the fertile intellectual soil of Athens. The harsh code of laws instituted in 621 B.C. by his predecessor, the Athenian politician Draco (fl.late 7th Century B.C.), were repealed by Solon who then codified Athenian laws in the prevailing atmosphere of Athenian democracy.

Solon also moved to limit the power of the entrenched Athenian oligarchy by extending citizenship to those who previously had been disenfranchised. And then, by the power vested in him as sole Archon of Athens, Solon succeeded in creating a judicial court of citizens and in reforming the election of magistrates, thus propelling the city-state of Athens into the first true democracy.

The champion of Athenian democracy, Pericles (c.495-429 B.C.), foremost amongst the statesmen and politicians of his day, not only carried Athenian democracy to a pinnacle of splendor but also patronized the arts and sciences, elevating them to new heights. Athens flourished during his long years of leadership, producing its finest architecture, sculpture, and dramatic plays.(2,22) Pericles commissioned Phidias (c.500-432 B.C.), one of the greatest architects and sculptors of antiquity, to construct public works and sculptures, the greatest monuments of the city. [19] Pericles opened government posts to all citizens, based on both politics and merit, and irrespective of social status. He attracted men of fame and genius to Athens, not only Phidias as we have mentioned but many other great figures of antiquity, including the dramatist, Sophocles (496-406 B.C.), whom he befriended. At the time, Sophocles was already established as one of the three foremost Greek poets of the period. Pericles also befriended the philosopher

[19] Phidias also constructed the leviathan Athena-Parthenos in Athens and the colossal statue of Zeus at Olympia, both structures in ivory and gold. The latter was one of the Seven Wonders of the Ancient World, of which only the Great Pyramids of Giza remain.(7)

Anaxagoras (c.500-428 B.C.). Anaxagoras, as you may remember, was a follower of Thales of Miletus and a teacher of the great peripatetic philosopher Socrates and the poet Euripides (c.480-406 B.C.). Anaxagoras taught that the universe was composed of matter containing elemental particles.(1,24)

Pericles built the Parthenon, completed the Acropolis, and presided over the rebuilding of the Athenian navy which established the naval supremacy of Athens over the other Greek city-states. It was said that Pericles, by sheer force of personality, established himself as the champion of democracy, of rule by the majority. He accomplished this task by ascending the ladder of power to become a paramount democratic leader and then controlling the assembly of citizens, the *Ekklesia*, taking power away from the *Areopagus* (after Ares, the god of war) – the supreme tribunal of Athens, which up to that time had been a council of the aristocrats.(2,22) In good time, Pericles had become the *Strategus* (general-in-command), a post from which he ruled for virtually 30 years.(24) Nevertheless, despite the credit due him it must be remembered that Pericles was not the first democratic leader. As we have discussed, Solon played a seminal and pivotal role, as did the Athenian statesman, Cleisthenes (fl.500 B.C.). Like Solon, Cleisthenes helped pave the way for democracy by successfully introducing democratic reforms in 508 B.C. and ending the rampaging civil strife beleaguering Athens by 506 B.C.

As you may also recall from history, Cleisthenes was known for his wise and commendable efforts to prepare Greece for the coming confrontation with the mighty Persian armies that threatened the independence of the Greek city-states in the late 5th Century B.C. He is also credited with the introduction of the practice of ostracism, or banishment, as judicial punishment for discredited politicians or vanquished political opponents.

Yet it was with Solon's election as Archon of Athens in 594 B.C. that the Western political axiom that government be effected *by written law and that both the people and the rulers should obey those laws* was formulated and implemented leading to the principles of a constitutional republic. Nevertheless, whilst in Rome this type of constitutional republican government was instituted and nurtured by the rule of law, in Athens and elsewhere in Greece, the path led towards either democracy or tyranny. Even in Athens, the birthplace of democracy, there were many long periods of interruptions of democracy by tyrannical rule which thwarted liberty, bred populism, and instigated mobocracy and lawlessness.(25) In the end, it was up to the Romans to solidify constitutional government in the form of a republic, whilst Athens succumbed to the arbitrary winds of majority rule (citizens only) which proved conducive to an impractical and unwieldy government, best exemplified in the Athenian justice system [20] and subject to conquest by a determined foe.

Nor was Pericles the last democratic leader, for we have records of

---

[20] Athenian democracy was in many cases carried to extremes. For instance in jurisprudence, judicial power was vested directly in the Athenian citizenry, and for this purpose, 6000 men were elected annually to act as judges and jurors; in most judicial (court) cases at least 500 men were needed to reach a verdict considered free of prejudice!(2) In this regard, the words of the American patriot, Alexander Hamilton (1755-1804), come to mind. He wrote in 1788, "Real liberty is neither found in despotism or the extremes of democracy, but in moderate governments." As is plainly clear from the *Federalist Papers*, the moderate government he referred to was "a republican government."

Demosthenes [21] (384-322 B.C.), a much celebrated Greek politician and lawyer, who continued to deliver brilliant oratory in support of Greek independence and democratic principles up to the period of the Macedonian conquest, and henceforth the beginning of the Hellenistic period under Macedonian leadership.

A New Way of Thinking

The search for basic truths led the early Greek philosophers to natural observations, as well as to the first hints of the need for scientific experimentation. During the early classical age of Greece, Anaximander, a pre-Socratic Greek philosopher (c.634-c.546 B.C.) believed that the universe evolved from the interaction of mutually repulsive and at the same time, mutually attractive elements (24); he is also reputed to be one of the first persons ever to perform an experiment to measure time and to predict the changes in the seasons of the year.(27) From his philosophic investigations are derived the modern concepts of the indestructibility of matter, as well as concepts anticipating the theory of evolution and physical laws of astronomy.(1)

We will have more to say about the Greek philosophers in Chapter 3 of this section, but for now, let us move forward in time to the Hellenistic period to discuss another philosopher who dealt with the physical sciences. And here we are referring to Eratosthenes (c.275-c.195 B.C.), cited for his ingenious calculations by Dr. Carl Sagan in his book, *Cosmos*.

Eratosthenes – a Greek astronomer, geographer, and director of the great library of Alexandria – correctly deduced the circumference of the Earth at 25,000 miles utilizing simple mathematic calculations and the principles of geometry. In the 3rd Century B.C., he compared the shadow length cast by a stick in Syene in northern Egypt with that cast by a stick in Alexandria at the Nile delta at noon and found it to be 7 degrees. He then compared the angular distance between Syene and Alexandria (800 km). And since 7 degrees is 1/50th of 360 degrees, he then correctly estimated the circumference of the Earth to be 40,000 km, which is approximately 25,000 miles.(27) He also devised a world map, measured the Earth's tilt, and calculated the distance from the Earth to the Sun and to the Moon.(1)

For his part, Anaxagoras, whom we have already met as a friend of Pericles, believed in an all-pervasive conscience that provided order to the physical world by combining particles and held that matter was defined by the predominance of one element. Most importantly, all matter was composed of elemental particles upon which the mind acts to produce the images that we see in the physical world.(1,24)

Yet, there were also sophists in classical Greece who questioned whether truth existed or was merely a matter of personal conjecture. Ionian philosophers

---

[21] Demosthenes was a pioneer in Athenian jurisprudence. Since under Athenian law, lawsuits were argued and decided in the presence of 500 jurors, and the verdicts were rendered by simple majority vote (established by Solon two centuries earlier), antagonists argued their own cases or hired others to plead their cases in court for them. There were no judges, and no regard was paid to precedents set in previous decisions. Demosthenes, being a master orator, was in great demand by litigants who would hire him to write their pleading speeches or to argue their cases in court. Perhaps one of the first genuine lawyers of antiquity, Demosthenes was so much sought after, that in time he was even known to write speeches for clients on both sides of the same legal dispute.(9)

argued that the universe was knowable and that nature had regularities that allowed its secrets to be decipherable by man's intuition. Nature had rules that even she had to obey, and therefore, she was not entirely unpredictable. The Greeks believed that even though the world was created from *chaos*, a new orderly universe had emerged called the *cosmos*.(27) This zeitgeist – characterized by curiosity, inquisitiveness, and a thirst for knowledge – paved the way for unprecedented progress in the fields of philosophy, astronomy, mathematics, and medicine.

THE GREEK HISTORIANS

A word about the great Greek historians of this period is also in order, for without them, much would have been lost by the widening chasm of time. And first amongst them is Herodotus (c.484-420 B.C.), the Father of History, born in the Ionian city of Halicarnassus, home of another one of the fabled ancient Seven Wonders of the World, the Mausoleum of Halicarnassus. Herodotus traveled to Egypt, Syria, and Mesopotamia. He was awed by the splendor of Egyptian civilization. With admiration, he described the Great Pyramids of Giza as well as Egyptian customs that he observed. He also traveled in Italy and journeyed to faraway territories around the Black Sea and the Caucasus.(28) As you will remember from previous chapters, we know much about Egyptian and Mesopotamian medical practices from Herodotus' observations recorded in the accounts of his travels in those regions.

Two other celebrated Greek historians who have likewise enriched our knowledge of antiquity were Thucydides (c.470-396 B.C.) and Xenophon (c.430-345 B.C.), both of whom are considered reliable historians, not only because of the attention to detail and substantiated accuracy of their writing but also because of the weight of credibility given to their narratives since they were active participants in many of the events which they described and cited.[22] Thucydides, for example, participated in the early period of the Peloponnesian Wars (431-404 B.C.) and fought on the Athenian side in that ancient and devastating conflict.(24) His experiences form the basis for his magnum opus, *History of the Peloponnesian War.* In the *Anabasis*, Xenophon, likewise recorded the account of the 10,000 Greek mercenaries (including himself) who served in the armies of a rebellious Persian King. The *Anabasis* painstakingly recounts the ill-fated expedition and the trials and tribulations encountered during the long historic march from Mesopotamia to a Greek sanctuary near the Black Sea where they sought refuge.(22)

---

[22] Herodotus is considered by many authorities as having often times been too gullible in the acquisition of historic information.

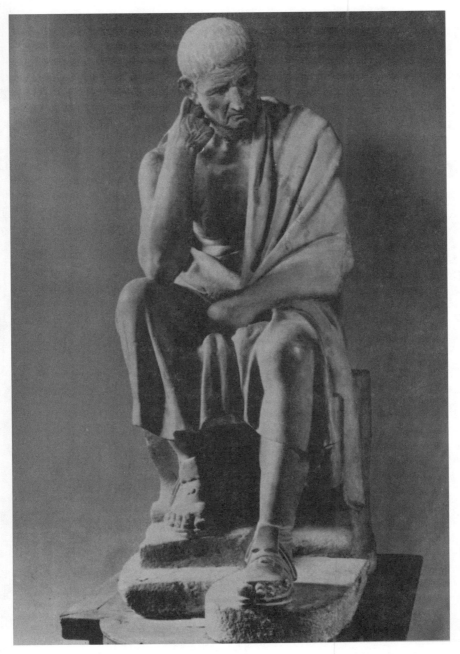

Plate 8 – Aristotle (384-322 B.C.) seated and pensive. Son of a physician, he was versed in all fields of knowledge. Roman copy of a Greek sculpture thought to represent the great philosopher. Plazzo Spada, Rome.

CHAPTER 7

THE GREEK PHILOSOPHERS

Philosophy is doubt.

Michel de Montaigne (1533-1592)

As we have observed in our discussion on the philosophers who dealt with the physical sciences, Greek scholars believed that even though the world was created from chaos, a new orderly universe had sprung, called the cosmos. We also observed how the philosophic ethos for learning and the zeitgeist of ancient Greece paved the way for progress in all areas of learning, particularly, the disciplines of philosophy, astronomy, mathematics, and medicine.

Fortunately for Western civilization (and the world), the fountainhead that was Athenian civilization was not destined to be undone by the Macedonian conquest of Greece, but on the contrary, it was boosted by such an event. When Philip of Macedonia (reigned, 359-336 B.C.) defeated the combined forces of the Greek city-states led by Athens and Thebes at Chaeronea in 338 B.C., instead of dismantling the Greek example of civilization, he fortified it and thereby paved the way for his son, the cosmopolitan Alexander "the Great." This great conqueror not only admired the best qualities of Greek culture, but under his leadership using his newly founded city, Alexandria as a beacon of learning, he spread Greek civilization throughout the known world. Then in 146 B.C., after the conquest and assimilation of most of the Hellenistic world by the triumphant legions of the Roman Republic, the survival and predominance of the Græco-Roman legacy was assured by the power that was Rome.

With this background, let us discuss the Greek philosophic basis for the biologic sciences, particularly rationalist Greek medicine – an art and a science based on experience, objective observation, and deductive reasoning.

THE PYTHAGOREANS

The birth of theoretical science may be traced to Greek intuitive thinking, especially Ionian reasoning and the critical observation of natural phenomena.(30)

The first scientist to come to us from history we have already mentioned (albeit, in a footnote), and he is the philosopher known as Thales of Miletus (c.634-c.546 B.C.). He came from a city in Asia Minor near Samos across the Aegean Sea. Thales learned from ancient Egyptian and Babylonian writing. This ancient knowledge was distilled into personified wisdom by Thales who was able, for example, to make mathematical calculations and use it to predict eclipses and other natural occurrences. For the first time, mathematics was used to explain natural observations and to verify scientific postulates. Thales proved many geometric theorems and posited the origin of the world, without invoking divine intervention from the immortals at Olympia.

Another Ionian philosopher, Democritus (c.460-370 B.C.), invented the word *atom* which takes its roots from the Greek for "unable to be cut." From his writings, it can appropriately be inferred that atoms were the ultimate matter of the universe. He explains, "nothing exists but atoms and the void."(27) He was a friend of Hippocrates and a contemporary of both Socrates and Herodotus.

The most influential Greek philosopher in the 6th Century B.C. was Pythagoras (580-498 B.C.) who came from the Island of Samos, also part of Ionia. He emigrated from Samos to the colony of Crotona in southern Italy to flee the wrath of the tyrant, Polycrates.(31) And it was Pythagoras who deduced that the Earth was a sphere and coined the word *cosmos* to denote a workable, harmonious universe, the opposite of chaos.(27) He and his followers were unusual philosophers in that they genuinely believed that mathematics and mysticism were inextricably intertwined. But after all, this was 6th Century Greece, when and where every imaginable idea could be contemplated – and exotic, esoteric, and inscrutable theories and philosophies abounded.

The 6th Century B.C. was indeed an unusual century, a century marked by great intellectual achievements in the Western world and universal religious fervor elsewhere in the East. As you will remember from our narrative, this was the century of Zoroaster in Persia, Confucius in China, Jewish prophets in the Holy Land, and Prince Siddhartha Gautama (Buddha) in India. Now, to this list of revered personalities, we can add Pythagoras of Samos and Thales of Miletus. And let us not forget either the semi-legendary fablist Aesop (c.620-560 B.C.), supposedly a Greek slave, nor the poetess Sappho (c.610-c.580 B.C.) of the Island of Lesbos, who enriched the folklore and literature of Greece during this century.

During his lifetime as well as in the ensuing centuries, Pythagoras influenced not only mathematics and philosophy but also science and medicine. Of particular interest to us is the Pythagorean student, Alcmaeon (fl.500 B.C.), who was the first person that we know in history to have dissected the human body.(14,27,31) He identified the brain as the seat of the intellect, an idea accepted by Hippocrates but contended by Aristotle. Alcmaeon also founded the science of embryology.

The Pythagoreans were also inexplicably obsessed with the size, shape, and volume of solids and geometric figures. They believed, for example, that the sphere was the perfect three-dimensional object because all the points on the surface were equidistant from its center. The word "quintessence," in fact, derives from the theoretic existence of a fifth solid object, the fifth essence, presumed to compose the substance of celestial bodies. Centuries later, Sagan would write, "the Pythagorean idea of a perfect and mystical world, unseen by the senses, was readily accepted by the early Christians...."(27) The Pythagoreans' abstruse and mystic concepts would indeed be reconciled with later Christian dogma during the early period of the Christian church.

The Pythagorean notion of a perfect and mystical world also influenced the later Neoplatonists and theosophists, not just the early Christian church leaders. It was this philosophic synthesis that forged the seemingly age-old concept that, whilst the Earth itself may not have been all that perfect, the heavens and the firmament were pure, clear, heavenly, and divine.(27)

The Pythagoreans also espoused strong views on health and disease which have been said to have significantly influenced Hippocrates and, to a lesser degree,

Galen. For example, Pythagoras' theory of mathematics influenced Hippocrates in his formulation of his *Critical Days* doctrine. Moreover, Pythagorean doctrine promoted hygiene, strict diet (for example, meat was taboo), gymnastics and exercise, and the use of herbal medicines.(31,32) The second part of the Hippocratic Oath is known to have been heavily influenced by Pythagorean principles concerning ethical standards in the patient-doctor relationship. For instance, the Pythagoreans went beyond the usual standards of medical practice to endorse the novel deontologic concept that the physician had an obligation not only to render care but also to protect his/her patients from the patients' own mischief, ignorance, and self-destructive habits. A Greek physician was also obliged to protect his patients from societal injustices as well.(32)

SOCRATES

The Greek philosopher Socrates (c.470-399 B.C.) has been regarded as one of the wisest men of all times, although he left no writings of his own from which today we could render objective judgment. Amongst his accomplishments, was a method of learning consisting of questions and answers as well as proposition and argument – the "Socratic dialogue" – designed to question established assumptions. Unlike sophists who questioned whether truth existed, Socrates not only affirmed it but also predicated it to be essential for a "perfect life."(24,33)

Most of our knowledge of Socrates comes from his famous pupil, Plato, and from the memoirs of Xenophon. Socrates was famous in his own time for his intellectual acumen and his dialogue, but it is said that he neglected his own personal affairs to argue in public places such metaphysical themes as the meaning of virtue, justice, piety, knowledge, and to seek the meaning of wisdom, the nature of one's own existence, and proper moral conduct. His Socratic dialogue or dialectic method of seeking knowledge consisted of asking questions of his students and then examining the implications of their answers.(1,2) The epitome of knowledge and virtue for Socrates was the exalted concept of self-knowledge, and thence, his famous aphorism, "know thyself." Not everyone in Athens liked the skepticism of his dialogues or took his method of teaching seriously. For instance, his dialogues and ideas were burlesqued by the Greek satirist Aristophanes (c.448-c.380 B.C.).(1)

Apollo's Oracle at Delphi declared Socrates "the wisest of all men" (reciprocating, Socrates avidly believed in the veracity of the counsel of the Oracle). In fact, one of the maxims inscribed on a column in the fore-temple at Delphi was Socrates' most famous aphorism, *nosce te ipsum*, "know thyself," a lofty ideal which may have been behind William Shakespeare's (1564-1616) well recognized maxim, "To thine own self be true."

But in 399 B.C., Socrates was ultimately arrested, tried, and convicted of corrupting the youth of Athens and espousing religious heresies. It is now believed that his criticism of the sophists and the Athenian political and religious institutions of his time, coupled with his alleged influence upon the Athenian leader and general, Alcibiades (c.450-404 B.C.) – who had betrayed Athens during the Peloponnesian War against Sparta – were behind the arrest and conviction. Indicted and condemned to death by an Athenian democratic court of citizens, Socrates refused all attempts to save his life and willingly drank the cup of poison, hemlock, given him for his execution.(1) His trial and ordered execution left an indelible impression on his pupil Plato, who not only discussed the trial and death of Socrates in various writings (e.g., *Apology, Crito, and Phaedo*), but also was influenced by the events leading to Socrates' death to question the wisdom of democratic rule; instead, Plato urged government by an enlightened elite.(33,34)

Drs. J.P. Dolan and G.R. Holmes have correctly written that, "of all the branches of human knowledge then existing (including mathematics and natural science), medicine is the most closely akin to the ethical science of Socrates." Moreover, these authors write, "Socrates's doctrine of ethical knowledge (on which so many of the arguments in Plato's dialogues turn) would be unthinkable without that model of medical science to which he so often refers."(32) We are referring here to that model of medical science that embodies the pursuit of a rigorous self-imposed code of ethics, the attainment of knowledge, and the utilization of that knowledge for the benefit of humanity.

PLATO

In c.387 B.C., the Greek philosopher Plato (427-347 B.C.) founded near Athens the most influential and prestigious school of ancient Greece, the famous *Academy*, where he taught until his death.(1) Plato is considered one of the fathers of Western thought because of his writings on political philosophy, theology, ethics, and morality. He is said to have written 36 books.(33) In the *Republic*, he proposed that the best government is that of an oligarchy made up of an enlightened elite – a supreme guardian class – possessed with vision and beneficent ideology. This ruling elite would have equality of the sexes and would be chosen by intellectual ability and merit, rather than by birth or station.(33) He believed in the just rule of government by "the best and the wisest"; and, as if to underscore this point, his writings are distinctly imbued with a revulsion for democratic rule and democratic institutions which he correctly (at least historically) believed had a tendency to degenerate to mob rule, injustice, and tyranny.(34)

Interestingly, the scholar Michael H. Hart points out that despite his rational arguments, there is no civil government, past or present, that has as yet explicitly adopted Plato's principle of an ideal republic. Nevertheless, some authors have pointed out a striking similarity between the self-perpetuating hierarchy of the Catholic church in medieval Europe and the structured government of Plato's elite. And there are similarities. For instance both Plato's ideal republic and the Catholic church hierarchy have in common the underlying motive of altruism and idealism and are concerned with the idea of good, the welfare of society and public service, rather than wealth, self aggrandizement, or pragmatism, at least in principle, if not in practice.(16) It was perhaps no coincidence then, that the early Christian church led by such theologians as St. Augustine of Hippo was able to reconcile early on Christian dogma with Plato's social philosophy.

Here again, the writers Dolan and Holmes accurately describe the image of the medical profession in classical Greece as exemplified by Plato. They write:

Plato speaks of doctors and medicine in such high terms that, even if the early medical literature of Greece was entirely lost, we should need no further evidence to infer that, during the late fifth and fourth centuries before Christ, the social and intellectual prestige of the Greek medical profession was high indeed. Plato thinks of the doctor as the representative of a highly specialized and refined department of knowledge and also as the embodiment of a professional code rigorous enough to be a perfect model of the proper relation between knowledge and its practical conduct.(32)

Nevertheless, as Professor S.R. Benatar points out, the medical profession had always had its critics. Even Plato had two criticisms of the physicians of his day: "One was that doctors treated the slaves as carefully as they treated free men or philosophers, and the other, that doctors treated patients including sick philosophers, like slaves!"(35)

ARISTOTLE

Aristotle (384-322 B.C.) was perhaps the most influential, if not the greatest, philosopher of all times. He was born in Macedonia the son of a physician in the court of King Philip of Macedonia. Implicit in his writing is Aristotle's attitude that natural processes, human life, and institutions are subject to careful observation, thought, and critical analysis. The universe is not controlled by chance, magic, or the caprice of the gods, but by natural laws that can be studied, ascertained, and explained by careful observations of natural events or deduced by simple experimentation. Conclusions can therefore be made by empirical observations and logical reasoning rather than by superstition and mysticism. In short, Aristotle was to the natural, social, and political sciences what Hippocrates was to medicine.

Aristotle was a prolific writer. He is credited with writing 170 books, of which 47 survive today.(33) His erudition was astounding, his works constituting a veritable encyclopedia of scientific knowledge in all areas of human endeavor: the natural sciences, including biology, botany, and zoology; the physical sciences, encompassing geography, geology, physics, and astronomy; the medical sciences, including medicine, embryology, anatomy, and physiology; the social sciences, notably education, psychology, economics, theology, politics, rhetoric, metaphysics, and above all, ethics and logic in which he excelled supremely.(36) He was conversant in all fields of learning of his day – and, as Hart points out, preeminent in science and philosophy.(33)

Aristotle studied at the Academy under Plato and later formed his own school, *The Lyceum*, in Athens. In 342 B.C., Aristotle became the private tutor for the son of Philip II, the powerful King of Macedonia. Aristotle's 13-year-old pupil would one day be known to the world as Alexander the Great. As tutor and advisor to Alexander, Aristotle also influenced the course of history. For example, he exhorted Alexander's troops to practice hygiene and sanitation in their camps, to boil water before drinking, and to bury their dung away from their camp.(37) He thus, perhaps, contributed to Alexander's armies' invincibility.

During the Middle Ages, Aristotle was simply referred to as "the Philosopher." In truth, he was the premier philosopher from antiquity through the

Renaissance and remains extensively quoted and studied to this day. As a student of nature, Aristotle was more interested in facts than in ideas. He wanted to know things as they were, not as they should be in an idealized world. In epistemology, he espoused the Hippocratic method of systematic observations of nature and formulated an extensive classification of living organisms using this approach.(36) Unlike Plato who proclaimed that the highest virtue of man is the idea of good, Aristotle counseled the "Golden Mean: virtue in moderation, the mean between opposite vices." The ethical code of Aristotle was not the lofty Socratic goal of self-knowledge or the Platonic idea of good, but the cultivation of moderation.

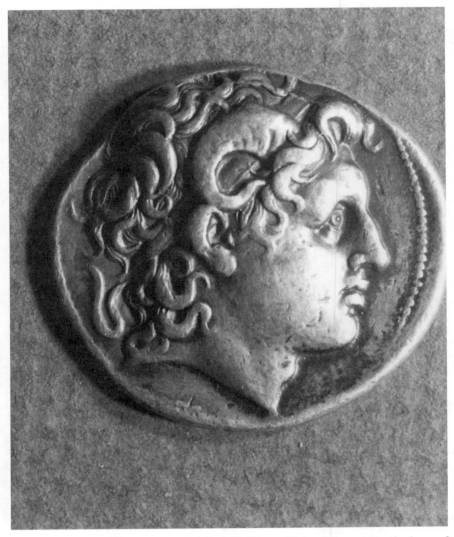

Plate 9 – Alexander the Great (356-323 B.C), King of Macedon, wearing the horn of
Ammon. Silver tetradrachm issued by Lysimachos, Alexander's former bodyguard and
King of Thrace (297-281 B.C.) Author's private collection.

CHAPTER 8

ALEXANDRIA AND
HELLENISTIC CULTURE
(323 B.C.-30 B.C.)

The final test of a leader is that he leaves behind in other men the conviction and the will to carry on.

Walter Lippmann (1889-1974)
Liberal journalist

ALEXANDER THE GREAT

And so it was destined to be that in 336 B.C., Alexander would become King of Macedonia at the tender age of 20. His father, King Philip II who had many enemies, had been assassinated. Alexander had previously complained to his father that there would be no kingdoms left for him to conquer, since Philip had already conquered his share of surrounding territories and had even crushed the rebellious Greeks at the Battle of Chaeronea in 338 B.C. [23]

After Philip's assassination, the Greek city-states led by Athens seized the opportunity and rebelled. Assuming political and military power in Macedonia, Alexander (356-323 B.C.; King of Macedonia, 336-323 B.C.) acted decisively and proved his military genius by regaining ascendancy over all of Greece with his lightening raids in battles. In victory after victory, he defeated the armies of one Greek city-state after another. Then, after conquering all of Greece and placing the rebellious city-states again under the Macedonian yoke, Alexander felt ready for the Persian campaigns. Without hesitation he marched his army into Asia, crossing the Hellespont [24] and entering Persian territory. With his highly disciplined but much smaller army, he then attacked the colossal Persian empire, the mightiest empire of his day. This was the same Achaemenid empire that, as you will remember, had been founded by Cyrus the Great (c.600-529 B.C.) two centuries earlier. The vast empire was now ruled by King Darius III (ruler, 338-330 B.C.).

Along the route of his march, Alexander and his Macedonian army defeated allies of the Persians or their surrogates. He then was left to face the huge army of Persian warriors led by Darius himself. But Alexander could not be stopped. The Persians were defeated, despite their numerically superior army, at the battle near the river Granicus in Asia Minor in 334 B.C., and at the Battle of Issus in 333 B.C. Alexander also captured the important Phoenician cities of Tyre and Gaza and conquered Egypt in 332 B.C., and whilst in the Nile delta, founded Alexandria. He then entered Mesopotamia and again defeated Darius III at the

---

[23] The Greeks, after much debate about the intentions of Macedonia, had finally been incited to defend their liberties and their country by the orations of Demosthenes (384-322 B.C.).

[24] This is the ancient name of the strait of Dardanelles that separates Europe from Asia in Turkey, and with the Sea of Marmara and the Bosporus, it connects the Black Sea to the Mediterranean Sea.(1)

Battle of Arbela in 331 B.C. Alexander had indeed struck with his Macedonian dagger at the heart of the Persian empire.

His victory over Darius III at the Battle of Arbela was decisive, and for all practical purposes, ended the Persian-Achaemenid dynastic reign which had ruled the Persian empire from 539 B.C. The empire officially ended in 312 B.C. Persia then went through a series of monarchic and dynastic rules of which the most prominent were the Parthians and the Sassanids (312 B.C.-A.D. 637), until the final conquest by the Islamic holy warriors, the Arabs, and the establishment of Islam as the major religion in the Middle East and North Africa.

Alexander then resumed his dream of world conquest and led an invasion into the valley of the Indus River by crossing the steep-sided Hindu Kush mountains, passing through the Khyber Pass;[25] he then entered and marched virtually unimpeded into northern India in 326 B.C. He won the Battle of Hydaspes, but his soldiers, tired of wars of conquest (after all, they had reached the farthest extent of the known world), refused to go further. Alexander reached the Indian Ocean and sailed his army up the Persian Gulf. He then marched his men through the desert and back to Babylon where he died of a fever at age 33 in 323 B.C. – at the palace and throne of Nebuchadnezzar.(1,2,22,24,33)

AN EMPIRE DIVIDED AND THE MACEDONIAN AFTERMATH

After Alexander's death, his empire was splintered amongst his trusted lieutenants: Ptolemy I (d.284 B.C.) ruled Egypt (becoming pharaoh in 305 B.C.) and established the Ptolemaic dynasty – the Macedonian dynasty that ruled Egypt from 323 to 30 B.C.; General Seleucus became Seleucus I, King of Babylon, founding the Seleucid dynasty that ruled Syria and much of the Middle East from 312 to 64 B.C.; Antigonus II (reign, 277-239 B.C.) became King of Greece and Macedonia. [26]

The Hellenistic world founded by Alexander and cultivated by his successors, notably the Ptolemies in Egypt, remained divided. Nevertheless, the cosmopolitan Hellenistic world created by Alexander and embodied in the city of Alexandria served as a conduit to divulge Greek culture and promote the achievements of Hellenistic art, science, and philosophy – achievements which were to endure for 300 years.

[25] The narrow and precipitous mountain pass is located today on the Pakistan-Afghanistan border. Since antiquity, this narrow pass was used as the western route to India. Besides Alexander the Great, the Mongol conqueror, Tamerlane (c.1336-1405), used this canyon pass to invade India. Today the pass links via tunnels, highways, and a railroad – the cities of Peshawar, Pakistan with Kabul, Afghanistan.(1)

[26] This period was by no means quiescent. A major civil war broke out in Macedonia for control of Macedonia, Greece, and the rest of Alexander's empire amongst the *diadochi*, the successors to Alexander, who fought a bitter and bloody struggle in which Alexander's mother, Olympias, in 316 B.C., Alexander's widow, Roxana, and their son perished in 311 B.C. Amongst the *diadochi* were Cassander, King of Macedon (316-297 B.C.); Antipater, regent of Macedon (334-323 B.C.); Pyrrhus, King of Epirus (c.318-272 B.C.); Antigonus I and his son Demetrius I (reign, 301-292 B.C.) and Antigonus II (reign, 277-239 B.C.). The brutal internecine warfare split the empire and drained Macedonia of wealth and resources until the rule of Antigonus III (reign, 229-221 B.C.) who restored order and regained Macedonia's hegemony. Thus, stability was regained for a time, with the empire split amongst the descendants of Ptolemy, Seleucus, and Antigonus. Nevertheless, with a new power rising majestically on the horizon, Macedonia was never to regain its military supremacy. The Macedonian kings, Philip V and Perseus, were ultimately defeated in the Macedonian Wars (215-168 B.C.) by that new power, Rome. Macedonia was, in fact, the first province of the Roman Republic, annexed by Rome in 146 B.C.(1)

Although in Egypt, Ptolemy I and his successors nurtured and embellished the majestic city with a splendid library and an elaborate museum which bode the glory of antiquity, the fact remained that the empire built by Alexander had been torn asunder and would remain splintered. Moreover, these kingdoms continued to be rivals, and their political and military rivalry contributed to their eventual declivity. Despite the cultural splendor of Alexandria, the Hellenistic world would weaken and devoid of its former military vigor would soon be threatened by a new power and a most formidable foe – Rome.

With the risk of digressing excessively from our current discussion, namely Hellenistic culture, allow me to relate the aftermath of the decline and fall of Macedonia, the torch-bearer of Greek (Hellenic) culture, and of necessity, introduce the new rising power in the Mediterranean: After the Second Punic War (218-201 B.C.) in which Rome defeated Hannibal (247-183 B.C.) and the Carthaginian empire, Greece and Macedonia, then weak and divided (c.200 B.C.), fell prey to the Roman war machine and were eventually annexed as Roman provinces and assimilated by Rome.

After the Third Punic War (149-146 B.C.), just as advocated by the Roman statesman Marcus Cato "the Elder" (234-149 B.C.), Carthage was destroyed (146 B.C.). As you may remember, Cato the Elder was the famed orator and politician who – despite his "devotion to the old Roman principles of life, honesty and courage" – concluded all his speeches with the statement, *delenda est Carthago*, "Carthage must be destroyed."[1,2]

The Roman Republic with its disciplined legions now ruled supremely in the littoral Mediterranean, and her neighboring states were either, willing or induced, to be Rome's allies, or forced to be "under Roman protection."[2] Now, let us go back and discuss the intellectual zeitgeist of Hellenistic culture centered in Alexandria and the great events of civilization that took place before the rise of Rome.

ALEXANDRIA – A JEWEL ON THE NILE

As we have learned, Alexandria was founded by Alexander the Great after his conquest of Egypt in 332 B.C. Even after Alexander's death in 323 B.C. in Babylon, Alexandria continued to grow and prosper for the next 300 years under Ptolemy I and his successors.

At its pinnacle of glory, this dazzling and cosmopolitan city was indeed the hub of learning and the center of civilization and therefore, it was no wonder that the great scholars and scientists of the age flocked to Alexandria from all parts of the known world to work and contribute to the body of learning.

The splendorous city became home to the most celebrated library of antiquity which was estimated to contain 750,000 volumes of handwritten papyri scrolls.

Alexandria was also the sight of one of the ancient Wonders of the World, the Pharos of Alexandria, the most famous and majestic lighthouse of the age.[27] This ancient wonder, built by Ptolemy II, stood an imposing 440 feet high with a ramp ascending to the summit where the ever-burning signal fire blazed.(23)

[27] From this magnificent structure the scholarly journal of the medical honor society, Alpha Omega Alpha (A.O.A.), takes its name: *The Pharos*.

Founded at the Nile delta, the great Alexandria was not only the hub of cultural learning but also a center of commerce in the ancient world. Regarding the Ptolemies, Hellenic culture, and the founding of this marvelous city, the medical historian V. Robinson wrote:

Alexander's chief monument is the city he founded and forgot – Alexandria. In the division of the spoils, the shrewdest of his generals, Ptolemy Soter, possessed himself of Egypt. He had been conspicuous in the conquest of Afghanistan and India, and wedded a Persian princess at Alexander's desire. The Ptolemies became so intimately identified with Egypt, that we are apt to forget that they were Macedonians. We read of the Egyptian dark-skinned Cleopatra: we know little about her skin, but we do know she did not have a drop of Egyptian blood in her. The Ptolemies were extremely consanguineous, and married only each other. As for the first Ptolemy, according to contemporary gossip, he was the half-brother of Alexander; if not, he could have been, for Ptolemy's mother had been the mistress of Alexander's father. Macedon was a part of the Hellenic world, but geographically it stood on the outskirts of Greece, and culturally was admittedly barbaric – hence its sensitiveness to Greek opinion. Ptolemy as a Macedonian ran true to tradition: since triumphant Macedonia always paid intellectual homage to Athens, Ptolemy began transforming Alexandria into a second Athens.(39)

And with regard to Ptolemy II (c.308-246 B.C.; ruler, 285-246 B.C.) and Alexandria, Robinson likewise notes, "His successor, Ptolemy Philadelphus, of frail physique, but equally enthusiastic over his various mistresses and the glory of Hellenic culture, actually made Egypt's capital the center of Greek learning and the playground of the world...."(39)

Fortunately for mankind, the Ptolemies were obsessed with learning and the desire to promote the growth of Hellenistic culture. They strove assiduously and ardently to advance their library and museum in Alexandria, whilst simultaneously promoting prosperity with trade and commerce in Egypt. Robinson further related:

The early Ptolemies were noted for their collection of books and their women; the finest houses in the town were owned by courtesans....The third of the line, Ptolemy Euergetes, confiscated every book that tourists brought to Egypt – returning to the owner a copy of the work – and he secured, by purchase or trickery, the original manuscripts of the classics from the Athenian Archives.

Moreover, the Ptolemies monopolized the manufacture of papyrus – paper for which all Greece clamored. The Alexandrian library grew until it contained three-fourths of a million papyrus-scrolls.(39)

Thus, it is no wonder that scholars of all nations flocked to Alexandria and made it their home. Robinson's wonderful vignette of Alexandria and its library concludes:

The Alexandrian library was only a part of the Alexandrian museum....It was not a museum as we employ the term, but a university which at one time enrolled 14,000 matriculants. [There were] extensive gardens for botanists, menageries for zoologists, observatories for astronomers, laboratories for chemists and physicists, while the anatomical school for physicians was equipped with dissecting rooms....And thus the first modern university is the University of Alexandria.(39)

The library of Alexandria was partially destroyed during a terrible conflagration in 47 B.C. at the time of the reign of the romantic queen of Egypt, Cleopatra (69-30 B.C.). The catastrophe coincided with the state visit by the Roman general and dictator, Julius Caesar (100-44 B.C.). Alexandria recovered and continued to be a major center of culture, trade, and commerce, but it never regained its former glory. It steadily declined following the annexation of Egypt by Rome under Augustus Caesar (63 B.C.-A.D.14), and the defeat of Mark Anthony (c.82-30 B.C.) and Cleopatra at the decisive naval Battle of Actium in 31 B.C. in which Augustus' trusted friend and lieutenant, the admiral Agrippa (fl.40-30 B.C.), led the Roman forces.

The library was finally burned to the ground in A.D. 641 by Arab zealots during the Islamic onslaught and conquest of Egypt. The conquest of Egypt at the height of the impressive Mohammedan victories put a definitive end to the remnants of ancient Egyptian culture, covering with a pall of gloomy silence the vestige of an entire civilization.

HELLENISTIC SCIENCE AND MEDICINE

Alexandrian science in general and medicine and surgery in particular, with their emphasis on learning and experimentation, resulted in an unprecedented accumulation of knowledge which exemplified the achievements of the Hellenistic Age.

Alexandria kept the torch of learning burning from 332 B.C. until the last twinkle of light was quenched, by which time its knowledge had been consumed not only by the Græco-Roman world including the Byzantine Empire but also, if I may use poetic license, inscribed in the collective consciousness of the world thanks to Rome and her legacy.

Although Alexandria barely survived through Roman times, and its dazzling glare had diminished to a glimmer by the 4th Century A.D., the knowledge and distilled wisdom of ages past lingered. And, although I was referring previously to such priceless intangibles as knowledge and wisdom, material possessions, books, and art treasures were also preserved in the storerooms of its library and museum until its final destruction in A.D. 641.[28]

The gifted scholars who continued to work in Alexandria between the 1st and 4th Centuries A.D. continued to achieve scientific advances, though at a steadily decreasing pace. During these centuries (especially, the first two), it was glorious Rome, and not Alexandria, that held the attention of the Western world.

Nevertheless, the achievements of Alexandria in sundry areas of learning and human endeavor, such as physics, astronomy, geography, mathematics, biology, philosophy, and even the applied sciences such as medicine and engineering were not to be surpassed until the advent of the Renaissance, 15 centuries later.

---

[28] Explorations of the catacombs of Alexandria have unearthed marvelous works of arts reflecting a strange synthesis of Greek and Egyptian civilization (i.e., paintings of the Egyptian jackal-god Anubis in Greek garments). The catacombs are also believed to contain the tombs of Alexander the Great and the prophet Daniel.

Amongst the many scholars in Alexandria were physicians such as Herophilus (fl.290 B.C.) and Erasistratus (c.330-250 B.C.) who dissected the human body and taught anatomy, physiology, and medicine, and mathematicians such as Euclid (fl.c.300 B.C.) and Archimedes (c.287-212 B.C.).

Archimedes founded the school of mathematics in Alexandria, but he is perhaps better known today as the one who designed various mechanical devices and formulated such principles as the simple lever. He also devised more intricate machinery using pulleys and even complex engines whose mechanisms have been lost to us from the pages of history. Moreover, his discoveries on mechanics laid the foundation for the science of hydrostatics and the concept of specific gravity used both in engineering and in medicine. Archimedes, the Greek mathematical genius, the story goes, is alleged to have uttered, "give me a lever and I will move the world."(2)

Of singular interest is the amusing story whereby the great mathematician, upon suddenly arriving at the solution to a mathematical conundrum whilst still partially submerged in the bathtub of his home in Syracuse, reportedly raised himself up – and still wet and naked – ran into the street yelling, *Eureka, Eureka*: "I have found it!" He had suddenly come up with the ingenious idea that determined the amount of gold in the crown of the King of Syracuse (in Sicily) by reasoning that submerged objects placed in liquid media should displace their own volume of liquid and have their corresponding weight diminished by an amount equal to the weight of liquid displaced – this is the concept of density, the weight per unit density of an object as opposed to the total weight of the object.(24,33)

Archimedes was killed during the successful Roman attack on the independent Greek colony of Syracuse during the Second Punic War in 212 B.C. The Greek colonists unwisely had sided with the Carthaginians in that war.

For his part, the mathematician Euclid not only postulated a number of mathematical theorems but also deduced many fundamental elements and axioms of geometry. For his theorems, he formulated orderly proofs that are still known and used today by students of geometry worldwide. His great work, *The Elements*, written in Greek, resulted in the rational systematization of geometry - Euclid geometry. Euclid also seemed to have been possessed of a dry sense of wit. Whilst toiling with a difficult mathematical problem and being asked by Ptolemy I about the nature of his intense labors, he is said to have retorted, "there is no royal road to geometry."(24,33)

We should not forget to mention Hipparchus (2nd Century B.C.), the Greek astronomer and mathematician who accurately observed the stars in ancient time and discovered the equinox. He compiled a star catalogue listing over 850 stars, giving their position and apparent brightness in magnitudes. This catalogue would be invaluable to later astronomers.

We have already discussed Eratosthenes, the 3rd Century B.C. Greek astronomer, geographer, and mathematician who with simple tools and the use of logic proved, rationally and mathematically, that the Earth was round, a sphere and its circumference, approximately 25,000 miles.

Alexandria, the heart of Hellenistic culture in the ancient world, was also home to engineers such as Heron (fl. 1st Century A.D.), the inventor of such machines as gear trains and steam engines. An engineering genius, Heron even anticipated the science of robotics and made complex models towards that end.

Alexandria was also home to the scholar Claudius Ptolemy (fl. 2nd Century A.D.), who theorized and then constructed a geocentric mechanical model of the world. In his model, he postulated his theory of the motions of the planets with the Earth at the center of the universe (c.A.D.150) This geocentric model held sway for 1,500 years until our physician colleague, Nicolaus Copernicus (1473-1543), convincingly overturned this theory, placing the sun at the center of our solar system, the heliocentric model of planetary motion. Copernicus' conception of the solar system, developed during the Renaissance, became a theory that revolutionized the world.

Within the context of the theories about the solar system, it must be noted that although Aristarchus (310-230 B.C.) had previously proposed a heliocentric theory in antiquity based on astronomic observations and calculations, Claudius Ptolemy's geocentric theory prevailed in convincing the world and unfortunately this erroneous theory, buttressed by his carefully constructed mechanical models, was the one incorporated into the body of knowledge in later centuries. It was Claudius Ptolemy, and not Aristarchus, who influenced the world up until the time of Copernicus in the Renaissance.

In Alexandria, medicine was well represented by Herophilus (fl. 290 B.C.) after whom the torcular heterophili (the posterior confluence of the intracranial venous sinuses) is named. He is considered by many authorities, and with good reason, to be the Father of Anatomy. We have mentioned his contemporary, Erasistratus who likewise is considered by some scholars of medical history to be the Father of Physiology. Erasistratus invented the urinary catheter, an ingenious devise used in the treatment of urinary retention. The important empiric school of thought in medicine was also formally formulated in Alexandria. It espoused medical observation of the patient by the physician prior to the initiation of treatment, and asserted that the "trial and error" method of obtaining medical knowledge was essential to successful medical practice.

After the death of Hippocrates in 370 B.C. and up until the founding of the medical school in Alexandria (c.320 B.C.), medicine continued to flourish and its banner was carried by devout physicians belonging to different sects or schools of thought including Praxagoras of Cos (fl. 340 B.C.), who was the first to recognize that arteries pulsated and veins did not. Unfortunately, he drew the wrong conclusion from that observation. He posited that the veins contained blood and arteries contained air, perhaps based on examination of postmortem material. Although Aristotle had made no distinction between arteries and veins, he nevertheless correctly asserted that the vessels which he called arteries contained blood and not air. Praxagoras, however, further postulated (again erroneously) that arteries pulsated because of the air, pneuma, within them. It is because of this false belief that the word artery (meaning "air containing") is used to describe the thickened blood vessels that carry oxygenated blood away from the heart in the systemic, and de-oxygenated blood in the pulmonary, circulation. Similarly, *tracheia arteria* was used to describe the cartilaginous "air-containing" tube in pulmonary anatomy. Today, it is the plain trachea. It would not be until Galen's discoveries in physiology almost four and a half centuries later that Praxagoras' error would be corrected.(40)

THE TRANSITION FROM A HELLENISTIC TO A GRÆCO-ROMAN WORLD

As we have seen, after the death of Alexander in 323 B.C., Ptolemy I and his successors nourished a magnificent city with a splendid library and museum –

components of a veritable university which blossomed to variegated colors of
glorious resplendence.

By the time of Ptolemy III, the magnificent library of Alexandria contained 500,000 to 750,000 volumes and boasted to possess books from all parts of
the known world. For obvious reasons, scholars, including astronomers, poets,
mathematicians, and physicians, were all attracted to this hub of learning, culture,
and center of civilization.

Alexandria and its Hellenistic culture served as a two-way conduit
between Greek civilization and the outlying Eastern cultures. Nevertheless, by 30
B.C., the rising star was Rome. Rome was to absorb much of the theoretical and
practical knowledge and put it to good use in her domain.

The Romans extracted ideas from this melting pot of Hellenistic and cosmopolitan culture and built upon it an empire. The Roman physician and surgeon
Aulus Cornelius Celsus (25 B.C.-A.D.50), as we shall see, was for medicine, science, and bioethics, what Marcus Tullius Cicero (106-43 B.C.) was for philosophy,
law, and legal ethics, and what Cato the Younger (95-46 B.C.) [29] was for republicanism and morality in politics. They all served as conduits of ideas from the ebbing
Alexandrian and Hellenistic world and its Eastern outskirts to the emergent Rome
and her radiant Empire. From this admixture of cultures and ideas came a corpulent
Græco-Roman civilization which would become even stronger with the addition of
a still inchoate Judeo-Christian tradition.

The Roman *medicus,* Celsus, wrote *De Medicina* (A.D.30), the oldest
Græco-Roman medical treatise after the *Corpus Hippocraticum*, and the first
Roman textbook of medicine concerned with the treatment of diseases with diet as
well as with drugs and surgery. As a result of *De Medicina's* exemplary clear literary style, Celsus was bestowed with the title of *Cicero Medicorum*. His book, lost
during the Middle Ages, was rediscovered in Milan during the Renaissance in 1443,
becoming one of the first medical books to be printed and widely circulated.(41-43)

In his book, Celsus, understanding the medical necessity for human dissection in the procurement of medical knowledge, writes:

> *Moreover, as pains and also various kinds of diseases arise in the more internal
> parts, they hold that no one can apply remedies for this who is ignorant about the
> parts themselves; hence it becomes necessary to lay open the bodies of the dead
> and to scrutinize their viscera and intestines....For when pain occurs internally,
> neither is it possible for one to learn what hurts the patient, unless he has
> acquainted himself with the position of each organ or intestine.(41)*

We will return to Celsus later. For now let us mention one last profession
besides law, politics, and medicine which also flourished during this epochal but
transitional period. I'm referring to architecture. Foremost in this field was the
Roman architect, Pollio Marcus Vitruvius (c.90-c.20 B.C.), whose *De Architectura*
is the only architectural andengineering masterpiece to survive from antiquity.(1,28)

---

[29] Cato the Younger, great-grandson of Cato the Elder, was devoted to the ideals of the early Republic and conservatism.
He was said to be honest and incorruptible and a genuine follower of Stoic philosophy that placed him above reproach.
As a loyal follower of Pompey the Great, in his struggle against the populist Caesar, Cato the Younger committed suicide at Utica, sometime after learning of Pompey's defeat at Pharsala in 48 B.C., bidding his followers to make peace
with the victorious Julius Caesar.(1)

Though his work may have had some influence upon European architects during the Medieval period, his designs and writings did not become immensely popular until after they were published with commentaries and illustrations during the Renaissance (between 1486 and 1511). The rediscovery of this classic work "ushered in the revival of the classical orders in Italian Renaissance architecture."(1)

Moreover, it was from Vitruvius' writings that Leonardo da Vinci (1452-1519) extracted many of the engineering concepts sketched in his celebrated notebooks. For example, da Vinci's ubiquitous *Vitruvius Man* is derived from the descriptions left by this brilliant architect of antiquity and immortalizes both the Renaissance artist and the Roman architect. The work is the sketch of a man with outstretched hands, which, in this position, become perpendicular to his feet which are closed together. The figure thus portrayed describes a perfect square, which when superimposed on the same individual, now with raised hands and feet spread apart, forms a perfect circle: the quintessential physical and spiritual man, the man possessed of Pythagoras' celestial fifth essence.

Leonardo da Vinci's sketch of the *Vitruvius Man* is today widely circulated, adorning books, prints, and pamphlets of the Renaissance artist, who remains much more popular than the still obscure ancient architect who inspired him.

PART THREE: ROME

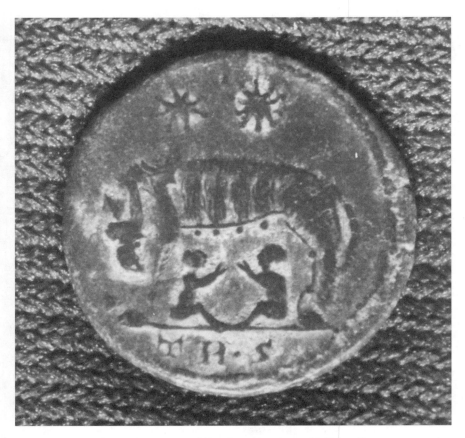

Plate 10 – Romulus and Remus suckling from the she-wolf. "Roma" commemorative
bronze coin c.A.D. 330-346. Author's private collection.

CHAPTER 9

ANCIENT ROME

Rome was not built in one day.
John Heywood (1497-1580)

THE MYTH

Most textbooks give 753 B.C. as the traditional date for the founding of Rome by the mythologic twins, Romulus and Remus. According to legend, the twins were born to the Roman god of war, Mars, and one of the Vestal Virgins. The baby boys were abandoned in the wilderness and brought up by a she-wolf that suckled them and nurtured them to health during their vulnerable infancy. Though legend says that the twins founded the city of Rome together, they later quarrelled and Romulus (after which Rome is named) killed Remus. The story, imbued with the usual philosophic duality of myth and prophecy of antiquity, presaged that as punishment for the sacrilegious act of fratricide, nascent Rome built upon the Palatine Hill, would grow and prosper to become a mighty and dazzling city that, in due time, would rule an impressive and glorious empire – but as atonement for the unspeakable crime, the power of Rome would only last a thousand years. The unforgivable sin of fratricide would ultimately bring down the City Upon the Hill, which otherwise had been destined for glory.

So, it did not come as a total surprise to many of the citizens of the Empire when, nearly a millennium after the founding of Rome, the feared Attila the Hun, King of the Hunnish hordes (reigned, A.D.434-453), prepared to march on the Eternal City. The Roman citizens prepared and braced themselves for the worst and expected nothing less than divine retribution from the "Scourge of God" – as Attila had been christened by a bemoaning priest who had witnessed the pillaging and plundering of the marauders on the outskirts of the Empire.

Another story attributes the founding of Rome to the Trojan hero Aeneas, a story which is described in Virgil's great epic poem, *The Aeneid*.(1) *The Aeneid* traces the saga of the indomitable Aeneas and his band of compatriots who managed to flee after their defeat at the hands of the Greeks and the sacking of Troy.(2) After a long, arduous, and hazardous journey, they reach their destiny at the outskirts of the "Seven Hills," and upon the Palatine Hill, they chose to found the fateful city of Rome.

As destiny would have it, during her first two and a half centuries, Rome was ruled, not by Latin Romans, but by the harsh, despotic Etruscans. In the early 6th Century B.C., the Etruscan royal family was headed by King Lucius Tarquinius Superbus (Tarquin the Proud). In 510 B.C., King Tarquinius Superbus would finally be overthrown by the people he had previously subjugated, the Romans, who then abolished the monarchy and founded the Roman Republic.

THE ROMAN RELIGION

By night an atheist half-believes in God.
> Edward Young (1683-1765), from The Complaint, or Night
> Thoughts on Life, Death and Immortality (1742-1745)

The religion of the early Romans was polytheistic, characterized by the worship of a myriad of local deities, the personification and deification of ideals,[30] and also by syncretism – a predisposition to assimilate other cultures' belief-systems and their religions. Because of their syncretistic attitude, the Romans eventually adopted many of the Greek gods as their own, and in time replaced many of their own local deities with the worship of the great Olympian divinities. The anthropomorphic Greek gods were thoroughly assimilated: Zeus became Jupiter; Aphrodite, Venus; Artemis, Diana, etc. Roman religion was in fact so adaptable, tolerant, and syncretistic that it easily identified its divinities with foreign deities to the extent that it incorporated into its pantheon incongruous divinities and deities from faraway places, whether allied kingdoms or subjugated peoples. Even centuries later during the declivity of the Empire, three of the most popular religions or rather quasi-religions, mystery (usually secret) or health cults, were of foreign origin, and these lasted well into the Christian era: The cult of the primal goddess, Isis-Hygeia; the dreaming and healing cult of the temples of the Asklepiads; and the revered Oracle at Delphi of the god Apollo.

THE DELPHIC ORACLE

The Delphic Oracle, like Greek religion, was assimilated by the Romans and deserves some elaboration as to its origin, purpose, and eventual decline, for it exerted tremendous influence in the Græco-Roman world. Although we have already mentioned the Oracle at Delphi from one perspective of Greek religion, I would now like to share with you a bit more information about its origin, c.2000 B.C., and about its closing, in the 4th Century A.D. during the declivity of the Roman Empire and the rise of Christianity.

The Delphic Oracle stands at an awe-inspiring chasm close to where the Pleistos river flows into the Gulf of Corinth on the southern flank of Mount Parnasus. Its white marble columns stand 2300 feet atop a precipice of white rocky cliffs where the "navel of the Earth" was said to be fissured by a deep geologic cleft. Legend relates that from this precipice and chasm of the earth, the high-priestess of the Oracle ordered the fablist Aesop to cast himself to precipitous death for the sin of sacrilege and defiling Delphi c.500 B.C.(3)

According to Professor Norma L. Goodrich of Claremont Colleges, Delphi was previously named Pytho, after the Nubian priest who presided there,

---

[30] The personification and deification of ideals in Roman religion included *fortuna* for the deity representing fortune, *dignitas* for dignity, *justicia* for justice, *pax* for peace, *pietas* for piety, *felicitas* for happiness, etc., which were frequently represented on the reverse side of Roman coins. Nevertheless, these personifications and deifications of highly venerated Roman ideals never quite reached the divinity status afforded their gods and goddesses.

before Apollo took possession of the Oracle c.1500 B.C.[31] The Pytho (or python) was assigned to the Greek Oracle by the dynastic queens (and high-priestesses) of Egypt. His purpose was to guard the sacred Castalian Spring found therein. Nevertheless, the black warriors of Upper Egypt were defeated by Apollo and his patriarchal warriors and, according to Professor Goodrich, "the direct link between Egypt and Delphi was severed." The Pythia was left dependent upon Apollo and his "solar" Greek Indo-European warriors who settled and conquered Greece. Apollo killed Pytho at Delphi near the sacred Castalian Spring c. 1500 B.C. Yet even before Pytho, Gaea,[32] the Earth-Mother goddess, may have been the first Pythia and her daughter, Themis, the queen of oracles.(3)

In honor of the slain Pytho, the high-priestesses of Delphi took their name of Pythia. The Pythia, nevertheless, was no ordinary prophetess, for she resided and presided over the antediluvian "navel of the Earth," considered the geographic center of the Earth and the most powerful and revered Oracle of antiquity. Even the *Omphalos*, the prophetic navel stone, was said to be housed there in the service of the Pythia.(3)

The ancient pilgrims who worshipped there had to undergo sacraments and rites of purification before they were allowed in the holy site. They also gave offerings before they traveled up the Sacred Way to the temple. The Eternal Flame of Greece burned at Delphi, and its inner sanctum, which Goodrich instructs us was due west past the eternal flame, led to the rear and most sacred portion of the temple where the "towering cult statue of Apollo stood in gold."(3)

The Pythia resided in the most sacred underground chamber, where she was believed to rest her head on the *Omphalos* during the recitation of her prophesies. In her book, *Priestesses*, Goodrich mentions that the Pythia would enter into a prophetic trance, a state which could have resulted from the inhalation of mephitic fumes coming from deep fissures in the subterranean chamber or from the chewing of laurel leaves or the inhalation of the smoke of incensed laurel leaves. Whilst "ecstatic revelations" and "prophetic trances" might have been Asian (Minor) in origin, the oracles so articulated were, nevertheless, considered divine words sent and uttered by the Pythian priestess from God.

According to Goodrich, "the Pythia practiced self-induced hypnosis, hypnogogic reverie and dreams as useful paths to self-knowledge."(3) And Plato, in his *Republic*, called the Pythia, "our national divinity," for the Pythia, as head of the Oracle of Delphi, exemplified two important routes for the acquisition of knowledge: intuition as a way of self-knowledge and revelation as a way of divinely revealed knowledge.

Nevertheless in Roman times, the Oracle was at the disposition of Rome. So much so that in A.D.69, Plutarch, who was one of two priests at Delphi, traveled to Rome to plead for the restoration of the Oracle (which had been sacked by Emperor Nero). And in A.D.117, the Roman Emperor Hadrian planned the full restoration of Delphi but his plans never came to fruition.(3) The Oracle remained functional up to the time of Emperor Julian "the Apostate" (emperor, A.D.361-363).

---

[31] According to mythology, in the words of Professor Goodrich: "This transpired following the great flood, which inundated the earth to such a depth that even one of the cliffs over Delphi there on Mt. Parnasus was submerged. After the waters receded, a great chasm lay below Delphi. That was when Themis became queen and High-priestess of the Oracle. When Apollo saw that divinely prophetic words were issuing from this chasm, he decided to kill Pytho, claim the shrine, and become a prophet himself."(3)

[32] In the study of myth as pointed out by Professor Goodrich, "priestesses take the name and identity of the goddess they serve, and dress in her prescribed, traditional costume."(3)

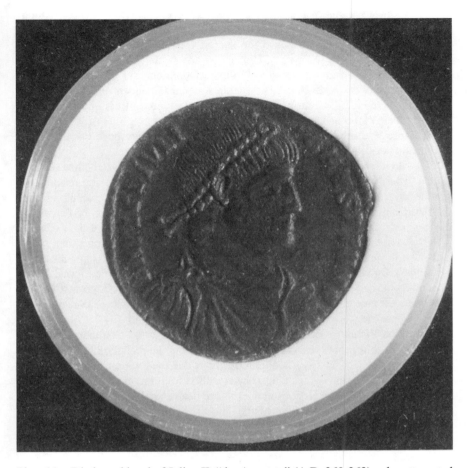

Plate 11 – Diademed head of Julian II, "the Apostate" (A.D. 360-363), who attempted to restore paganism to the Empire, but died in battle at age 33. Silvered bronze follis. Author's private collection.

In fact, the last oracle was delivered to the physicians attending Emperor Julian the Apostate in A.D. 362.[33] Emperor Julian had tried unsuccessfully to restore the Roman pagan cults and suppress the newly-sanctioned Christian church. He was the last Byzantine ruler to attempt to resurrect the old Roman religion (after Christianity had already become the official state religion). The oracle delivered to the emperor's physician urged, "tell the emperor that the temple has fallen to the ground, that bright Apollo no longer has a roof over his head or prophetic laurel, or babbling spring. Yes, even the murmuring water has dried up."(4)

Like Greek religion, Greek medicine was assimilated by the Romans. Yet, the majority of physicians in the Empire, though separated into many different medical sects, were composed mostly of Greek practitioners because the Roman citizens considered the medical profession below their dignity. In fact, it was Cicero (106-43 B.C.) the gifted Roman lawyer and eminent orator, who considered medicine a noble profession for commoners, but even he still considered politics, rhetoric, law, and philosophy to be the appropriate endeavors leading to the dignified professions for aristocratic Roman citizens. Cicero played a leading role in the introduction of Greek thought and philosophy to ancient Rome. Along with the great Greek philosophers, notably Plato, he played a pivotal role in the formulation of religious philosophies that influenced Western thought. Both Plato, who believed in divine revelation, and Cicero, who believed in the need for self-knowledge, asserted the necessity for the fusion of these concepts before one could know oneself, or the divine mind of God. Thus, the Pythian or Socratic maxim, "know thyself," through Plato and Cicero came to influence Islam, "he who knows himself knows his Lord," and Judeo-Christian theology, "know thy soul, and thou wilt know the Lord."(5)

THE GODS, GODDESSES, AND CULTS

Legend proclaims that the worship of Æsculapius was first brought to Rome in an attempt to contain a horrible epidemic assailing Rome in 290 B.C. The Romans were said to have pleaded for help to the Oracle at Delphi, which in response, advised consultation with followers of the mythologic Greek physician Æsculapius at one of his temples. According to Goodrich, the Romans consulted the sacred *Sibylline Books*; she writes: "When a pestilence decimated the Romans in 292 B.C., the [*Sibylline*] *Books* instructed them to send for the healer Asclepius; and one of his 'snakes' (priests) came over to Rome two years later. War had delayed his departure."(3) According to mythology recorded by Ovid (c.43B.C.-c.A.D.17), the Roman poet and author of *Metamorphoses*, Æsculapius transformed himself into a serpent, traveled by ship to Rome and there divinely ended the horrible plague. The cult of Æsculapius and temple medicine endured for centuries. So much so in fact, that medical historian Dr. Steven Metzer maintains that the cult of Æsculapius in the Græco-Roman world continued to compete successfully with Christianity until well into the 5th and 6th Centuries A.D.

[33] Although in mythology, the Delphic Oracle thrived in Mycenean times (i.e., both Agammenon and Odysseus went to Delphi c.1200 B.C.), the golden age of the Oracle, according to Goodrich, was the period between the 8th and 5th Centuries B.C. Yet, centuries later, the Pythia via Apollo was said to have foretold in A.D.79 the eruption of Mt. Vesuvius.

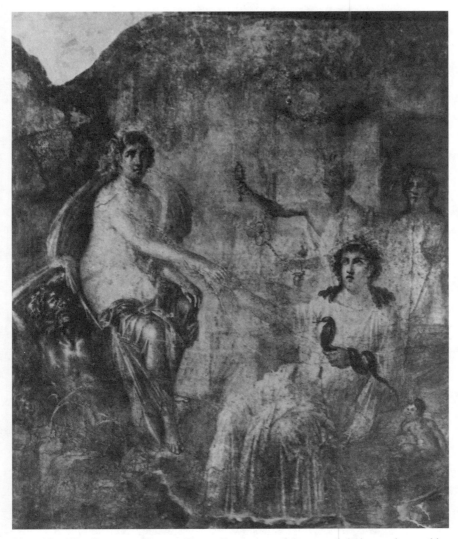

Plate 12 - *The Coming of Io into Egypt*. Depiction of the nymph being welcomed by the goddess Isis-Hygeia from the Temple of Isis in Pompeii. Museo Archeologico Nazionale, Naples.

Early Romans subscribed to *animism*, that is, they attributed to natural phenomena or inanimate objects the conscious life of a supernatural being or deity. Therefore, they worshipped sundry gods and a myriad of local deities associated with nature such as the winds, streams, forests, and harvesting, as well as, household and fertility goddesses, as in the most primeval of cultures. Later, after the Hellenistic conquests, the Romans adopted the Greek gods and goddesses by identifying them and assimilating them as their own, by the process which we have outlined previously, *syncretism*. As you would remember we also mentioned how they adopted Venus, the Greek goddess of love who became Aphrodite; Hades, who ruled over the dead in the Underworld, was called Pluto by both the Greeks and the Romans; Phoebus Apollo, son of Zeus, considered "the most Greek of all the gods"(4) remained Apollo; Hermes, Zeus' messenger, with his winged sandals and his magic wand became Mercury; Jupiter replaced Zeus as the supreme god at Mount Olympus, and Diana, Apollo's twin sister and chief huntress of the gods, substituted for the Greek Artemis. Last but not least, was Pallas Athena, daughter of Zeus alone, given birth via parthenogenesis, and born full grown and in full armor. So incarnated and armed, she sprang from Zeus' head and became the Roman goddess Minerva, the protector of civilization – a heavy burden, even for a goddess.

The Romans also adopted esoteric Oriental religions and arcane Eastern cults such as the cult of Mithras, a cult very popular with the soldiers of the Roman legions, especially those serving on the outskirts of the vast empire. Another popular cult was the Egyptian cult of Isis which in Græco-Roman high circles became the cult of Isis-Hygeia. The cult of Isis-Hygeia was as popular with the upper classes as with the lower classes.

Nevertheless, under the auspices of the powerful Roman Emperor Constantine I, "the Great" (emperor, A.D.306-337), Christianity grew steadily throughout the Empire. Constantine I even presided over the Council of Nicaea in A.D.325, by which the Nicene Creed was adopted by the church. Then under Theodosius I, "the Great" (emperor, A.D.379-395), Christianity was made supreme. Pagan sects were persecuted, and Christianity was proclaimed the state religion. Under the leadership of these two strong emperors, the Roman Empire was twice unified and resurrected – only to repose finally and irreversibly, at least the western part, as we shall see, after the apocalyptic plague of the 6th Century.

Besides the treatments rendered at the temples of the Asklepiads, only the cult of Mithras and the cult of Isis provided Christianity with any serious rivals in the healing-religious arena of the Roman Empire.(1)

The cult of Mithras was of Persian origin and was linked to the Zoroastrian concepts of the duality of light and darkness, and the perpetual struggle of good (God) and evil (Satan). Yet it also consisted of primitive rituals – the taurobolium – which involved the sacrificing of bulls followed by baptism of the initiates with the blood of the gored animals.

The cult of Isis-Hygeia blended eastern Egyptian attributes with Greek aesthetic health ideals, whilst providing more pabulum for the initiates: the reassurance of a future life, whilst resurrecting the old primal concepts of Earth-Mother goddess rituals. It also provided a nexus between the exotic mysticism of the Egyptian past, the philosophic inquiries of the Greeks, and the realities of the practical Roman world. These two cults provided the much sought-after and needed rewards of an afterlife, yet they lacked the hierarchical organization and body of priests needed for the conversion and assimilation of large segments of society. Only Christianity – with the comfort that it provided to the masses during troubled times, enforced by the young, aggressive, missionary spirit of the Christian priests – had the propensity and vitality to ultimately triumph during the dark descent that was the decline and fall of the Western Empire.(1)

Christianity was triumphant because its evangelical gospel not only preached man's immortality, promised the blissful rewards of heaven, taught universal love, and other noble Christian concepts, but also satisfied man's age-long fascination with consoling liturgical rituals and his innate need for obeisance of a fulfilling religious as well as ethical and moral code. These Judeo-Christian attributes were too appealing to be ignored by the masses of people in need of spiritual guidance during the various recrudescences of feelings of anguish and despair that were, with good reason, so prevalent in the turbulent 5th and the apocalyptic 6th Centuries.

THE CUMAEAN SIBYL AND THE LEGEND OF THE VESTAL VIRGINS

A word about the Cumaean Sibyl is in order, as she was considered by many authorities the High-priestess of Rome, and through her Oracle, she exerted considerable influence over Rome and her territorial possessions, especially during the centuries of the early Republic. Legends recorded by both Virgil and Livy proclaimed that the vicinity of Cumae received its first prophetess at approximately the time as the founding of Rome in 753 B.C. It is believed that Mount Etna in Sicily, under tectonic pressures, burst open previously dormant volcanic rents, resulting in the deep earth fires, "the red fumaroles of the Flaming Fields" of Cumae.(3) Cumae, incidentally, is situated on the Italian peninsula in the north bend of the Bay of Naples, where the ancient Greek geographer Strabo[34] believed that it served as a refueling station for Greek colonists on their way to Tangier or Cádiz.(8) Cumae is the coastal land near Circe's Promontory and Calypso's Isle recounted in *The Odyssey*. It was also near one of the entrances descending into Tartarus, the lowest region of Hades where the wicked are doomed to eternal torment.

The Cumaean Sibyl, like her counterpart at Delphi, delivered prophetic or instructive oracles which were sung or recited in verse. The story, as compiled by Goodrich, goes on to say that an old woman came into the presence of the Etruscan king, Tarquinius Superbus, to sell him the nine books, the *Sibylline Books*, containing the prophecy of the destiny of Rome and the world. He hesitated, and only later, offered to buy the last three remaining books. By then, it was too late for him and for the Etruscan kingdom, for we know how the Romans overthrew the despotic Etruscans and set up their model Republic.

And later, during the Second Punic War, Goodrich writes, "the situation of Rome grew most precarious in the spring of 217 B.C., when the African commander

[34] Strabo (c.63B.C.-A.D.21) was the prolific Greek geographer and historian who traveled widely, recording observations and making sketches of the exotic places that he visited. Out of his 47 books quoted by later scholars only a few are extant. His most complete, *Geographia,* contains a cornucopia of historic, geographic, and cultural data, a veritable fountain of ancient knowledge including treatises on the geography of the Mediterranean, littoral regions, as well as hinterlands of Europe, Asia, and Africa.(7)

Hannibal moved out of winter quarters to finish his so-far highly successful conquest of Rome. That Spring, in both Italy and Sicily, the heavens warned of impending death."(3) Indeed, the Carthaginian general inflicted defeat after defeat on the Roman armies as he moved toward Rome. Then in 216 B.C., he inflicted the most serious defeat on Rome, at Cannae, a veritable disaster for Rome, but for the Carthaginian general Hannibal, one of the most brilliant military victories in history. Rome appeared doomed. It was at this time that, Goodrich relates, "the Cumaean Sibyl finally ordered people to go sit at the crossroads and pray to Triple Hecate, and, last of all, to bring from Asia the Black Stone of Mother Cybele, and then Cybele herself, as their protectress in this great emergency."(3)

Goodrich decries the fact that up until the 20th Century[35] the veracity of the existence of the Cumaean Sibyl was questioned, despite the fact that St. Augustine himself believed that there was a sibyl who spoke words derived from God, and Michelangelo "painted them beside the prophets on the vault of the Sistine Chapel, at the Vatican in Rome."(3)

But what about the Vestal Virgins, the priestesses who kept the protective fire in the hearth of Rome? The story of the mythic Trojan princess, Rhea Silvia, was related by both the historian Livy and the poet, Ovid, and it gives us some insight into this holy priesthood of Rome. The maiden Rhea Silvia is associated with the origin of the Vestal Virgins as recounted by Goodrich. She had been reared by her father, a Latin king who claimed to be a descendant of the Trojan hero, Aeneas. He had raised her in the priesthood of the Vestal Virgins to preclude her from one day having a male heir who, legend had declared, would claim his kingdom. As things turned out, however, Rhea Silvia was raped by the Roman god of war, Mars,[36] as she went to the river to fetch water; and in time, she gave birth to the fateful twins: Romulus and Remus.(3)

Through the centuries the Vestal Virgins were, as their name implies, expected to remain virgins and to keep the eternal flame of Rome ablaze. And for the most part, they did – for the destiny of Rome depended on it.

A ROMAN REPUBLIC OR A GREEK DEMOCRACY?

The worst inequality is to try to make unequal things equal.
Aristotle (384-322 B.C.)

As we have already intimated, in the 6th Century B.C. Rome was still an unimpressive Latin city on the Italian peninsula on the Left (east) Bank of the Tiber, whilst Athens was already in full bloom, carrying the torch of Western civilization. Even today, 2500 years later, the relative contributions of Athenian democracy and the Roman republican form of government to the origin of our own American constitutional republic remain intermixed and undiscernible to the average American. Perhaps the topic is too hot for handling, deemed best ignored by

---

[35] In the early 20th Century the Italian archaeologist Giuseppe Consoli-Fiego, after performing extensive excavations alongside the Bay of Naples, unearthed and revealed the site of Cumae, and the Cumaean Sibyl was established as the plausible High-priestess of Rome, "and as a member, one priestess after another, of a priesthood venerated for centuries by Romans."(3)

[36] Mars in Greek mythology is known as Ares. The month of March is named after this powerful Roman god of war.

those who know, and a non-issue by those who don't.[37] Yet it is an important distinction that needs to be brought forth and discussed, as we continue to move leftward in the political spectrum on our relentless neo-Fabian march toward global socialism in the closing decade of the 20th Century.

It is imperative that the citizenry, particularly the embattled medical profession, possess a basic knowledge of history, law, and political science, just as trial lawyers possess more than a passing interest and a cursory knowledge of medicine, surgery, and medical practice. Moreover, citizens in general and physicians in particular should have an idea of the consequences inherent in the changes that are taking place today in our political system. Perhaps it is worth remembering at this time the wise words of Louis D. Brandeis, a former Supreme Court justice (1916-1939), who wrote that the most important office was that of the private citizen – a truism that should remind us of our civic duties and political obligations to remain ever vigilant of the winds of political change.

Today, our own form of government is rapidly undergoing a metamorphosis from a constitutional republic (and representative democracy), based on a foundation of individual self-reliance and private philanthropy, to a socialist democracy, based on the raw power of an ever-increasing omnipotent government authority and an amoral, amorphous, statist, and exuberant bureaucracy that, in a Faustian transaction, claims to provide security in the form of cradle-to-grave services to the countless dependant masses in return for their dignity, autonomy, and liberty. Though these changes have gradually been taking place in American society for over 70 years, the metamorphosis toward a socialist democracy has been palpably accelerated in the last 25 years. This social transformation is almost more akin to Karl Marx's vision of world socialism (despite the fall of communism) than to the delaying tactics of Roman general Quintus Fabius Maximus Cunctator, "the delayer," from which the British Fabian Society takes its name.[38] Along with these drastic societal changes there have been significant changes in health care and the practice of medicine and it is within this context – namely, the historic precedents set between changing political systems and the practice of medicine [39] – that we want to approach this timely subject. First (as always) allow me to digress to recount a bit more pertinent history.

In ancient Greece, as we have noted, Solon's election as Archon of Athens in 594 B.C. opened the door for substantive political changes in Athenian democracy. Solon was able to militate for the acceptance of his bold concept, that government be effected by written laws and that *both the people and the rulers obey those same laws*.(9) Thus, the Archon of Athens began implementing the leading principles of a constitutional republic in the fledgling Athenian "democracy," whilst instituting economic and general reforms destined to reconcile the different factions – aristocratic, commercial, and the various other popular groups vying for political and/or economic power in Athens. His Athenian constitution was based on nearly universal citizenship and constitutional reforms which, again, were more akin to the

---

[37] Still others consider the issue settled by the fact that the gap between the terms "mass democracy" and the "constitutional republic" form of government (the latter equated with a representative democracy) has been bridged by the term denoting a "constitutional" or "mixed democracy."

[38] The Fabian Society promoted socialism by slow, evolutionary change rather than by the radical revolutionary class struggle advocated by the German socialist philosopher, Karl Marx (1818-1883).

[39] In fact, the recent unveiling of the American Health Security Act of 1993 (September 22, 1993) presages momentous changes for American medicine.

rule of law of a constitutional republic than outright majority rule of a popular democracy. Moreover, the country was to be administered and governed by the rule of constitutional and legislative law. The laws were to be written and codified so they would be known and obeyed by all citizens.

Here we must pause and reflect, for we have encountered two basic and brilliant principles of constitutional government that protect citizens from abuse and usurpation of power by their own government. Moreover, these principles protect all citizens – individuals as well as members of minority groups (ethnic or otherwise) – from the excesses and abuses of the majority. These important tenets, proclaiming that laws be written and applied equitably to the people and rulers alike, are also of paramount importance because they thwart tyranny and curb the monopolistic tendency of government to accumulate power. The application of justice by the rule of law to protect the individual citizen as well as members of unprotected minorities such as physicians, businessmen, and other professionals from the arbitrary power of government and the tyranny of the majority, cannot be overemphasized, for it represents the very essence of a constitutional republic.

Paradoxically, as Rome began her progression in 510 B.C. from a small Latin kingdom in Italy to a grand republic, Athens, for her part, began her move from the constitutional principles set down by Solon to the concept of simple majority rule and mass democracy, thence subject to periods of populist absolute rule at the whim of a majority whose sentiments and opinions were labile and susceptible to the sophistry and charismatic oratory of populist demagogues or ambitious political tyrants.

Thus, as Rome moved from the outset towards a more stable government founding a marvelous republic in 509 B.C. (the year after the Etruscan monarchy was overthrown) and lasting almost without interruptions for nearly five centuries, Athenian democracy went through several cycles of dictatorship and tyranny.[40]

It was then up to the nascent Roman Republic to implement long-lasting constitutional reforms and codify the laws so that they could not be easily scuttled by the whim of tyrants claiming to speak (and sometimes actually speaking) in the name of a volatile, impassioned majority. As we know from mob psychology, charismatic leaders can incite the masses by appealing to some of man's most primitive and dark instincts: fear and hatred.

As we have seen, Greece, weakened by warfare amongst its city-states, notably Athens and Sparta, and afflicted by devastating pestilences, was conquered by a determined foe, King Philip II of Macedonia in 339 B.C. For a time, Macedonia upheld Greek culture, but ultimately, beset with divisiveness, lack of respect for discipline, law, and order, the once glorious Greek civilization and the Hellenistic world of Alexander fell, only to be assimilated by the power of Rome. Many of the Greek institutions and facets of Greek culture, such as the arts, religion, philosophy, etc., but not her laws or military, were absorbed by the rapidly expanding Roman world.

---

[40] The dictatorial rules of Pisistratus (612-527 B.C.) and his sons Hippias and Hipparchus – and even the rule of the Athenian statesman, Cleisthenes (fl.510 B.C.) – provide vivid examples as well as insight into the tenuous demarcation between populist democratic leaders and outright tyrants. "Like many champions of the poor, Pisistratus was no man of the people, but a dissident aristocrat," a tyrant who seized the opportunity to reach coveted power.(1) Likewise Cleisthenes, considered a founder of Athenian democracy, ruled as a virtual dictator (especially after 506 B.C.) after he had expanded his power base by "democratic" reforms.

THE GLORY OF THE REPUBLIC (509 B.C.-49 B.C.)

We are in bondage to the law in order that we may be free.
Cicero

As we have already mentioned, in 510 B.C., the last Etruscan king of Rome, Tarquinius Superbus, was overthrown by a popular Roman uprising, hence the following year, 509 B.C., has come down to us in history as the traditional year for the founding of the Roman Republic.

Towards this lofty goal of establishing a republic, the Roman Senate, in 454 B.C., sent a commission to Athens to peruse the legislation implemented by Solon. And later, upon the commission's recommendation, the Roman assembly formulated a set of new laws for Rome, codified in the celebrated *Twelve Tablets*, the written constitution of the fledgling Roman Republic, which as the American statesman Robert Welch stated, "remained for 900 years the basic laws of Rome."(9) These basic constitutional laws survived despite the creation and imposition of the Roman Empire (between 31 and 27 B.C.). In fact, upon Augustus Caesar's (emperor, 27 B.C.- A.D.14) investiture, one of the first acts decreed by the emperor was to restore all the constitutional safeguards of the Republic. This act would be associated with economic stability and prosperity, and the wise political administration of the provinces, not to mention the enforcement of the *Pax Romana* which resulted in the golden age of Rome.

The point is that the foundation laid by the Republic and the tradition of abiding by the rule of law remained in effect well after the Empire had formally replaced the Republic in 31 B.C.(1,7,9) In fact, as late as A.D.160, a Roman citizen named Gaius wrote, "all law pertains to persons, to property, and to procedure."(9)

To prevent the accumulation of power in any one branch of government, the Roman constitution provided an elaborate system of check and balances. And to further protect the people from government tyranny, just as our Founding Fathers designed the Bill of Rights, the Roman Republic established the office of Tribune in 350 B.C. to safeguard the rights of the citizenry from their own intrusive government.(1,9)

The young republic was founded on a firm foundation and solid ground. It was possessed of religious tolerance, economic freedom, and political liberties. Fortified with these just principles, it would grow and expand and in due time, defeat the colossal maritime commercial power of Carthage in the First Punic War (264-241 B.C.) to gain Sicily. Later, in the Second Punic War (218-201 B.C.), Rome, the Eternal City, would even survive the disastrous Battle of Cannae[41] – a bloody defeat inflicted by the brilliant and audacious Carthaginian general, Hannibal (247-183 B.C.).

And although later in the history of the Republic there would be divisive political debate and sometimes outright violence, as in the affair of the Gracchi brothers,[42] the republican form of government during the span of four centuries would prove superior to all other forms of governance, including Athenian mass democracy or dictatorship.

---

[41] In that Roman debacle, 45,000 Roman soldiers were killed in a single afternoon in 216 B.C.
[42] Tiberius Sempronius Gracchus (d.133 B.C.) was elected Tribune in 133 B.C., and his younger brother, Gaius Sempronius Gracchus (d.121 B.C.), followed him in that office from 123 to 121 B.C. Both brothers were social reformers who resented the accumulation of wealth by the *nobiles* and sought to redistribute wealth. Toward this end, they supported the Sempronian Law for the redistribution of public lands. Both were killed in street riots.(1,7)

The situation in Rome changed with the influx of newcomers into the Republic and the instigation of class hatred and warfare by aspiring populist demagogues. Predictably, a major civil war ensued from 88 B.C. to 86 B.C. fueled by a social conflict that worsened an already parlous situation. The divisive conflict was led by two outstanding but also ambitious Roman generals: Marius (155-86 B.C.) and Sulla (138-78 B.C.). The class hatred that fueled this civil war was particularly unfortunate because the Romans had enjoyed opportunities and civil liberties unprecedented in history. Moreover, though the populace was divided between the *patricians* (from the Latin *pater* for "father") representing the old aristocracy, and the *plebeians* (from the Latin *pleo*, for "the masses") representing the rest of the population, the latter was composed not only of workers and peasants but also the more affluent merchants all of whom had prospered under the Republic. The truth is that, by in large, the entire population had gained and prospered from the Roman political liberties (natural rights of citizenship), economic freedoms (free enterprise, land and property ownership rights), and social mobility.[43] In fact, by the 3rd Century B.C., the plebeians had won political equality with the patricians, and it was their virtual synthesis that produced the prosperous Roman community that enjoyed the political, social, and economic benefits of a constitutional republic. So much so, in fact, that it was in this milieu that a new class, the *nobiles* ("the nobles"), deriving their power from their own individual effort and acquired wealth, became the predominant ruling class in society afforded by the ladder of Roman social mobility.

Yet, in the last century of the Republic, unfortunately, there was enough class strife and social unrest – injudicious attempts by lenders at collecting insolvent debts, unsettled land disputes ultimately resulting in the brake-up and redistribution of large tracts of land referred to as *latifundia*, and the incitement of the masses by populist demagogues – to provide the necessary ammunition to instigate sufficient discord and to foment enough anarchy to lead inexorably to the fall of the Roman Republic. In fact, some historians, including Will Durant, have argued that it was instigated "class warfare not Caesar who killed the Roman Republic."(9) And for those who call attention to the existence of slavery in Rome and her territories, we must point out that as iniquitous as this institution might have been, slavery in the ancient world was universal and Rome, in this regard, was no exception. She too believed in the old adage, that to the victors belonged the spoils of the enemy.

In 72 B.C., Spartacus (d.71 B.C.), a Roman gladiator, led a large slave insurrection which, although short-lived, shook the foundation of Roman society. This slave rebellion was the last major slave revolt in ancient Rome, but the serious event would nevertheless remain etched in the memory of the Romans. The insurrection was finally squelched in 71 B.C. by the Roman generals Crassus and Pompey the Great,[44] with the ensuing crucifixion of 6000 captured slaves including the leader of the rebellion, Spartacus.

Judged by the standards of her age, the Roman Republic was a fair, just, and highly successful political experiment in constitutional government. The

---

[43] And thus the pride inherent in the phrase, *Civis Romanus sum*, "I am a Roman citizen."

[44] This was Marcus Licinius Crassus (d.53 B.C.), the general and later the third member of the First Triumvirate with Julius Caesar and Pompey the Great. His family began as an old plebeian family that rose to be a *nobile* family by the efforts of Crassus and his father Lucius Licinius Crassus (d.91 B.C.), "a noted orator and lawyer much admired by Cicero."(7) On the other hand, Pompey the Great (106-48 B.C.) was Julius Caesar's rival and the champion of the republican forces in the Senate between 54 to 48 B.C.

noblest ideas of political governance had been put successfully into effect. She had eclectically siphoned the best ideas of Athenian democracy, learned warfare tactics from the Spartans, ascertained maritime routes and the principles of commercial entrepreneurship from the Carthaginians – distilling all this knowledge into wisdom tailored to befit the practicality of the Romans. The Roman Republic also provided the abstract ideals and the tangible benefits of individual liberty and civil protection for its citizens, including property and inheritance rights for women. Slaves were excluded, of course, although in those days slaves included Greek teachers, philosophers, and even physicians who continued to practice their vocation as "enslaved" professionals. The word "slave" did not connote quite the same meaning as it did centuries later. However, one might speculate and even convincingly argue that the degree of enslavement does approach most closely the situation that American physicians are poised to face in the very near future.

The Roman Republic was much more successful and efficient than Athenian democracy, and for women and ethnic minorities provided infinitely better opportunities. Moreover, Athenian mass democracy was frequently plagued by interruptions in democratic rule, government paralysis during times of political turmoil, and inefficiencies in the function of daily government. Oligarchy, anarchy, and mobocracy all plagued and hindered Athenian democracy which was, therefore, only destined to be a brightly-lit torch of very short duration. It was not conducive to the long-term progress, stability, prosperity, and security that was needed for the guardian of Western culture and civilization. This task of guardianship and bearer of the torch of Western civilization was fittingly left to the Roman Republic, and later, the Roman Empire.

Even under the leadership of Athen's most deserving champion, Pericles (c.495-429 B.C.), the Athenians succumbed to the tragedy of the Peloponnesian Wars (431-404 B.C.) which ended with victory for militaristic Sparta – with not only agony and defeat for aesthetic Athens but also the institutionalization of tyranny in the birthplace of democracy. Ultimately, because of Rome and the wisdom and the power that she represented, Athenian philosophy, as well as the Greek arts and sciences, would survive and be preserved for posterity. Likewise, the military tradition and spirit of the defeated Spartans would fortify the already martial essence and resilience of the victorious Romans. Rome, the city on the Palatine Hill, would be suffused with both the aesthetic qualities of Athens and the martial spirit of Sparta, destined to hold the reins of Empire for another five centuries.

At *prima facie*, the fate of the Roman Republic *per se* was foreclosed with the advent of Gaius Julius Caesar (100-44 B.C.) who crossed the Rubicon River on January 19, 49 B.C., and marched on Rome in triumphal success. His exploits, including his victories in Gaul, defeat of the Senatorial armies, and his final victory over Pompey at Pharsala in 48 B.C.[45] had sealed the fate of the Republic, at least in part. Julius Caesar's assassination on the steps of the Senate building in the Roman Forum on the *Ides of March* (March 15, 44 B.C.) was the price he paid for dooming the Republic. Nevertheless, this turmoil was only the symptom of the inner disease which had undermined Rome's foundation – namely

---

[45] Gais Julius Caesar, who was born into an old patrician family of Rome, was a populist leader, a member of the democratic or popular party of Rome. As *Pontifex Maximus* and with the help of scholars, Julius Caesar reformed the calendar in 63 B.C., which henceforth became known as the Julian calendar. Crassus had already been killed after his army had been defeated and routed by the Parthians at Carrhae in Mesopotamia in 53 B.C.(7)

the abuse of power that had taken place in a republic which had finally degenerated into raw lust for power by military leaders, greed and avarice manifested by the ruling classes, and most importantly the *sine qua non* for the death knell of the Republic (or any constitutional republic, past or present), the class envy fomented by populist politicians who deliberately created an atmosphere where class warfare and hatred in society unctuously insinuated itself like a malignant disease. A deliberate catastrophe had been instigated and created in the name of the people, all because, as Lord Acton's well-known aphorism so clearly states, "power tends to corrupt and absolute power corrupts absolutely."

Miraculously, it seems the foundation of the Roman Republic was stronger than expected. Despite the founding of an empire, republican institutions persisted and for the first two centuries, constitutional principles remained in practice. The semblance of the rule of law and republican principles would survive until formally repudiated by the edicts of Diocletian in the 3rd Century A.D. It was the dictatorial emperor, Diocletian (emperor, A.D. 284-305), who ended all forms and semblances of republican government in the Empire and eliminated local self-government in the provinces. Although Diocletian was extremely successful militarily – not only did he restore law and order and beef up the army, but he also reclaimed Britain for the Empire in A.D. 296, and defeated and subjugated the Persians in A.D.298 – still, his economic policies were a dismal failure. He created a welfare-driven, collectivist, totalitarian state, with himself as absolute ruler. He levied exorbitant taxes on the population and instituted draconian wage and price controls, taking great pains to be as equitable and as fair as possible, yet predictably, his economic reforms resulted only in the equitable distribution of misery amongst the population. Diocletian was a powerful ruler and despite the formation of his Tetrarchy, a system by which two "senior" Augustus and two "junior" Caesars ruled different districts of the Empire, by sheer personality he continued to pull the strings of government in matters of interest to him.[46]

The Republic, then, served the Roman citizenry well for nearly five centuries. Moreover, it was during the time of the Republic that Rome extended herself well beyond the city boundaries to most of the Italian peninsula and then through the littoral Mediterranean. Like the United States, it was during the years of strict republican rule that Rome extended her frontiers and grew faster, to assimilate with unprecedented tolerance, people from other ethnic backgrounds, religions, and cultures. It was the well-disciplined, citizen-armies of the Roman Republic that defeated the well-paid but heterogenous and largely mercenary armies of the maritime and commercial Carthaginian empire. The same Roman legions of citizen-soldiers later conquered the independent Greek city-states, and in the wake of these conquests, first assimilated, and later propagated Greek culture. Much of what is considered the best in Greek traditions, philosophy, art and architecture, as well as myth and religion, were also absorbed by the Romans.

The Roman Empire extended its boundaries further, but it was the legacy of the Roman Republic, governed by the rule of law and served by her

---

[46] Diocletian took the extraordinary step of abdicating and summarily retired to his castle near Salonae in 305 A.D.; still from time to time, he would advise the Tetrarchy about matters of state when his counsel was sought, as during the political upheaval and crisis precipitated by Emperor Maximian's (joint emperor, A.D.286-305 and A.D.307-308) return to power aided by his son, Maxentius (breakaway emperor, A.D.306-312). Diocletian intervened and confirmed Maximian's previous abdication and loss of imperial power.(10)

well-disciplined citizen-army as her instrument of law (force), which effected this policy and enforced the *Pax Romana* for nearly two centuries, thereby bringing much wanted peace and security to the Western world.

It may be worth repeating that the mighty, seemingly invincible, disciplined Roman legions of the Republic were composed of citizen-soldiers, in the way of the celebrated Roman citizen Cincinnatus. Cincinnatus was the embodiment of the quintessential Roman citizen-soldier patriot. Twice he performed his duty: putting aside his plow to lead the Roman army as "dictator."[47] Once he was appointed by the Senate to serve the Republic which was in imminent danger from a foreign enemy and he, as a loyal soldier, was chosen to lead the war effort, which he dutifully performed. When the crisis passed, Cincinnatus promptly returned to his farm and resumed his plowing. On another occasion, he was called to duty to put down a domestic insurrection. Again, he performed his duty, putting down the revolt and when the danger passed, he returned to his farm, and as before, quietly resumed his plowing.(1,7)

It was the wise and witty Benjamin Franklin (1706-1790) who I believe was thinking of the history of the Roman Republic – our predecessor in political history and model of government – when he responded to a question posed to him by an inquisitive lady at the completion of the proceedings of the Constitutional Convention in Philadelphia in 1787. The lady asked, "What have you given us, Mister Franklin?" and he replied, "A republic, ma'am, if you can keep it."(9)

---

[47] In those days the duty of the "dictator" was to serve the Republic as commander of the army for short periods of time. Cincinnatus (Lucius Quinctius; fl.5th Century B.C.) served as consul in 460 B.C. and "dictator" twice in 458 and 439 B.C.

CHAPTER 10

ROME AND HER EMPIRE

Love conquers all.

Virgil (70-19 B.C.), Eclogues

Time heals what reason cannot.

Seneca the Younger (c.3 B.C.- A.D.65), De Ira

THE ROMAN MEN-OF-LETTERS

The Augustan Age and the tumultuous times immediately preceding it (1st Century B.C.) were a remarkable period of recorded history, which saw, amongst other things, the blossoming of literature such as drama, (especially satire), prose, and lyric and epic poetry. The inauguration of this majestic age began when a frightened Roman Senate voluntarily voted to bestow upon the triumphant Octavian,[48] grandnephew and heir of Julius Caesar, the title of "Augustus" in 27 B.C. This heralded the beginning of a new age, a new Imperial Age, marked by Augustus' 41-year reign and the beginning of the *Pax Romana* that would last, arguably with a few interruptions, up to the reign of Emperor Marcus Aurelius, or perhaps even more precisely, until the assassination of the young emperor, Severus Alexander (reigned, A.D.222-235), whose death denoted the rise in the tide of anarchy in the 3rd Century A.D. [49]

The stability of the Augustan Age made possible the flowering of the arts and the blooming of the work of the *literati* of the age. This resurgence in learning, especially in philosophy and literature, had actually begun during the last gasps of the Republic, but had been interrupted by the upheaval of the social and political civil wars of the 3rd Century A.D. Philosophy, logic, and rhetoric were discussed in open market places including the Roman Forum. The Greek philosophies of Zeno (c.495-c.430 B.C.) and Epicurus (341-270 B.C.) – Stoicism and Epicureanism, respectively – were introduced and discussed during the Republic and widely circulated amongst the upper classes and *literati* within the Empire.[50] These philosophies contributed significantly to the melding of Greek ideals with Roman practicality. Although the Romans did absorb many Greek philosophic concepts and their sense of aesthetics, the Romans also had their own accomplished philosophers and poets.

Among these we find Horace (65-8 B.C.), the Roman lyric poet and satirist.

---

[48] Octavian (63 B.C.- A.D.14; 1st Roman emperor, 27 B.C.- A.D.14) became *de facto* ruler of the Roman Empire after his victory over Mark Antony and Cleopatra at the naval Battle of Actium in 31 B.C.

[49] Julia Mamaea, the mother of the young emperor Severus Alexander, was said to have been the real power behind the throne.

[50] Stoicism maintained that all reality is material and molded by a universal and pervasive force that is divine. Epicureanism held that the ultimate reason for existence and the highest good was pleasure attained by happiness, serenity, and the absence of pain.(7)

Horace, you will remember from Latin studies, urged his fellowmen, *Carpe diem, quam minimum credula postero* ("Seize the day, put no trust in the morrow"). Yet, in reference to advancing age and impending retirement, he also exhorted: "Dismiss the old horse in good time, lest he fails in the lists and the spectators laugh."(11)

There was also the poet and philosopher, Lucretius (c.99-c.55 B.C.), who wrote a didactic book of poetry consisting of six volumes, *On The Nature of Things*. In this masterpiece, he described and commented on the philosophies of Epicurus and Democritus, who deeply influenced his works. Lucretius believed in the transcendental and existentialist concept that consciousness ended with death and that there was no immortality of the soul.(7,12)

And then there was the poet Ovid (43 B.C.- A.D.17) who wrote the celebrated mythical masterpiece, *Metamorphoses*, a collection of stories written in hexameter verse. Ovid was the master composer of elegiacs, of which the most celebrated are his erotic poems, such as *Amores* and *The Art of Love*. He was banished by Augustus in A.D. 8 to Tomis near the Black Sea because of the "immorality" of some of his poetry; in exile, he continued to write verse until his death.(7,12)

Virgil (or Vergil;70-19 B.C.), the greatest of Roman (Latin) poets and a favorite of Augustus, wrote the epic poem *The Aeneid*, picking up in Latin where Homer left off in Greek. *The Aeneid*, Virgil's magnum opus, is an extraordinary narrative in hexameter verse that represents the veritable crowning achievement of the literary epic. In this work, Virgil recounts the trials and tribulations of the Trojan hero, Aeneas, after the fall of Troy. Virgil's Aeneas "is a paragon of Roman virtues – familial devotion, loyalty to the state, and piety."(7) The heroic poem, contained in twelve books, relates Aeneas' epic adventures and ordeals following the defeat of Troy, his escape from the doomed city with his followers, through his torrid affair with the Carthaginian Queen Dido [51] to the founding of Rome.

During the Middle Ages, many thought Virgil was a magician, because he was believed to have been possessed with vast and forbidden knowledge.(13) Yet, we know he was a Roman patriot and that the purpose of his writing was not to gain such dubious distinction in posterity, but to produce a national epic, a monumental literary work to exult the grandeur of Rome and to rejoice over the presaged and perceived glorious and patriotic destiny of the Roman Empire.

The great philosopher of the 1st Century A.D., Lucius Seneca "the Younger" (3B.C.-A.D.65), as tutor to Nero and informal advisor to Nero's mother, Agrippina (II),[52] came to be virtual ruler of the Empire during the first years of Nero's reign. Like Cicero, Seneca the Younger leaned toward stoic philosophy. Moreover, he wrote intriguing and enthralling tragedies saturated with grandiloquent rhetoric. Yet not forgetting his stoic philosophic inclinations, his drama was imbued in stoic overtones and deliberately set in gloomy surroundings, as in the case of his successful play, *Medea*. Centuries later, Seneca's tragedies would profoundly affect Renaissance drama.

---

[51] Dido was the mythologic queen and founder of the city of Carthage. She loved Aeneas, and when he left her to continue his journey and fulfill his destiny, she killed herself, her body consumed on a funeral pyre.

[52] The first Agrippina (I) was mother to the perverted Roman emperor, Caligula, whilst Agrippina (II) was mother to the infamous Roman emperor, Nero. Agrippina II was also the fourth wife of the Roman Emperor Claudius, whom she poisoned, but only after she had first secured for Nero (her son by a previous marriage) the position of successor to Claudius.

Seneca is also known for his sentimentality, pithy sayings, and humanistic reflections: "No untroubled day has ever dawned for me," and on further introspection on the subject of man's attempt to escape from adversity and perhaps even his own shortcomings, "Night brings our troubles on the light rather than banishes them." In regards to will and human susceptibility to vices, "Drunkenness is nothing but voluntary madness," and on man's destiny and the order of things, "Fate rules the affairs of mankind with no recognizable order," and "Failure changes for the better, success for the worse." His profound sayings reflect life experiences that touch all, "It is often better not to see an insult, than to avenge it," and on the transcendental subject of justice, "Injustice never rules forever"; and "Cruelty springs from weakness." On the eternal subject of reaching and attaining truth, "Time discovered truth." In regards to the opportune theme of, or rather, the lack of individual responsibility and accountability, "Vice can be learned, even without a teacher."(11)

Ultimately, Seneca, the great philosopher, committed suicide amidst accusations of treasonous conspiracy. The act of committing suicide in the face of such charges was considered a sublime act by the Romans.(7) In a later section, we will return to Seneca the Younger and cite him in reference to his contributions to medical ethics.

Lucius Seneca "the Elder," (c.54 B.C.- c.A.D.39) father of Seneca the Younger, is best known as a great connoisseur of the art of rhetoric. His works were centered on the history and way of life of the upper classes during the reigns of Emperors Augustus and Tiberius (reigned, A.D.14-37). Tiberius, the son by a previous marriage of Augustus' wife, Livia Drusilla, is known to history for his able administration of affairs of state and preservation of the imperial frontiers. Tiberius, as you would remember, continued Augustus' policies of preserving peace and prosperity, even in the most distant provinces of the Empire. Through the writings of Seneca the Elder, we learn much about this period, not only history, but also the art of rhetoric and oratory.(12)

During this period the Roman historian Livy (59 B.C.- A.D.17) wrote with patriotic fervor his life's work, *Books from the Founding of Rome*, a monumental history describing with great zeal the expansion of Roman power in Italy and the battles of the heretofore, seemingly, invincible legions of the Republic as Rome faced the vicissitudes of the winds of war against the power of Carthage. Livy recounts how after a horrendous war, the Romans finally defeated the great Carthaginian general Hannibal, vanquishing the commercial power of Carthage. Livy then relates in particulate detail Rome's story of reaping the spoils of victory after the Third Punic War, with the seizure and possession of Carthage's maritime empire of the eastern Mediterranean. Livy's tomes consisted of 142 books of which 35 are extant. His annals begin with the traditional date of the founding of Rome in 753 B.C. and ends with the period of the indomitable Roman general, Drusus Germanicus (38 B.C.-9 B.C.), who inflicted several military defeats upon the marauding Germanic tribes, although as we shall see, even he failed to subdue the Teutonic tribesmen permanently.

Livy exalted the glory of the Roman Republic which he so eloquently described as a "free nation, governed by annually elected officers of state and subject not to the caprice of individual men, but to the overriding authority of the law."(14) Emperor Augustus was a benefactor of the arts and letters, and as such, a patron of Virgil, Ovid, Livy, and Horace.

Amongst historians we also find such Roman Men-of-Letters as Pliny The Elder (A.D.23-79), who was a tremendous storyteller and a great encyclopedist. During the Middle Ages, he was still considered the ultimate authority in all areas of learning from history to medicine. An intrepid naturalist, he died whilst observing and recording the events in the wake of the eruption of Mt. Vesuvius near the provincial city of Pompeii in A.D.79.

And of course, there was the historian Suetonius (c.A.D.69 - c.122), imperial biographer, who wrote the *Histories of the Twelve Caesars*, a work filled with interesting anecdotes and unique tidbits of information on the imperial families to which he was privy.(15)

Cornelius Tacitus (c.A.D.55 - c.117) wrote realistic histories of the Empire and its rulers. His *Histories* cover the years from Nero's death in A.D.68 and Galba's reign (A.D. 68-69), to the assassination of the brutal Domitian in A.D.96. His *Annals* cover the reign of Tiberius, but unfortunately only parts of the reigns of Claudius and Nero survive. Tacitus' republican sentiments and his distaste for the Empire are implicit in his writings, particularly in his *Annals*. Moreover, he was a harsh critic of contemporary Roman society.(7,12) Many of his aphorisms, given the unchanging quality of human nature, are still relevant today: "Things forbidden have a secret charm."(11)

The Romans not only excelled in Latin and rhetoric but also in politics and statesmanship. Amongst these notables we find Marcus Tullius Cicero (106 B.C.- 43 B.C.), the greatest of all Roman orators, as well as an eminent jurist, politician, Stoic philosopher, and letter-writer.(16,17) The noted rhetorician Quintilian (c.A.D.35-c.95), author of *Instituto Oratoria*, discussed the formal education of an orator and compiled scholarly critiques of previous Greek and Roman writers.(7,12) He also tersely, sarcastically, and wittily wrote, "A liar should have a good memory," and proclaimed, "The obscurity of a writer is generally in proportion to his incapacity."(11) He was said to have had common sense to urge the necessity for good taste and moderation.(7)

We have already mentioned Marcus Vitruvius (fl.1st Century B.C.) whose encyclopedic volumes in Roman technologic knowledge, *De Architectura*, was printed (after its rediscovery) in Venice in 1511. This book was an engineering masterpiece that denoted the advanced state of Roman technical knowledge in architecture and general engineering. One of his works, denoting both physical and metaphysical insight, provided a humanistic paradigm envisioned in antiquity which centuries later would be immortalized in Leonardo da Vinci's *Vitruvius Man*.

But what about the physicians of this period? Let us return to the Roman *medicus*, Aulus Cornelius Celsus (25B.C.-A.D.50), the outstanding physician who was also a scholar of great repute, and deservingly so. Celsus' surgical text, *De Medicina*, rediscovered by Pope Nicholas V (pope, 1447-1455) in a library in Milan during the Renaissance, contains the first accounts of controlling and stanching hemorrhage during surgery (surgical hemostasis) by the use of ligatures; it also includes a description of lithotomy (surgical evacuation of urinary tract stones) as performed by the noted lithotomists of his time using the lateral surgical approach. Herniotomy (hernia repair) is also discussed.(18) We also find the earliest discussion of plastic surgery techniques including the detailed repair of traumatic mutilations. After its discovery, this celebrated book was printed and reprinted and became the authoritative text for the medical scholars of the period. *De Medicina* earned Celsus the title of *Cicero Medicorum*, "the Cicero of the physicians."(18) This work, considered his magnum opus, is a compilation, a veritable encyclopedia, of medicine and surgery which was cited by both Pliny the Elder in his *Naturalis Historia* and Quintilian in his *Instituto Oratoria*.(12,18-20)

Celsus believed in the importance of "hands-on" medical practice as opposed to book learning; thus understandably, he emphasized experience in medical practice, "...it is true that nothing contributes more to rational treatment than experience."(19) He firmly believed that experience was the primary method of learning medicine and becoming a good physician – an unusual plea for a Roman *nobile*. Celsus, as an aristocratic Roman physician, asserted that medicine should be undertaken by talented Roman citizens as an honorable profession and not left solely to the province of the conquered servile Greeks.

Of interest to the reader should be the insightful perspective on Celsus and the Roman *nobiles* written by the medical historian, Dr. Betty Spivack, particularly regarding the prevalent misconceptions imputed to the ancient Roman nobility in recent times. Spivack writes, "Roman patricians were not a parasitic group of esthetes, who lolled around in their villas, gorging themselves. Roman patricians undertook extensive public and private responsibilities, serving as diplomats, governors, legates, army officers, legislators, lawyers, as well as filling many other significant roles."(19)

Spivack correctly points out that the deeply ingrained dual notion of "Hellenophilia-Romanophobia," which early in this century was especially prominent, "still exists to a remarkable degree today."(19) This perception, of the Greeks as the sole philosophers and innovators and the Romans as copiers and emulators of culture, remains alive and well today in the liberal mindset of Western academia. Never mind the tremendous infrastructures - be it roads, bridges, aqueducts, or such architectural marvels as the Roman Forum with its Colosseum and triumphal arches, and the Pantheon – all of which are still standing and dazzling in resplendence, built by the Romans possessed of supreme technologic knowledge for their time. All of these wonders we often take for granted without giving them thought and without extolling the virtues and lauding the sacrifices and accomplishments of those who came before us, blazing the path of Western civilization as they went, pioneers in time – for such is the reigning liberal myopic zeitgeist of our precarious times, long on opinions and assertions, short on history and facts.

Although aristocratic Roman landowners, such as the encyclopedist, Pliny the Elder, and the master politician and orator, Marcus Porcius Cato (234-149 B.C.), exemplified the Roman practical sense of self-sufficiency and may have even practiced family medicine (21) within the context of *Pater familias*, Spivack argues with good cause that these *nobiles* should be differentiated from Celsus, who was a true professional physician and surgeon. She thus quotes Celsus, the surgeon: "...while one having experience can bleed very swiftly, it is more difficult for the ignorant; for the veins are next to the artery and sinews (or nerves). Thus if the scalpel touches the sinew (or nerve), spasms follow and the patient is cruelly maimed. And an incision of the artery neither clots nor heals; sometimes, in fact, it causes the blood to erupt strongly. If there has been vigorous cutting of the vein itself, the ends are compressed and blood is not forthcoming. But if the scalpel is plunged in timidly, it only cuts the outer skin and not the vein. Occasionally, it may even be hidden and not easily discovered. Thus, many things make this difficult for the unknowledgeable, while it is very easy for the experienced practitioner."(20)

It should also be noted within the context of the presently evolving ethics that, unlike the old Babylonian-Greek ethics of not accepting hopeless cases or refusing to treat patients with poor prognoses, Celsus went ahead and treated difficult cases after obtaining informed consent from patients and families, especially if the intended therapy was deemed dangerous or risky. Ahead of his time and being the superb surgeon that Celsus was, it was therefore no wonder that Theophrastus Bombastus von Hohenheim (1493-1541), the famous Renaissance physician, would christen himself "the equivalent of Celsus," Paracelsus, thirteen centuries later. And as the reader will discover in the closing chapters of this book, that would be an honor not totally undeserved.

THE GRANDEUR OF IMPERIAL ROME

The slave begins by demanding justice and ends by wanting to wear a crown.
Albert Camus

Civil war ensued following the assassination of Julius Caesar on the steps of the Senate building in the Roman Forum on the Ides of March, and after the dust of civil war had settled, the political ascendancy of Octavius (Augustus Caesar, 63 B.C.- A.D.14; 1st Roman emperor, 27 B.C.-A.D. 14), was assured and the all but inevitable transformation of the Republic to Empire was a virtual and certain reality. Octavius, Julius Caesar's grandnephew and adopted son, had the title of *Imperator*, [53] meaning "commander," conferred upon him by the Senate in 29 B.C., and later in 27 B.C., he was bestowed with the title, *Augustus*, which he dutifully assumed and which meant "exalted" or "revered." Moreover, he also assumed the title of *Pontifex Maximus* (a title first given to Julius Caesar) which made him not only the supreme political and military leader of the Empire, but also its paramount religious leader. His full appellation accordingly, was *Imperator Caesar Augustus*, though he was said to have preferred the more modest title, *princeps*, which meant "first citizen" – his traditional title as republican leader.(1,7,12,22,23)

Nevertheless, Augustus, for all his titles, preserved the underlying republican institutions which had been firmly embedded in Roman traditions, such as governance by the rule of laws, whilst safeguarding the rights of Roman citizens. Moreover, he initiated a period of stability in public functions and private affairs "including a growth in wealth and economic opportunity" that permeated all walks of Roman life.(12,22-24) His superbly adept administration of the provinces, allowing for self-rule, assured consolidation of the Empire. Moreover, the military remained disciplined and strong, able to ward off the nordic barbarians and capable of enforcing peace throughout the Empire, a *Pax Romana* which in turn ushered in a golden age for Rome.(10,12,15,22-24)

As with the Republic, the might of imperial Rome was embodied in the morale, that is, in the *esprit de corps*, the structural integrity and discipline of her

---

[53] The Latin, *imperator*, is the etymologic root of the word "emperor."

well-trained and well-led imperial legions. And throughout this period of relative tranquility and prosperity, the *Pax Romana* imposed Roman peace in the Western world and kept the frontiers of the Empire impenetrable to the barbarians. Yes, the borders were preserved and maintained, and law and order achieved, even at the farthest outposts of the Empire by the pride of Rome: the Roman legions.

Emperor Augustus kept the Germanic tribes in check at the northern frontiers on the Rhine and the Danube, and the Parthians at bay on the eastern front. During his reign, except for one instance which we will discuss at length later, there was no credible force, event, or rival power to challenge the might of Rome. What is more, Rome's republican traditional institutions survived almost intact, despite changes in the laws and the implementation and enforcement of the various imperial decrees. Much of Rome's republican form of government remained in place and engendered stability and continuity in the Empire up to the 3rd Century A.D. The Roman republican traditions, defended by her proud disciplined legions, preserved the integrity of the Empire until the 3rd Century, when military morale collapsed and a series of debilitating civil wars wreaked havoc within the Empire. Even when debauchery and corruption were rampant at the highest level of government, because of the perverse or incompetent rule of some (fortunately transitory) emperors, the Roman government continued to carry on the affairs of government efficiently, and to preserve peace and tranquility throughout and law and order within, the Empire.(24) Yes, Rome survived such nefarious emperors as Caligula (emperor, A.D.37-41) and Nero (emperor, A.D.54-68). Caligula made his horse a Senator and himself a god. Nero, it has been said, fiddled (or recited his newly composed poetry) whilst Rome burned in the fire of A.D. 64, and then after accusing the Christians of the infamous deed, began the notorious Roman persecutions of Christians.

The hopeless victims were thrown into the gladiatorial arenas of the Roman Colosseum to be mutilated and killed by lions or other wild and ravenous beasts. Nero even had his mother, Agrippina II, murdered in A.D.59 and her body dissected to satisfy his own morbid curiosity of human anatomy. And as the reader will remember, it was also Emperor Nero who accused and inculpated his former teacher and mentor, Seneca the Younger, and others in a conspiracy against him. The other alleged conspirators were executed. Seneca was allowed to commit suicide. Finally, a popular revolt erupted, and the citizenry were able to rid themselves of this perverse emperor. Nero was forced to commit suicide – his last words, "What an artist the world is losing in me."(7)

Rome also survived the reigns of other infamous rulers such as the barbarous Domitian (emperor, A.D.81-96), son of the very capable military leader, Emperor Vespasian; and the brutal Commodus (emperor, A.D.180-192), son of the pious Marcus Aurelius.(10,15,23,24)

It is, therefore, a tribute to those old venerable Roman institutions, such as the concept of the rule of laws, the natural rights of citizens, the integrity of the family, etc., along with other praised and specified virtues of the Roman Republic such as justice, courage, and temperance which endured from the time of the Republic to salvage and sustain the Empire during those decadent reigns. Moreover, to the Romans we also owe such intangible ideals as peace through military strength, and the development and preservation of such stabilizing republican institutions as the Roman Senate, members of which could not be easily swayed by the winds of populism and political expediency, but rather, members who were inspired and guided by the cause of just laws and the rule of laws, as embodied in the spirit of Cicero who wrote:

> *[w]hat is right and true is also eternal, and does not begin or end with written statutes....From this point of view it can be readily understood that those who formulated wicked and unjust statutes for nations, thereby breaking their promises and agreements, put into effect anything but "laws." It may thus be clear that in the very definition of the term "law" there inheres the idea and principle of choosing what is just and true....Therefore Law is the distinction between things just and unjust, made in agreement with that primal and most ancient of all things, Nature; and in conformity to nature's standard are framed those human laws which inflict punishment upon the wicked but defend and protect the good.(25)*

It was this republican tradition and sense of fair play and justice which kept the Empire running relatively smoothly, even and in spite of the excesses of many over-indulged emperors and the eruption of various imperial crises that afflicted Rome from time to time. In fact, by the 5th Century A.D., as pre-saged by the legend of Romulus and Remus, the Roman citizenry had begun to accept what seemed to be the inevitable: the impending fall of the Empire, as divine retribution for Rome's original sin of fratricide. And so it went, that by the time of Attila the Hun's arrival on the decadent Roman scene, Rome was by then expecting and bracing for the worse, the painful fulfillment of a nightmarish but inevitable destiny.

Many illustrious scholars of Roman history have hypothesized as to the reasons for the collapse of Rome. For example, the famous historian Edward Gibbon (1734-1794), writing in the late 18th Century, blamed what he considered "the softening influence of Christianity."(24) He contended that during those waning days of the Empire, citizens were more preoccupied with the afterlife and salvation of the soul, than with the inherent duties and civic responsibilities of Roman citizenship. The heart of his thesis asserted that, by weakening the will of the citizenry and by braking the discipline of the Roman legions with such ideals as universal brotherhood and Christian charity, Christianity greatly contributed to the fall of the Empire in the West. Therefore in Gibbon's estimation, the Christian ideals of universal love, compassion, and charity were the real culprits behind the fall of Rome.(24)

Others have proposed a teleologic explanation such as that the Western Roman Empire had carried out its vital purpose which was the acceptance, and thence, the consolidation and spread of Christianity; once this task was consummated, Rome had fulfilled her primal and ultimate mission, and the Empire could now crumble to dust, destined to final dissolution.(26)

Still others have suggested more rational, even medical and scientific, explanations seeking to explain the reasons for the fall of the Empire in the West. Some have blamed chronic lead poisoning for the decadence and collapse, since the Romans used lead tools and cooking ware and utensils made of that poisonous heavy metal.[54] Others have blamed diseases such as malaria [55] that cause anemia with chronic lassitude and recurrent attacks of prostration, fever, and chills – chronic symptoms that would have weakened the Roman constitution, thereby making the population vulnerable to famine, pestilential disease, conquest, and even death.(27) According to the medical writers, Frederick F. Cartwright and Michael D. Biddiss, the fundamental reason for the decline and fall of Rome was the catastrophic effects of malaria, which they maintain was as significant, if not more so, than the invasion of the Goths and Vandals. They recount how the fertile land around Rome went out of cultivation as the small farmers, sick and exhausted, abandoned the tilling of the land, and to make matters even worse, moved in great numbers into overcrowded Rome, bringing with them malarial fever. [56]

According to these authors, the Germanic tribesmen were not only reaching military parity with Rome, but their northern birth rate was also rising, whilst Rome's was falling steeply as a result of the severe form of malaria then afflicting the Roman citizenry in the more temperate southern climates. Moreover, these authors write: "By the fourth century A.D., the mighty fighting power of the legions was no longer Italian; not only men but officers too were drawn from Germanic tribes. Possibly malaria, rather than decadent luxury imported from the East, accounted for the slackness of spirit which characterized the later years of Rome."(27)

Yet others have correctly deduced, supported by a massive body of evidence, that military collapse played a fundamental roll.(1,10,26,28) The sheer pressure exerted upon the Empire from the increasing hordes of barbarians wreaking havoc amongst the populace, ravaging the land and ruining crops, and finally breaching the Empire's borders at multiple points was simply overwhelming. These facts can be added to the reality that there were already substantive numbers of barbarians within the gates of the Roman Empire, many of whom had not been fully integrated into Roman society, yet they participated in farming, commerce, government subsidies, even the military, where some of them commanded Roman forces in the field. This reality, coupled with the fact that the Germanic tribes were fast approaching military parity with Rome, indeed makes the military explanation of the fall of the Western Empire seem not only plausible but inevitable. Nevertheless, although a military explanation was an important factor and may have been the most significant precipitating cause for the collapse of Rome, it is inconceivable as the sole explanation for the fall of Rome and the Western Roman Empire.

Most likely, an already internally weakened empire subverted within the gates by over-centralization, corruption, burgeoning bureaucracy, and rampant authoritarianism (1,29,30), and now battered from outside the gates by waves of Germanic tribes assaulting the walls, figuratively and sometimes literally, exerted overwhelming pressure and wrought the death knells to an already declining empire.(1,10,26,28) Economic collapse was already an unfortunate reality, first as a result of the reigning anarchy, recurrent infestations with pestilential diseases, and

---

[54] It is now well known that lead accumulates insidiously in the body at low doses, until it reaches toxic levels and causes harmful effects in man. In high doses, it can cause acute symptoms such as paralysis, seizures, and rapid death, expecially in children.

[55] Malaria is an infectious protozoan disease caused by the parasite *Plasmodium* and transmitted by the Anopheles mosquito. It is a recurrent disease of the tropical and subtropical regions of the globe. The word is derived from the Italian, *malaria*, "bad air."

[56] These writers neglect to mention the effect of the failed economic policies of Diocletian, which precipitated those same events and are discussed in Chapters 13 and 14.

the near-military collapse of the 3rd Century A.D. Later, as we have intimated and will discuss more thoroughly in the pages to come, the authoritarian and totalitarian policies of Emperor Diocletian, although leading to a reinvigoration of the military, would also lead to a worsening of the economic situation because of regimentation, increased centralization, bureaucracy, welfarism, and the predictable mass migration to the cities of farmers and both skilled and unskilled laborers in search of government subsidies and entitlements, rather than land to be tilled and work to be performed.

The economic policies, growth of government bureaucracy, and cultural degeneration that took place during this time is eerily similar to the untenable situation that we are rapidly approaching in America today.(30) Without a doubt, there are uncanny parallels which we will explore and expand on in the later chapters of this section. For now, let us just say that the crumbling and disintegration of the Western Roman Empire eventually resulted in a new reinvigorated Christendom, the emergence of a political and military feudal society, and an economic and manorial system – all held together by the power of the Church. And it may truly be said that the Western Roman Empire following its collapse, like a phoenix, rose from the ashes of the chaos of the Dark Ages, transformed and ready to infuse the "all exhausted latinized" citizenry with the new blood of the newly-christianized Germanic barbarians (26), forming a *novus ordo seclorum,* which in time, would be made up of distinct nations sputtering forth with renewed energy and vigorous spirituality, rallying behind the banner of the Christian church.

CHAPTER 11

THE LEGACY OF REPUBLICAN GOVERNMENT

The Republic is the only form of government which is not eternally at open or secret war with the rights of mankind.
                                                            Thomas Jefferson (1790)

The preservation of the sacred fire of liberty, and the destiny of the republican model of government, are justly considered as deeply, perhaps as finally staked, on the experiment entrusted to the hands of the American people.
                        George Washington (First Inaugural Address, April 30,1789)

The central theme fundamental to the rules of society is the concept of the rule of law. At least in principle, a republic is governed by clearly written laws formulated by a government that is limited in its powers and formed with the consent of those it governs. [57] In this system of government, members of society obey the laws so as to foster a climate conducive to prosperity, whilst preserving individual liberty and safeguarding the rights of citizens. The laws are fair and just so that they, in turn, are respected and obeyed by all. Written laws embody the tenets of natural rights and the negative concept of laws which protect individual citizens and members of minorities, who otherwise are subject to oppression from the unrestrained tyranny of the majority. Protection of the rights of all citizens is imperative in a republic because of the known tendency of most governments, including both monarchies and social democracies, to usurp power from the citizenry. Unlike republics, which allow for representative democracy and sometimes even "direct democracy," and which are ruled by written (constitutional) laws, social democracies are always ruled by an elite, pluralistic or otherwise, subject to the arbitrary wishes of the majority, and thus, as we are clearly finding out, are extremely sensitive to the winds of social or political change and particularly, political expediency.

In a classic republic, laws are implemented with the consent of the governed and are not so easily subject to the shifting winds of political expediency or the evanescent whims of the expectant but poorly informed masses, only the exigencies of the overwhelming legions of well informed and vigilant citizens; yet the basic traditional rights of individual citizens are always protected. In constitutional republics/representative democracies, individual rights are delineated to protect the

---

[57] Despite the governments of countless nations calling themselves "republics," in actuality very few nations in existance today are truly republics. One exception that comes to mind is Switzerland. Yet such media pundits as an associate editor of the influential magazine, *The Economist*, has called Switzerland a direct democracy because of Switzerland's use of referenda so that "any law proposed by the government must be submitted to a vote of the whole people."(31) The constitutional republic of Switzerland makes it possible for the people (a politically informed and vigilant citizenry to be sure) (32) to exert influence on the government by constitutional means namely referenda, or "direct democracy," if you will - and not the other way around. So that it takes much more than simple majority vote to overturn the Swiss Republic, or for that matter, abolish private property or institute draconian gun control measures as has taken place in many of the European social democracies.

individual from the arbitrary growth and monopolistic power of government or the capricious wishes of the incited, uninformed majority. For example, contractual agreements, lawfully and voluntarily entered into by the parties involved, are not considered just isolated business transactions, but binding civil contracts that the government is bound to respect. Rules of evidence are followed in the courtroom and in other matters of jurisprudence, just as the rules of law are honored in matters of individual rights, politics, or government.

In a republic, a written constitution protects the individual rights of its citizens. Basic (traditional) rights such as life, liberty, property, and the pursuit of one's life interest, occupation, and avocation are protected, for these basic rights are considered to be derived from God or Nature. Basic traditional rights are believed to be derived from natural rights or inherent to the human person in an enlightened secular state such as ancient Rome, or granted by the Creator in God-fearing nations, such as that forged by the Founding Fathers. These basic traditional rights transcend the state and cannot be revoked by majority rule.(25)

As Professor Charles E. Rice of Notre Dame Law School reminds us, "One does not have to believe in God to recognize that natural law requires that the power of the state be limited."(25) Moreover, basic rights, embodied in reason and natural law, were of paramount importance in the formulation of laws in ancient Rome. To underscore this fact, Rice quotes Cicero who wrote: "Law is the distinction between things just and unjust, made in agreement with that primal and most ancient of all things, Nature; and in conformity to Nature's standard are framed those human laws which inflict punishment upon the wicked and defend and protect the good."(25)

Suffice it to say that in those blessed and/or enlightened states in which constitutional republics are the rule, "life, liberty, property, and the pursuit of happiness," whether assumed to emanate from divine right or natural rights, are nevertheless guaranteed by a government with limited power, and ultimately, enforced by a vigilant and informed citizenry. In a democracy, at least theoretically, absolute majority vote rules; therefore, laws and perceived rights, whether written or not, may be modified and legislated to conform to the whims and wishes of the majority. Likewise, basic traditional rights (natural rights) may be qualified out of existance or abolished.

In recent times, the disorganized majority with little regard for precedents set by law (as in ancient Greece) has yielded a significant degree of influence and power to coalitions of special interest groups (pluralistic elites) and government-favored minorities which have come to wield considerable and disproportionate power relative to their numbers. Powerful special interest groups then have acted in unison with populist demagogues to incite their constituents to militate for changes that selectively benefit them, at the expense of the individual citizens. Moreover, the rights of individuals and members of the not-so-favored minorities have suffered. Ultimately, these groups (such as physicians, small businesses, and entrepreneurs) and the fruits of their labors are placed at the disposal of the majority or its surrogates, the aforementioned coalitions of government-favored groups (such as consumer groups, labor unions, and large businesses already in collusion with government) that carry inordinate political clout, and in Orwellian fashion, are more equal than others. To make matters even worse, these politically connected (and often obstreperous) groups in cahoots with government have been increasingly successful in achieving their desired social ends at the expense of those with less political clout. A good example of this phenomenon is the politization of the AIDS epidemic, an epidemic which should have been confronted head-on as the public health menace that it is, with doctors allowed to confront this malady using traditional public health methodology. On the contrary, AIDS has been, and still is, treated as a socio-political issue where political expediency, rather than public health and science, is paramount. This subject will be revisited in our section on medical ethics.

In a social democracy, a simple majority effects policy and legislates drastic changes in the law depending on the popular mood and majority expectations. The government provides entitlements and bestows welfare rights upon those who have political clout or those it knows it can web into its malevolent trap of government dependency (as in welfare recipients), or sense it can incorporate into its own parasitic body (as in government bureaucrats).

Republics require that its citizens be well informed and vigilant, lest government takes away not only what it has given, [58] but also those natural rights such as life, liberty, and property, to which it has no claim or authority. As we reflect upon the ancient past and draw parallels to the present age, it becomes obvious that eternal vigilance is essential to citizenship and the preservation of basic traditional rights. In 1790, John Philpot Curran asserted that, "The condition upon which God hath given liberty to man is eternal vigilance; which condition if he breaks, servitude is at once the consequence of his crime and the punishment of his guilt." And in 1815, General Andrew Jackson (1767-1845), later U.S. President wrote, "The brave man inattentive to his duty, is worth little more to his country, than the coward who deserts her in the hour of danger."

Although today politicians, academicians, and the media have blurred the differences between a democracy and a republic, the subtle differences should be noted, for painful lessons of history denote that a constitutional republic (or representative democracy) that is not properly nurtured is lost by civil strife and class warfare, to either tyranny and oppression, as eventually transpired in Rome, or lost to mobocracy, as occurred in ancient Athens. An informed and vigilant citizenry should be wary of ambitious politicians and populist demagogues who practice the old Machiavellian craft of *divide et impera*, "divide and conquer," by fomenting class warfare, or by employing subterfuge and deceit, or by granting benefits and privileges to one group to curry their favor, whilst taking from another. In the days of the late Roman Republic, this meant giving to the mob what did not belong to them in exchange for political power. Today, it means giving to the numerically, financially, or vocally influential groups at the expense of others, who in the Orwellian sense are less equal, and thus not as influential. Individual citizens, despite their numbers, frequently acquiesce to the various redistribution of wealth schemes, or fail to exercise their basic rights out of ignorance, complacency, acquiescence or actual complaisance, out of media indoctrination or arm-twisting submission by which many of us are coerced into the giving mode of forced socialist compassion, or out of the sense of helplessness, pessimism, or the sense of inevitability that this crucial decade so far portends. The

---

[58] This is a good point at which to recall the words of the eminent conservative Republican Senator from Arizona, Barry Goldwater, who said, "That which the government has the power to give, it can also take away."(11)

consequences of citizen inactions have resulted in the failure to promote the genuine general welfare of the nation, the loss of the once distinct American sense of self-reliance, the relinquishment of individual initiative, responsibility, and accountability, with the deterioration and adulteration of cultural values – in short, the loss of a myriad of desired characteristics of citizenship, erstwhile promoted by republican values.

THE CONCEPT OF THE LAW

The state – the great fiction by which everybody tries to live at the expense of everybody else.
Frederic Bastiat, The Law (1850)

Man is by nature a political animal....At his best man is the noblest of all animals; separated from law and justice, he is the worst.
Aristotle, Politics, I, c.322 B.C.

It was based on the Roman legacy of natural rights and constitutional government that the French patriot Frederic Bastiat (1801-1850), in his monumental little book, *The Law*,[59] asserted that the power of government was limited to protecting the natural rights of citizens and equated the rule of law to the attainment of justice. Bastiat, his health declining from the ravages of consumption (tuberculosis), wrote his masterpiece immediately following the excesses of the chaotic revolution of February 1848, when France was on the verge of relapsing into the socialism, egalitarianism, and collectivism of the French Revolution of half a century earlier. Undaunted, Bastiat wrote: "Each of us has a natural right – from God – to defend his person, his liberty, and his property. These are the three basic requirements of life, and the preservation of any one of them is completely dependent upon the preservation of the other two."(33)

Moreover, it was his belief that, "the law is the organization of the natural right of lawful defense. It is the substitution of a common force for individual forces. And this common force is to do only what the individual forces have a natural and lawful right to do: to protect persons, liberties, and properties; to maintain the right of each, and to cause justice to reign over us all. The Nature of Law is to maintain justice." Bastiat wrote that the law keeps a person within the balance of justice and imposes nothing upon the individual, but a mere negation of unjust actions. "[The laws] oblige him only to abstain from harming others. They violate neither his personality, his liberty, nor his property. They safeguard all of these. They are defensive; they defend equally the rights of all." Moreover, "...when the law, by means of its necessary agent, force, imposes upon men a regulation of labor, and method or subject of education or religious faith or creed – then the law is no longer negative. It acts positively upon people. It substitutes the will of the legislature for their own will."(33)

In short, from the aforementioned it can be logically deduced that when the services or labor of one person (as in the practice of competent and compassionate

---

[59] *The Law* was originally published as a political pamphlet in 1850 in the wake of the general revolutionary turbulence of 1848.

medicine by a physician) or one's property are taken by the state (as in the application of unconstitutional asset forfeiture laws to law-abiding citizens including again, physicians accused but not convicted of any wrongdoing), then we are not dealing with rights or justice, nor philanthropy, but legalized plunder, institutionalized servitude, oppression, and injustice.

Bastiat believed that socialism was legal plunder and that legal plunder was rooted in human greed and in false philanthropy. Moreover, he asserted that when the laws become perverted so that basic individual rights are circumvented, the government becomes an instrument of injustice which violates the negative concept of the law, "the purpose of the law is to prevent injustice from reigning." Accordingly, when the law becomes a positive concept, that is, when it becomes "an instrument of equalization insofar as it takes from some persons and gives to other persons," then it becomes an instrument of plunder and organized injustice.

In regards to legislation of law and morals, Bastiat exposed the socialists' *modus operandi*. With extraordinary clairvoyance he wrote:

> *But what do the socialists do? They cleverly disguise this legal plunder from others – and even from themselves – under the seductive names of fraternity, unity, organization, and association. Because we ask so little from the law – only justice – the socialists thereby assume that we reject fraternity, unity, organization, and association. The socialists brand us with the name individualist. But we assure the socialists that we repudiate only forced organization, not natural organization. We repudiate the forms of association that are forced upon us, not free association. We repudiate the artificial unity that does nothing more than deprive persons of individual responsibility. We do not repudiate the natural unity of mankind under Providence.(33)*

Bastiat argued that the socialists' goal is the subjugation of mankind to "philanthropic tyranny of their own social inventions." Moreover, showing great insight, Bastiat asserted that the doctrine of the social democrats is based on a triple hypothesis: "the total inertness of mankind, the omnipotence of the law, and the infallibility of the legislator. These three ideas form the sacred symbol of those who proclaim themselves totally democratic. The advocates of this doctrine also profess to be social." And as it regards the pursuit of redistribution of wealth as a form of social justice, Bastiat decried: "The mission of the law is not to oppress persons and plunder them of their property, even though the law may be acting in a philanthropic spirit. Its mission is to protect persons and property." He reminds us, further, "law is solely the organization of the individual right of self-defense which existed before law was formalized."(33)

If the law is used to establish an egalitarian philanthropic society, then it is perverted, because the sole end of the law should be the pursuit of justice. He writes:

> *If you exceed this proper limit – if you attempt to make the law religious, fraternal, equalizing, philanthropic, industrial, literary, or artistic – you will then be lost in an uncharted territory, in vagueness and uncertainty, in a forced utopia or, even worse, in a multitude of utopias, each striving to seize the law and impose it upon you. This is true because fraternity and philanthropy, unlike justice, do not have precise limits. Once started, where will you stop? And where will the law stop itself?(33)*

This road, I venture to interject, led to communism in China, in the Soviet Union, and in a third of the world during the tempestuous 20th Century. In our travels in uncharted waters, we are being lured by the sirens with their songs of socialism and collectivism, and if we are not careful, to the death of our republic. This, despite all the platitudes about the need for free markets and decentralization elsewhere on the globe. It is no secret that in spite of all this talk and the hours of lip-service devoted to free markets and democracy, America is headed to democratic socialism and the abattoir of global tyranny. If still in doubt, check the *Federal Register* and peruse the tens of thousands of pages of administrative decrees and unconstitutional regulations that increasingly regulate and control our lives.

And that is not all, in 1992, 40% of a typical American family's budget went into paying federal, state, and local taxes, more than food, clothing, and housing combined.(34) And this was before the largest tax increase in history was passed by Congress and signed into law by U.S. President Bill Clinton in 1993.

AN EVER VIGILANT AND INFORMED CITIZENRY

Enlighten the people generally and tyranny and oppressions of body and mind will vanish like evil spirits at the dawn of day.
                              Thomas Jefferson (1816)

"There is no free lunch," as the cliché says, yet, many people easily forget (or conveniently ignore) the fact that one cannot grant favors to a special group without taking from another, or that it is wrong for the government to abrogate individual rights such as liberty and property to give to others what it does not legally possess, or to use it perversely to bribe others without perverting the law and vitiating justice.

In a constitutional republic, individual rights such as life and liberty are "inalienable," whereas in a mass democracy, individual rights may be abolished or altered by simple majority vote. Alternatively, basic rights may be qualified out of existance so as to make them meaningless, as is the case of the United Nations International Covenant on Civil and Political Rights Charter, where the state retains the prerogative to abrogate the individual's basic traditional rights at its discretion.(35) That, of course, is not the case in the U.S. Constitution where basic rights are inviolable. [60]

Another important concept is private philanthropy. Here it is crucial to remember that compassion, beneficence, and true charity are qualities that come from the heart, instilled in the young within the purview of the traditional family setting with passion, learning, and understanding. These qualities cannot be legislated, judicially-ordered, or governmentally-mandated, that is, if they are truly voluntary. Moreover, we know that if the majority grants them, then they can also take them away whenever they want. All that is needed is a simple majority vote.

---

[60] Yet on April 2, 1992, five U.S. Senators passed this dangerous U.N. document in an unrecorded vote on the Senate floor (no one asked for a quorum). With no public debate and shrouded by the silence of the media, most Americans are not even faintly aware of the existence of this document and its perilous implications for their basic constitutional rights. For details see, *Global Tyranny...Step By Step* by William F. Jasper, Western Islands Publishers, Appleton, Wisconsin, 1992.

Likewise, the Founding Fathers agreed in the natural rights of citizens to life, liberty, and property and in the government's fundamental function for their protection. By "equality," the Founding Fathers did not mean equality of birth, wealth, intelligence, talent, or virtue. Inequalities in society were accepted as a natural product of diversity amongst people. It was definitely not the function of government to reduce these inequalities.(36)

The Founding Fathers also believed that the origin of government is a social contract amongst people who pledged to obey laws in return for protection of their natural rights. According to the political scientists, Drs. Thomas R. Dye and L. Harmon Zeigler, "The ultimate legitimacy of government – that is, sovereignty – rested with the people themselves...and the basis of government was the consent of the governed."(36)

These authors write: "The Founding Fathers believed in republican government....By 'republican government' they meant a representative, responsible, and non-hereditary government. But by 'republican government' they certainly did not mean mass democracy, with direct participation by the people in decision making."(36) Moreover, the structure of government – "its republicanism and its system of separated powers and check and balances – was also designed to provide protection of liberty and property. To the Founding Fathers, a *republican government* [their emphasis] meant the delegation of powers by the people to a small number of citizens whose wisdom...patriotism and love of justice will be least likely to sacrifice it to temporary or partial considerations."(36) In other words, government was entrusted to enlightened representatives whose political judgment would not be easily subverted by the volatile changing populist winds of the uninformed masses.

Perhaps the ultimate difference between a republican form of government and mass democracy is exemplified by the lynch mob analogy provided by *The New American* writer, Robert W. Lee: "In a democracy, whatever a majority wants it gets, and written laws and constitutions become mere window dressing....At a lynch mob, there is only one man against it. But when republican principles prevail, the sheriff intervenes to lay down the law, telling the mob that the victim cannot be hanged unless he is first proven guilty after a fair trial by a jury of his peers, and that he may not be held for excessive bail or compelled to testify against himself regardless of what the majority might desire."(37)

In a democracy then, the rights granted to special minorities often are transacted with Faustian overtones. All too often, these welfare rights or entitlements are conducive to subtle enslavement, whilst creating political dependency and instilling a false sense of economic security. Moreover, these entitlements are subject to resentment and to backlash from other groups or even from the majority who may not be recipients of those benefits – thereby, fomenting discord and instigating class warfare. The end result is civil strife in which no one benefits, except those aspiring to political power who instigated the conflict for their own benefit. It was this type of civil discord, class strife, and rife class warfare that incited the civil war during the 1st Century B.C. in the late Roman Republic, which had allowed herself to degenerate to unlimited (mass) democracy and virtually unrestrained mobocracy. In this light, Seneca the Younger considered, "democracy more cruel than wars or tyrants."(9)

It is worth emphasizing this fact, namely that the Roman Republic had in fact degenerated in the 1st Century B.C. to what today would be akin to a social democracy gone amok, in which populist demagogues were rampant, creating disharmony where there was once harmony, and chaos where there was once order in their quest for power. In fact, Cicero himself, who lived during these tempestuous years, asserted that these populist leaders were "bold and unscrupulous...who curry favor with the people by giving them other men's property."(9) These ambitious politicians led various warring factions which pushed the country over the precipice of overt civil war. It was this degeneration of the Roman Republic into a *de facto* mobocracy that permitted it to lapse into the chaotic fratricidal civil war, which ultimately, persuaded the various interests and influential citizens, the power elite, to forsake the Republic in exchange for stability, and to allow the political procession to proceed down the road of dictatorship.

Dye and Zeigler regard mass activism, "an expression of resentment against the established order, and it usually occurs in time of crisis, when a counter-elite, or demagogue, emerges from the masses to mobilize them against the established elite." Furthermore, "mass activism tends to be undemocratic [sic] and violent because masses do not have a strong commitment to established institutions and procedures. Populist values – nativism, intolerance of nonconformity, anti-intellectualism, religious fundamentalism, and egalitarianism – generally become the impetus of mass movements...."(36)

Thus, lessons of history predicate that constitutional republics/representative democracies (or mixed democracies) require that citizens remain ever vigilant to preserve their individual rights and the rules and procedures of law. Apathy and acquiescence by the law-abiding citizenry may result in the rise of populist demagogues who pretend to speak for the people, but instead are only interested in the selfish acquisition of raw power. Actions resulting from such demagoguery foment civil strife, because in its essence it takes from one group to give to another, instigating hatred and resentment. Class warfare invariably ensues, resulting in anarchy and chaos, situations that lead invariably to the disintegration of society as befell the Roman Republic, 2000 years ago. From amongst the demagogues in this obscene "battle royale," one strongman invariably emerges as the "savior" of the country, to which the people flock in droves, gladly surrendering their lives, their liberties and...their happiness.

And so it was that this very chaotic situation allowed a strong, charismatic man such as Julius Caesar to seize power. With anarchy the order of the day, the Roman citizens were ready to abandon their republican sentiments and accept dictatorship in exchange for the restoration of law and order. Thus by 49 B.C., the Roman Republic had come to an end, and Julius Caesar had become absolute dictator of Rome.(38,39)

Despite Rome's exemplary form of government, Americans, recipients of a republic barely 200 years old, do not seem to understand the fragility of a constitutional republic. And that being the case, that it must be carefully nurtured. Instead, we have strayed, lured by the songs of the sirens, songs whose lyrics exalt the illusory promises of egalitarianism and false security. So today we are sadly witnessing the gradual dismantling of our constitutional republic, and the building in her stead, a mammoth American-style brand of democratic socialism in which the rights of the individual are subordinate to the power of the state. Although all citizens are at risk, no segment of society has been made more keenly aware of this recently than American physicians.

Yes, it seems that we Americans are resolved to create our own brand of American socialism, never mind the demise of socialism, collectivism, and central planning elsewhere in the world. Nor is this utter collapse of socialist policies solely a phenomenon of hard-core socialist or former communist countries. Both the newly liberated nations of Central and Eastern Europe and the social democracies of Western Europe, including France, Great Britain, the Netherlands, and Scandinavia, notably Sweden – the darling of the soft Left – are clamoring unabashedly for free-market capitalism, and are on the retreat, whilst trying to save face, attempting to dismantle their socialist apparatus. We Americans should be humble enough to learn not only from our own mistakes but also from the mistakes of others. But it seems that we are too arrogant to do that. Foolishly, we have to give it a try ourselves. Using the state to effect egalitarian socialist policies, we find ourselves traversing perilous waters, adrift in a vast ocean of rules and regulations aboard a rudderless ship. Let us hope we can regain control, navigate safely, and find our way out of this global socialist ocean to reach our rightful and lawful destination.

We must remain ever vigilant to preserve our constitutional republic and preserve the features of our representative democracy where all citizens are protected from the incursions of government. We must heed Benjamin Franklin's 1759 admonition when he wrote: "They that give up essential liberty to obtain a little temporary safety deserve neither liberty nor safety."

Physicians, even those in the trenches of health care delivery, have a duty to set aside their reflex hammers and stethoscopes – like Cincinnatus who put down his plow – to join the fight to regain their civil rights. As individuals and as citizens of this great nation, they are inherently possessed of basic traditional rights, rights that must be salvaged to protect whatever constitutional safeguards therein remain. As members of a noble and venerable profession, physicians have a moral obligation to defend their individual rights and those professional prerogatives, such as the preservation of the patient-doctor relationship, intrinsic to their calling. Furthermore, they have a duty to defend their intangible possessions such as their hard-earned medical degrees, their right to practice medicine unencumbered by government, and their right to provide their professional services at fair market value. And for those who cannot afford their service, that is, for indigent patients, physicians have always been happy to provide charity medical care as something that came with the territory, something that came with the privilege of being a member of a compassionate, venerable profession.

Another problem that physicians face is that government, as we have already alluded, has to a significant extent been successful in transforming societal values. For example, where society once relished individual initiative, self-reliance, responsible risk-taking, and the entrepreneurial spirit of Americans, today these items are perceived as obsolete and irrelevant. Instead, society rewards government dependency, worships in the cult of victimhood, and expects life to be risk-free. And to the cult of victimhood, alleged victims are flocking in droves to partake and imbibe out of the troughs of deep-pocket "tormentors" (be they employers, product manufacturers, physicians, aging parents, or celibate priests) who must pay for the victim's shortcomings and other alleged abuses, real or imagined, of their previous benefactors.

We must stand up for fair play, constitutional and representative government, and the rule of law, or American society as we have known it would surely perish, scuttled by the demagoguery of opportunists joining the big leagues of a not-so-vague New World Order bent on giving us domestic socialism and global tyranny. "Megabucks" would be the name of the game (and those dispossessed of it would not be welcomed), and the players would be the corporate internationalists playing on a slanted field against small business and budding entrepreneurs. They would be assured of winning because they would be drafting policies and instituting monopolistic practices in collusion with government. If citizens acquiesce at this critical juncture, Americans would be subjected to the oppression of socialist global tyrants, not the liberation of Roman tribunes.

As John F. McManus, publisher of *The New American* observed, our Founding Fathers, the framers of our constitution wisely conceived our United States as a "constitutional republic – governed by the rule of law, not a democracy governed by the rule of the unrestrained majority. Because it is a system built on the recognition of the rights of the individual, its laws are directed at controlling government, not the people."(35)

The framers of the U.S. Constitution were wary of the power which even they had themselves created during the Constitutional Convention of 1787. Therefore, to further protect the personal liberties of the people from usurpation by government, they added the Bill of Rights, the first 10 amendments to the Constitution. It is doubtful that the U.S. Constitution would have been ratified in 1789 if a promise of adoption of a Bill of Rights had not been made. Thomas Jefferson, who was in Paris serving as U.S. Minister to France at the time of the Constitutional Convention, praised many of the features of the proposed constitution but lamented the lack of a Bill of Rights.(40)

The 5th Amendment to the U.S. Constitution, in addition to propounding the criminal defense rights, also protects the natural rights of citizens, so that they could not be "deprived of life, liberty or property without due process of law; nor shall private property be taken for public use, without just compensation." The 13th Amendment of 1865 ended slavery and involuntary servitude, while the 14th Amendment of 1868 was intended to end the after-effects of slavery in the South and included a clause providing that no state shall "deprive any person of life, liberty or property, without due process of law; nor deny to any person within its jurisdiction of the equal protection of the law" – which in effect incorporates and extends the doctrine and protection of the Bill of Rights of the individual to the states.

So the Bill of Rights was added later to the main body of the Constitution to protect individual liberties and the God-given or Nature-derived rights that the government guaranteed and was sworn to defend. Thus, the Founding Fathers conceived of our United States with a Bill of Rights to protect individual rights and liberty, and to limit the power of government authority. Moreover, to safeguard the rights of the accused in alleged criminal offenses, the accused party was (and still is) considered innocent until proven guilty. And from the setting and interpretation of judicial precedents there evolved legal principles not only to protect the citizens from the abuse of government but also to promote continuity and predictability in the legal system. In this fashion, such legal tenets as the precept that criminal convictions be based on "beyond reasonable doubt" – to protect the innocent, even at the risk of allowing an occasional "guilty" party to go free – was set forth and embraced by our judicial system.(25)

CHAPTER 12

THE PERILS OF THE REPUBLIC

Inferiors revolt in order that they may be equal, and equals that they may be superior.
Aristotle

    I will not describe further either the splendor of the Roman Republic at its apogee, nor the grandeur of the Empire at its zenith. Professional historians have with great zeal and sufficient documentation discussed the glory that was Rome. We will discuss, nevertheless, the perils of the Republic and the factors surrounding the decline of the Empire. It is important that we do this, because Rome, the city founded on the Palatine Hill, set down the moral standards that not only influenced Western thought, but in later centuries, preserved and fortified the Judeo-Christian tradition that was evolving in Western civilization. Rome also laid the foundation for the system of jurisprudence that later formed the basis of civil law in Latin nations, e.g., Italy, France, Spain, Portugal, and countries of Central and South America. Even English-speaking countries, such as the United States, England, Australia, and New Zealand, whose laws were based on evolving English common-law were influenced by the Roman civil system. As the world historians C. Brinton, J.B. Christopher, and R.L. Wolff note, "...they [English-speaking countries] too, have shared in the enduring ideals of equity and natural law bequeathed by Rome."(1) As these authors correctly point out, the tradition of "deciding cases according to the spirit of the law rather than the letter of the law" was a Roman concept. Influenced by the Stoics and Cicero, as we have pointed out, the Romans believed in the concept of "natural law," a higher law, above those created by the state, that was divinely inspired and applied to all men in all states by virtue of their humanity.(1) But what about the safety of the Republic that engendered these noble ideals? Was the Republic (and her ideals) always safe, or were there moments of danger stalking Rome and her legacy? The following chapter recapitulates those moments, encapsulated in "the Perils of the Republic."

GAUL

    Almost four centuries after the traditional founding of Rome in 753 B.C., and a little over a century after the founding of the Republic and the codification of the *Twelve Tablets*, Rome was attacked, overrun, occupied, and burned by fierce Gallic tribesmen. This humiliating event took place in 390 B.C. [61] The sacking of the Eternal City by the barbarians [62] was an event which left an indelible mark in the collective memory of the Romans.

    Next, I suppose, we should mention another semi-legendary enemy of the

---

[61] The famous Ransom of Rome, one thousand pounds of gold, was said to have been paid by Rome to the barbarians, who were later driven out of Roman territory and back across the Rubicon by the reorganized Roman defenders who had by then regained the initiative.

[62] *Barbarian* was the word that the Greeks used to call those who were non-Hellenic and who were considered to lack the culture and refinement of the Greeks. It was adopted by the Romans to refer to the fierce Germanic tribesmen bordering and frequently threatening the frontiers of the Empire.

Roman Republic, not because he posed an imminent or mortal threat to Rome, but because of his historic and almost mythologic fame and attributes. We are referring to Pyrrhus, King of Epiros (c.318-272 B.C.), who was called to Italy in 280 B.C. to defend the Greek colonizers of Sicily, fought the Romans, and "defeated" them in two battles (at Heraclea in 280 B.C. and at the battle of Asculum in 279 B.C.). However, the casualties inflicted upon his army by the disciplined Roman legions of the Republic were so horrendous that the victories were vacuous – the king himself proclaiming, "One more such victory and I am lost."(7,12) And thereby, we have the origin of the term "pyrrhic victory." King Pyrrhus was finally and decisively defeated by the Romans at Beneventum in 275 B.C., and a few years later, exited history when he was killed in a minor battle in Argos.

CARTHAGE

We will either find a way, or make one.
Hannibal

Rome found herself in great peril again in 221 B.C. when Hannibal (247-183 B.C.), the son of the great Carthaginian general Hamilcar Barca,[63] took command of the multi-ethnic, mercenary army of the maritime and commercial power of the North African city of Carthage. The conflict – the Second Punic War – began in 219 B.C., after Hannibal seized the Spanish city of Saguntum, a Roman ally; Rome then declared war on Carthage. Hannibal invaded Italy in a celebrated campaign and led his army in one battle after another reaping victory after victory. In 216 B.C., Hannibal annihilated between 35,000-45,000, Roman legionnaires, 7/8ths of the entire Roman army, in a single afternoon on the field of battle at Cannae. Cannae was a horrendous defeat for the proud and disciplined Roman legionnaires, the sword of the Republic, and a humiliating defeat for the capable Roman general, Paulus Varrus. The destruction of the Roman army at Cannae put the Republic, and Rome herself, in grave and mortal danger. Moreover, the loss of men killed at Cannae was so great that for the first time in recorded history, the women of the Roman Republic had, of necessity, taken charge of the civic and political affairs of Rome.

Women inherited vast amounts of wealth from their male kin who died at Cannae. Suddenly, they found themselves wealthy and independent. Unfortunately, many displayed their new wealth impudently and lavishly. This situation resulted in a backlash against the erstwhile, progressive social, economic, and political status of women in Roman society (i.e., property rights and inheritance laws). As a result, laws were passed by the elders of Rome to curtail the panoply of dazzling jewelry, carriages, and other effects that were being seen both in the Roman countryside and at urbane social gatherings. The passage of legislation (Oppian Law) curtailing the rights of women to conduct business transactions and tightening inheritance laws may be interpreted by strong proponents of matriarchy as an attempt by Roman elders to reassert the power of the Roman *Pater familias* system over the potential

---

[63] Hamilcar Barca was a celebrated hero who fought bravely and victoriously in Sicily during the First Punic War. He was said to have also "ruthlessly" quelled a mercenary revolt in 238 B.C.; he died in battle attempting to conquer Spain for Carthage in 237 B.C.(7)

threat posed by the emancipation of women. I have a less elaborate explanation, namely, that the imprudent exhibition of property wounded the patriotic sense of the Roman citizenry. Nevertheless, it is possible that given the parlous condition of the Romans at this time and the debacle at Cannae, Roman elders felt that their society was threatened and on the brink of reverting to matriarchy.(3,41) I would rather think that the thought of Rome reverting to matriarchy was illusory (at best, merely a momentary flashback to a romantic Neolithic, Earth-Mother goddess past)...if matriarchy ever existed.(42)

Nevertheless, with the Roman disaster at Cannae, for the first time since 390 B.C., Rome felt in imminent and mortal danger from the seemingly invincible Carthaginian army, led by the military genius, Hannibal. With his famous elephants, the dashing invader had crossed the Alps, overrun the Po Valley, and was marching relentlessly toward Rome.[64] The perilous state of affairs for Rome did not, in fact, end until Hannibal's brother, Hasdrubal, who was advancing to join and bring supplies and reinforcements to Hannibal, was defeated by the Roman consuls Nero and Livius at the Battle of Metaurus in 207 B.C.(26) Hannibal, with his men exhausted after more than a decade of fighting, and his lines of supply and communication cut, was ordered back to defend Carthage from the threat of the Roman general Scipio, who had invaded North Africa.(43) Finally, at the Battle of Zama in 201 B.C., Hannibal was decisively defeated by Scipio, who was later, in honor of this victory, suffixed with the title Scipio "Africanus."(26)

Legend, almost always romanticizing events which may have been rooted in historic fact, says that Hannibal, at the outskirts of Rome (sometime after the Battle of Cannae), was stopped from marching into the "defenseless" city by the pleading of an old woman, who turned out to be his former nanny, a woman who had attended him in his infancy. The story goes that she miraculously came from within the gates and prevented the Carthaginian onslaught. It is more likely that Hannibal, ahead of his supply lines and in desperate need of supplies, did not feel ready or strong enough to march on fortified Rome. He went on, instead, to southern Italy where he ravaged the countryside for 15 years and made allies against Rome. With the defeat of his brother, Hasdrubal, on the banks of the Metaurus river, his dream of capturing Rome was shattered and, according to the 19th Century historian, Edward S. Creasy, it was the Carthaginian debacle at Metaurus – not at Zama – that was one of the fifteen most decisive battles in world history.(26)

Ultimately in defeat, the great Carthaginian general was sacrificed by the city he had defended so well. He was forced into exile by commercial interests, the Carthaginian plutocracy (at the urgings of Rome). Finally, to avoid capture by the pursuing Romans, who evidently still feared and considered him a threat, Hannibal committed suicide by taking poison and died in Crete in 183 B.C.(1,7,12,26,43)

After the Third Punic War (149-146 B.C.), Carthage, which had never fully recovered militarily from the Second Punic War to even pose a semblance of a renewed threat to Rome, capitulated after a lopsided, three-year military confrontation with the new mistress of the Mediterranean, and was burned to the ground. The Romans had finally carried out Cato the Elder's request, *delenda est Carthago*, "Carthage must be destroyed." With Carthage destroyed, the old Phoenician empire

---

[64] Hannibal's army consisted of 40,000 troops and 38 war elephants, but it is estimated that he lost most of his elephants and 25% of his troops because of inclement weather during his crossing of the Pyrenees into southern France, and the Alps into northern Italy.(1,7,12)

already under the Roman yoke, the Hellenic world subdued (Greece was conquered in 200 B.C.), and the power of Macedonia thoroughly broken by 149 B.C., Rome now turned her attention to the northeast to face the inevitable and seemingly perpetual threat of the Teutonic tribes and other barbarians menacing the Republic.

PONTUS VS ROME

The popular Roman leader and general Gaius Marius secured his re-election as Consul of Rome on five occasions during the years 108-100 B.C., then he set out to and successfully repelled the Teutonic invasions, thereby providing security to Rome's territorialities and consolidating her gains. His campaigns lent further credence to the invincibility of the Roman army. Between 89 and 85 B.C., Lucius Cornelius Sulla, another prominent Roman consul, general, and leader of the conservative Senatorial faction, led the mighty Roman armies to victory in the East, defeating Mithridates VI (c.132-63 B.C.) in the first war between Rome and the King of Pontus. Mithridates had been and for some time to come would remain a veritable thorn in Rome's side, a perennial threat to Rome's interest in Greece and Asia Minor.

Shortly after Sulla's triumphal return, civil war broke out between the rival factions led by Marius and Sulla.[65] Sulla emerged victorious, became dictator of Rome (82-79 B.C.), and successfully restored "the machinery of government."(12) After his victories over both Marius and Mithridates VI, Sulla, a member of the patrician class, successfully restored law and order as he had promised, and even succeeded in rebuilding the eroded political power and prestige of the Senate.[66] Unfortunately for Rome (and the world), his authoritarian rule was an obstacle to republican principles and constitutional rule, for in the end, it ushered in further unrest, including Spartacus' spectacular slave rebellion that brought chaos to Rome and bloodshed to southern Italy for nearly two years.(1,7,12,44)

And as if all of these events at home were not enough, the troublesome Mithridates resumed his belligerence toward Rome and massacred 80,000 Roman citizens during a rampage in Asia. In this second war (83-81 B.C.), the King of Pontus threatened to march on Rome herself, after defeating several Roman legions stationed in Asia Minor. The troubles with Mithridates, who by now may be correctly called Rome's arch-enemy, did not come to an end until the third war (74-64 B.C.) when the Roman legions, this time led by Pompey the Great, decisively crushed the unruly king. In fact, even though Pompey had served as Consul of the Roman Republic in 70 B.C. and had established his military reputation by disbanding the Mediterranean pirates who had been a nuisance and a hindrance to Roman trade and commerce in the years 67 to 63 B.C., it was Pompey's crushing military defeat of Mithridates in 66 B.C. that culminated his career and brought him fame and glory. Seizing the opportunity, Pompey then made himself master of the East, marching on and conquering Palestine and Syria, extending his troops and the power of Rome as far as the Caspian Sea and the Euphrates river.(12,38,39,44,45)

---

[65] As mentioned in Chapter 9, in the context of class warfare and civil war, Marius and Sulla led the rival factions of the popular and Senatorial parties, respectively, in the divisive civil (social) war.
[66] Indeed, Sulla had previously re-established the rule of law and extended citizenship to all Italians by 89 B.C.(44)

THE FIRST TRIUMVIRATE

Totally defeated, Mithridates fled to the Crimea where he attempted unsuccessfully to poison himself, and when that failed in 64 B.C., he ordered one of his soldiers to dispatch him with a sword. Pompey the Great went up to join Marcus Licinius Crassus, who had achieved his own fame by defeating Spartacus and suppressing the slave rebellion. They were joined by Gaius Julius Caesar (100-44 B.C.), who after gaining popular support with the use of extravagant public expenditures and other populist democratic overtures, had abolished the government of the constitutional republic to form the First Triumvirate in 60 B.C.

Notwithstanding its short-lived existence, the First Triumvirate contributed significantly to the demise of the Roman Republic. And perhaps not surprisingly, all three strong men that composed this body polity, Julius Caesar, Pompey, and Crassus, lived and died by the sword.

In 53 B.C. at the Battle of Carrhae in Mesopotamia, Crassus' army was routed by the Parthians, and Crassus himself was said to have been "treacherously murdered."(7) For his part, Pompey parted with Caesar siding with the aristocratic Senate, which had attempted to prevent Caesar's takeover and the demise of the Republic. Pompey, in fact, became the champion of the Roman Senate and the defender of the principles of the Republic,[67] and for this task he was again popularly elected Consul of Rome in 52 B.C.

PANEM ET CIRCENSES

Caesar's victories in Gaul – recounted in his book, *On the Gallic Wars*, in which the celebrated words, *veni, vidi, vici*, "I came, I saw, I conquered," remain forever imprinted – were a looming and lethal threat to the power, prestige, and independence of the Roman Senate, and as events unfolded, the very existence and survival of the Republic. When in 50 B.C. the Senate ordered Caesar to disband his legions, the tribunes Marc Antony (82-30 B.C.) and Quintus Cassius Longinus (d.45 B.C.) disobeyed the wish of the Senate and vetoed the measure. They then joined Julius Caesar. Caesar, with the support of his legions and the backing of the two tribunes, assembled his army against the Senate. On the fateful day of January 19, 49 B.C., Caesar crossed the Rubicon and entered Italy, heralding a civil war in which his army ultimately prevailed against the forces of the Senate. He entered Rome in triumph. Fearing the wrath of the victorious Caesar, Pompey fled to Egypt, where he was defeated at Pharsala in 48 B.C. And whilst attempting to flee from North Africa, he was subsequently assassinated by orders of the intriguing and mystifying Cleopatra VII (69-30 B.C.), Queen of Egypt.

Gaius Julius Caesar ruled briefly but with immense popularity amongst the masses because of his proclivity toward demagogic oratory and popular reforms, including agrarian laws, housing accommodations, public projects and improvements, the extension of citizenship to subjects within Roman territories,

---

[67] The Roman Senate not only enjoyed great prestige but was also the most cherished of Roman government institutions. It exerted great influence over the affairs of the Republic as its political motto exemplified: *S.P.Q.R., Senatus Populusque Romanus* ("The Senate and the Roman People").(1)

and even government subsidies for certain goods and lavish public entertainment, *panem et circenses*. With these devices, he managed to seduce the populace. His unrestrained public expenditures, his land reforms, and his promise to pursue egalitarianism and wealth redistribution proved irresistible to the masses. Thus, he was endowed dictator for life in 44 B.C. The cherished Roman Republic had been given the *coup de grace* and now she lay there, exsanguinating. As the masses enjoyed their *panem et circenses*, a one-man dictatorship was being created supplanting the rule of law. The voice and vote of the citizenry had been effectively substituted for "bread and circuses" which amounted to grain subsidies for the populace and gory entertainment at the Roman amphitheaters (including the Roman Colosseum) for the distracted and cheering masses.

Julius Caesar preemptively made sure that the exploits of his military campaigns and his victories over the Gauls and Britons survived through his written accounts of the campaigns in his magnum opus, *On The Gallic Wars*, a veritable Latin prose masterpiece. Caesar's crossing of the Rubicon was an event of great significance in history, for with this seemingly romantic act of defiance, he had not only threatened and defied the aristocratic Roman Senate, but also the very existence of the Republic. And indeed, after defeating Pompey and crushing the Senate, he became absolute dictator of Rome, nevermind that as the prudent leader he was, he had refused the crown which had been offered him when he became dictator. Even with this vapid and disingenuous overture, his motives and intentions were clear and aroused great resentment amongst the republican factions in Rome. Republican partisans understood all too well Lord Acton's latter-day axiom about the corrupting influence of absolute power.

As Caesar's power became more totalitarian, it also became more intolerable for the Senate and for his republican enemies. Thus, on the Ides of March, 44 B.C., a group of Caesar's former friends and *protégés* led by Marcus Junius Brutus (c.85-42 B.C.) and Gaius Cassius Longinus (d.42 B.C.), stabbed him to death on the steps of the Senate in the Roman Forum. It should be noted that even though Brutus had sided with Pompey against Caesar at the Battle of Pharsala, Brutus had been pardoned by Caesar, and instead of punishment, had been given the governorship of the Cisalpine Gaul. Later, he was even appointed to be Caesar's governor in Macedonia, a prized province. So it was no wonder that upon seeing Brutus amongst the assassins, Caesar exclaimed, *et tu, Brute*?, "thou too, Brutus?"

Brutus, like Cassius, had genuinely sought to re-establish republican rule in Rome. They detested the usurpation of republican rule and the imposition of the absolute rule of a dictator, even if the dictator was the popular Julius Caesar. Despite succeeding in the assassination, the conspirators ultimately failed in the *coup d'etat*. The conspirators fled to Syria and then to Macedonia, where ultimately their combined armies were defeated by Octavian and Mark Antony at Philippi in 42 B.C. Cassius, thinking the battle was lost, committed suicide after the first engagement. Brutus and the rest of his accomplices, in defeat, also committed suicide.(7,12,38,39)

Despite the obvious dichotomy, the admiration of republican Rome by many who praised her for her simplicity, practicality, and stability, and condemnation by others who vehemently reproached her for her lack of sentimentality, spartan ways, and class distinctions, the immutable fact remains that the average Roman citizen, protected by the rule of law, constitutional principles, and a strong, disciplined army, lived better, enjoyed liberties, and benefitted from prosperity unequaled in the history of Western civilization during the five centuries of its existence.

It was not the aristocratic character of the Senate, or the insistence of the republican factions of abiding by constitutional principles and the rule of law, or even the class distinctions that characterized the earlier centuries that doomed the Republic. The prevailing wave of demagoguery, class envy, and the mobocracy that particularly afflicted the last century killed the Republic. Despite the shortcomings that befell both the Roman Republic, and as we shall see later, the Empire, the glory that was Rome, the City Upon the Hill, was unsurpassed in history – and yes, it lasted nearly a thousand years.

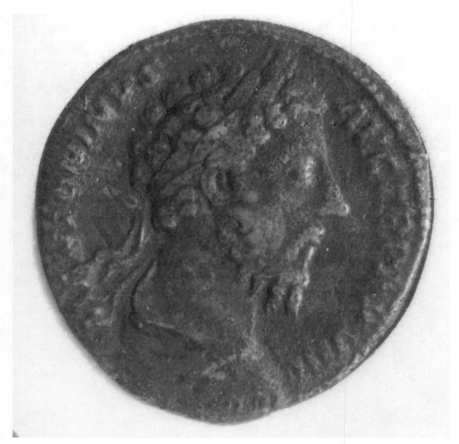

Plate 13 – Laureate head of Emperor Marcus Aurelius (A.D.161-180). Bronze sestertius. Author's private collection.

CHAPTER 13

THE PERILS OF THE EMPIRE

By gnawing through a dyke, even a rat may drown a nation.
Edmund Burke (1729-1797)

ARMINIUS AND GERMANIA

The Augustan Age that heralded the inauguration of the Roman Empire and brought an era of greatness was not without interruptions or distractions. For instance, even though Augustus Caesar was successful in preserving most of the boundaries of the Empire established by Julius Caesar, his attempt at creating a buffer state in Germania triggered a revolt of the Germanic tribesmen led by Arminius.

In A.D. 7, ominous tidings were brought to the emperor from the Germanic frontier. The shock waves were felt throughout the Empire, and even the usually calm Augustus was alarmed: the Germanic chieftain Arminius had defeated the seasoned and well-disciplined Roman legions under General Varus, thus preventing the conquest and subjugation of Germany by Rome. An entire Roman army had been annihilated by the fierce Germans. The disastrous defeat and decimation of three Roman legions under Varus in Germany foreshadowed the fact that no further attempts would be made by Rome to expand northward to conquer the Germanic barbarians. The debacle squelched all dreams of annexing Germany for the Empire. The Roman generals, Germanicus (d.A.D.19; brother of Claudius and father of Caligula) and Drusus Caesar [68] (14 B.C.- A.D.23; son of Tiberius), both relatives of Emperor Augustus, assailed the Germans in retaliation for the massacre of the Roman legions. Nevertheless, despite these later victories, Rome never again tried to subdue the Germanic barbarians and annex Germania.[69] Even Augustus himself became reconciled to the idea that, by their sheer numbers and barbarian ways, the Germans were unconquerable. From then on, the Roman Empire would preserve its northern border in those provinces, and its policy would be to contain the Teutonic tribes of the northern Rhine along the Danube-Rhine border, a frontier that the Empire would maintain for centuries (22,23). Thus, Roman practicality prevailed even in war.

QUEEN BOADICEA AND BRITANNIA

Rome also possessed Britain, a legacy of Julius Caesar who explored and briefly subdued her inordinate inhabitants in the years 55-54 B.C. The province of

---

[68] Drusus Caesar was later poisoned by Sejanus, Tiberius' minister.
[69] We should not fail to mention the Roman general Nero Claudius Drusus Germanicus (38-9 B.C.) stepson of Augustus and brother of Tiberius, who as his name Germanicus implies, also ravaged the Germanic barbarians both east and north of the Rhine, but failed to subdue the Nordic hordes permanently. He died in Germany.(7)

Britannia was formally consolidated into the Empire following the reconquest by Emperor Claudius (reigned, A.D.41-54) in A.D.43. The Celtic tribes, advised by their Druid priests, had again gone to war and been defeated. This time the Romans built dwellings and fortifications, settling in their country villas to colonize the seemingly pacified province.

But the subjugated Celts resented Roman rule, the imposition of taxes, the prohibition of human sacrifices demanded by their Druid priests, and other Roman measures. Finally, they were incited to act against the Romans. The triggering event was the exhortations of their Iceni queen, whose estate in Norfolk had been confiscated by Roman officials. Moreover, their queen had been striped naked and publicly flogged because of her obdurate defiance of the Romans. This latest opprobrium and intolerable Roman affront inflicted upon the Iceni queen could not go unpunished.

Thus, a bloody insurrection erupted and in A.D.61, the fierce and defiant Boadicea (or Boudicca), Queen of the Iceni, a Celtic-Druid tribe of Norfolk in southeastern England, led her Celtic tribesmen into a massive revolt against their Roman overlords. From her war chariot, Boadicea conducted the uprising which wiped out the local Roman population and garrison. Even the first Roman legions that arrived to re-establish order were annihilated. Regarding this episode, Winston S. Churchill wrote, "The slaughter which fell upon London was universal. No one was spared, neither man, woman, nor child. The wrath of the revolt concentrated itself upon all of those of British blood who had lent themselves to the wiles and seductions of the [Roman] invaders."(46) In the end, the imperial Roman legions led by the Roman governor, Suetonius Paulinus, prevailed and subdued the fearsome Celtic warriors. Boadicea took poison.(7,12,44-46)

The Romans held Britannia until A.D. 410, when the last legions were recalled to defend the rapidly disintegrating empire under young Emperor Honorius (A.D.393-423) who resided in Ravenna. At that time, however, the real power was wielded by the adept Germanic general, Stilicho.(24)

JEWISH REVOLTS WITHIN THE EMPIRE

With the capture of Jerusalem and the integration of the Holy Land into the Empire in the 1st Century B.C., the fiercely independent and monotheistic Israelites were placed under the Roman yoke. And whilst under that Roman yoke, three major Jewish revolts took place. Although there were intermittent pockets of resistance up to the time of the final Jewish Diaspora in A.D.135, these three revolts warrant some historic consideration. To enhance the understanding of these momentous events, a brief recapitulation of the history of Palestine – as the province was named by the conquering Romans during this period – is in order.

The conquest of Palestine began in earnest with the Roman general Pompey the Great in 65 B.C. He extended Roman rule and conquered Syria and Palestine; these provinces were then summarily annexed by Rome and added to the Roman Empire. Jerusalem itself fell to the Roman sword and was captured in 63 B.C. The Romans governed the provinces as usual, that is, allowing for the expression of local traditions and acceding to substantial regional autonomy.

We must also remember that during this time, Jerusalem was not only the political and spiritual capital of the Hebrews but also served "as the scene of Jesus' last ministry."(7) During the years following Jesus' crucifixion in the reign of Tiberius and the placement of Palestine under Roman "protection" in the years A.D. 66 to 70, the province became subject to the *Pax Romana*. The Hebrew population, however, found themselves encumbered by such "protective" restrictions and, seeking full autonomy, revolted against Roman authority.

Some scholars believe that in A.D. 68 or 69, as the Roman legions prepared to march on Jerusalem, faithful Jewish scribes fled the city to protect their library of sacred scrolls. These were the Dead Sea Scrolls that were found in 1947 (and in later years) hidden in clay jars in remote caves in the desert, and which are still under intense investigation by biblical scholars.

This Jewish revolt was crushed, and the rebellion ended with the destruction of Jerusalem by General Titus (emperor, A.D.79-81). At the head of his Roman army, Titus, a great tactician and military leader, accomplished a great military feat by leading his legions across the great desert of the Sinai Peninsula in barely five days. Titus then captured Jerusalem in A.D.70, at which time the Second Temple was destroyed, but it was not until A.D.73 that the last stronghold occupied by a group of Jewish zealots was assaulted, its walls breached, and the fortress taken by the Romans – the famed fall of Masada.

Titus, the great military leader, son of former loyal-soldier turned capable-emperor, Vespasian (emperor, A.D.69-79), ruled as emperor for only 3 years, from A.D.79 to A.D.81. Despite being a calculating and ruthless general when the need arose, once in power, Titus pursued a policy of conciliation and showed unusual tolerance to political opponents. He even ended the brutal treason trials that had commenced at his coronation.(10,12) He generously assisted the city of Pompeii after the disastrous eruption of Mount Vesuvius in A.D.79, as well as aided Rome by sending needed material and manpower to rebuild and refurbish the capital after a great conflagration that occurred during his reign.[70]

In A.D. 115, the Jews of North Africa including Egypt, as well as the island of Cyprus and the province of Palestine, again rebelled against the Romans. This time the Jewish uprising was quickly suppressed by the Roman emperor, Trajan (emperor, A.D.98-117). During his reign, Trajan, one of the greatest and most capable of Roman emperors, enlarged the Empire adding Dacia (Rumania) and much of the Parthian empire, which included Asia Minor and remnants of the old Persian empire in the Middle East. He went as far as to link Rome's northern frontiers, from Great Britain across the channel, to the Trans-Caucasus region and the Black Sea.

The final Jewish insurrection took place between the years A.D.132 and A.D.135 during the reign of the adept Roman Emperor Hadrian (emperor, A.D.117-138). The last of the major Palestinian-Jewish revolts was led by Simon Barkokba (also Barchocheba). It resulted in the final diaspora which followed in the wake of the crushing defeat of the Jewish rebels and the quelling of the insurrection in A.D.135.(44)

During the rules of the capable adoptive emperors,[71] Trajan and Hadrian, aside from the major revolts in North Africa and Palestine, the Roman Empire enjoyed an age

---

[70] Considered a benevolent ruler, Titus is one of the few Roman emperors for which the people openly wept upon hearing of his death. The Arch of Titus in the Roman Forum was erected by his brother, the despotic Emperor Domitian (reign, A.D.81-96), to commemorate Titus' conquest of Jerusalem.(7)

[71] The adoptive emperors were Nerva, Trajan, Hadrian and Antoninus Pius who hand-picked their successors by adopting as "son" the most capable Roman in the Empire, and thereby providing a smooth meritorious transition of rulers.

which again reached Augustan resplendence. Trajan was the adopted son and successor of Emperor Nerva (reigned, A.D.96-98), whilst Hadrian was Trajan's cousin and his loyal soldier and administrator. Hadrian, who turned out to be a brilliant commander, was in turn an adopted son and successor to Trajan. It may be said that Trajan conquered territories and Hadrian consolidated them into the Empire.

In this fashion, the frontiers of the Empire were expanded, reaching to the Euphrates as the Empire's eastern boundary, and to northern England as its northwestern boundary. Hadrian also built the 73-mile wall that bears his name to keep "barbarian Scottish tribesmen," the Scots and Picts, out of Britannia.(12) Trajan began and Hadrian continued the system of adoptive emperors which served the Empire well both politically and militarily, "the best and ablest man for the job," so to speak, groomed to serve as emperor.

ANARCHY WITHIN THE GATES

Ironically, this successful adoptive emperor system ended after the rule of the stoic philosopher-emperor Marcus Aurelius (reigned, A.D.161-180). As a stoic philosopher, Marcus Aurelius held that equanimity in the form of serenity and individual composure were the supreme goals of life. He asserted that this ideal state could be achieved by living in tune with nature, but it required the visions of wisdom, justice, fortitude, and temperance as dictated by reason. His philosophic thoughts were recorded in his book *Meditations*. Yet as emperor, Marcus Aurelius would spend 17 of his 19-year reign at the head of his army putting down wars and rebellions, fighting and pushing back the barbarian hordes threatening the Empire. Frequently, he or Lucius Verus (co-emperor, A.D.161-169) would hold the line against the Germanic tribes in the farthest reaches of the Roman territories or would quench rebellions in faraway restless provinces (10,24), no doubt, testing his stoic philosophy during those trying years.

It was also toward the end of his strenuous rule that we first detect the incipient threat (a hint) of the coming decline, for the *Pax Romana* was beginning to be no longer enforceable. In A.D.180, Marcus Aurelius was dead, and his brutal and irascible son, Commodus (reigned, A.D.180-192), was emperor. Commodus was said to have been "seduced into cruel and lecherous habits" by his companions. And when his reign became insufferable, he was assassinated at the instigation of the Praetorian Guard.(10)

A series of weak emperors followed, until Septimius Severus (reigned, A.D.193-211) finally re-established law and order. Unfortunately, this stability was short-lived, for with the end of the rule of the House of Septimius Severus, chaos reigned anew. For most of the 3rd Century, we witness a succession of crisis after crisis, from local revolts to overt civil wars. Insubordination of armies and assassination of generals and emperors was commonplace; military anarchy reigned and some provinces were left defenseless. For example, in A.D. 226, Artaxerxes overthrew the Parthian kingdom, resurrected Persian rule and then, taking advantage of the lack of security in some provinces of the Empire, attacked defenseless Roman possessions in the East.

In A.D.250, the Goths invaded Roman provinces, ravaging the land and wreaking havoc amongst the populace. Emperor Decius (reigned, A.D.249-251) not only suffered a humiliating defeat in battle at the hands of the Gothic invaders but was also captured and slain. In the wars between A.D.253 and A.D.260, various Germanic tribes including the Franks and the Alemanni also invaded such Roman possessions as Gaul, Spain, and Africa. The Goths then resumed their attacks in Anatolia and Greece.(10,24)

For its part, Persia under King Sapor conquered the Roman province of Armenia. Another emperor, Valerian (reigned, A.D.253-260), was captured and taken prisoner. Creasy summarizes the situation as "general distress of the Roman Empire."(26) The renown Roman historian, Michael Grant, calls it the "Age of crisis."(10) Sadly during this time, the reins of the Empire had fallen to the highest bidders; constitutional government and the rule of laws had been perverted, and for all practical purposes, forgotten.

And as history has taught us, in such perilous times the door stands open for a strong man who can again re-establish law and order, at any cost. The way was, therefore, paved for an absolute ruler, and his name was Emperor Diocletian (A.D. 245-313; Roman emperor, A.D. 284-305). His rule would be noted not only for saving the Empire from imminent military collapse but also for political and economic reforms, which, although based in part on security considerations for the Empire, were marked by centralization, collectivism, bureaucracy, and totalitarianism.

THE REIGN OF DIOCLETIAN

There is no question that the strong hand of Emperor Diocletian restored military order to the Roman legions and successfully defended the borders of the Empire. Diocletian moved quickly to solidify the borders of the heretofore disintegrating empire, restoring Britain as a Roman province (A.D.296) and subduing the Persians (A.D.298).(1,7,24) But these military gains and political successes at instituting law and order do not negate or exculpate the long-term damage inflicted upon the social fabric and the economic matrix of the Empire by his autocratic rule. His absolute rule imposed on the domestic front accelerated the corrosion of the metallic underpinning of the Empire. His reforms resulted in an Eastern-potentate type of centralized government and totalitarianism on a grand scale. For the first time, as historian-scholar, Fr. James Thornton points out, there is a deliberate attempt to eradicate the traditional Roman institutions and abrogate constitutional principles which had been established at the time of the founding of the Republic and preserved through the ages via codification and modification of written laws – preserved at least in principle, even through the civil wars and the painful period of transition to Empire.(30)

An overbearing centralized bureaucracy was created that wrestled power away from local government and the individual citizens, the *civitates*. In authoritarian fashion, Diocletian also increased the power of his appointed provincial governors whilst creating dozens of dioceses under "emperor-deputies" to, in turn, oversee the provincial governors. No one was above the suspicions of the emperor, especially when they had been appointed to execute his autocratic and bureaucratic reforms.(1)

In A.D.301, Diocletian instituted price and wage controls to stem the tide of inflation. His decrees to revive the economy and implement social policies are reminiscent of the Keynesian methodology used in 1973 by President Richard M.

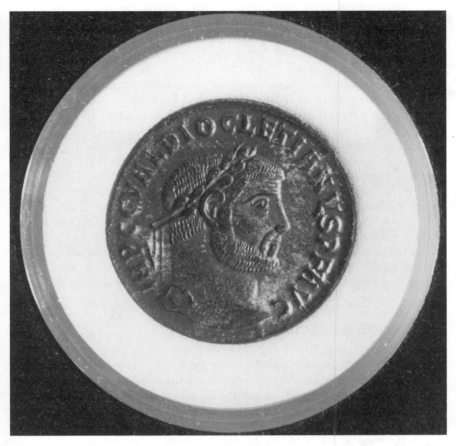

Plate 14 – Laureate head of Emperor Diocletian (A.D.284-305). Silvered follis. Author's private collection.

Nixon (U.S. President,1969-1974) to impose price and wage controls in America. Diocletian's imperatorial decrees sparked riots that were ruthlessly quenched an resulted in the institutionalization of the black market, with the inevitable rise of corruption in all segments and sections of the economy.

Benefits were given by the collectivist state for unemployment, whilst subsidies were distributed for farming and other failing segments of the economy. In return, every aspect of a Roman citizen's life was regimented, dictated, and controlled by the bureaucratic, and ultimately, totalitarian state. Heavy taxes were levied on individuals, property and land owners, artisans, tradesmen, and other self-sustaining working people (virtually anyone holding a job) in an attempt to refill the empty coffers of the state. Farmers became bound by law to the land, and for the first time, they became peasants, and then serfs in their own land.(30)

Likewise, to stanch the hemorrhage of manpower and to quell social unrest, Diocletian established a quasi-caste system in which not only farmers but also skilled workers, merchants, and even unskilled laborers were bound to their jobs in perpetuity; their trade was then passed on to their children on a hereditary basis. But this highly regimented, controlled economy was not the needed remedy for the ailing Empire. As events unfolded, the economic remedy turned out to be worse than the disease afflicting the Empire, even in its declivity.

Diocletian should be given legitimate credit for preventing or at least temporarily postponing (for one and a half centuries) the military collapse of Rome. He was successful in suppressing and containing the external forces pounding on the Empire's frontier. But on the domestic front, he may have accelerated the internal decadence afflicting Roman society. His absolute rule and his repeal of any enduring legacy of republican ideals undermined the remaining source of moral fortitude and the sense of political and economic freedom emanating from the republican institutions that had served Rome so well and for so many centuries.(1,7,9,10,24,29,30)

CHRISTIAN PERSECUTIONS

Ten major persecutions of Christians took place during a span of 250 years of governance of the Roman Empire. They followed the cruel precedent set by Nero c.A.D.65 to 69. Both Paul, the apostle to the Greek-speaking Gentiles, and Peter, chief amongst the original 12 disciples, met their end in A.D.68 during Nero's barbarous reign. Paul was beheaded. Peter was crucified. In A.D.70, whilst Christians were being persecuted under Emperor Vespasian, Jerusalem was being conquered by his son, Titus, and the rebuilt Second Temple was burnt to the ground. Then, during the brief but brutal persecution under Domitian, the younger son of Vespasian and brother of Titus, the apostle John, the last of the original 12 apostles, was proscribed to the Aegean island of Patmos, where in a series of prophetic visions, he is said to have received astounding revelations which resulted in his compilation of the enigmatic book of *Revelation*. This last book of the New Testament enunciates mystifying prophecies haunted by the terrifying inscrutable visions of multi-headed beasts, great armies maneuvering and fighting wars with horrifying new weapons of mass destruction, deadly pestilences, devastating famines, and surrealistic images of death.[72] The culmination is the Battle of Armageddon and the second coming of Jesus Christ.(47,48)

The persecution of Christians continued through the reigns of Emperors Domitian and Trajan. Trajan, unfortunately, considered Christianity sacrilegious and punishable for its refusal to accept the state religion, and even his otherwise enlightened successors, Hadrian and Antoninus Pius, continued the persecutions because they were popular, and sometimes demanded by the masses. There were persecutions during the otherwise exemplary reign of Marcus Aurelius, as well as during the stern rule of Septimius Severus. Fueled by popular support and instigated by the masses, the persecutions continued even during the fleeting reign of the Roman Emperor Decius, who was proclaimed emperor by his legions in A.D.249, and was later captured in battle and killed by his Gothic barbarian captors in A.D.251.

Nevertheless, the most barbaric and systematic persecutions were those inaugurated by a former military commander and one of the most powerful of all Roman rulers, the Emperor Diocletian. Diocletian's brutal persecution, the tenth and most systematic attempt to erase Christianity from the face of the earth, was unparalleled in history – hundreds of thousand of victims were exterminated in an unsuccessful attempt to extirpate, once and for all, the Christian religion from the Empire.(10,47)

DIOCLETIAN – THE AFTERMATH

So I should say that civilizations begin with religion and stoicism: they end with skepticism and unbelief, and the undisciplined pursuit of individual pleasure. A civilization is born stoic and dies epicurean.

         Will Durant

But back at the hub of power in imperial Rome, in A.D.285, Emperor Diocletian, in order to more efficiently rule the Empire and more effectively deal with the barbarian threat, divided the Empire into Eastern and Western sections, and created a new type of government, the *Tetrarchy*. The Empire was divided into four districts governed by two senior Augustus and two junior Caesars who were appointed by Diocletian. The recalcitrant barbarians, nevertheless, continued to pose a threat by applying mounting pressure at various points in the imperial frontiers.

Long after Diocletian's abdication, the Empire remained divided at its core between East and West, although it was twice reunited by strong and determined emperors: once between A.D.324 and 364, under the strong emperor, Constantine I, "the Great" (reigned, A.D.306-337), and again for a scanty 5-month period between A.D.394 and 395, under Theodosius I, "the Great" (reigned, A.D.379-395). With the rule of Theodosius I, the reunification was not only fleeting and transient but it was also officially the final one, for the Roman Empire's East and West would never again be formally reunited.

In summary, Diocletian, a strong and capable ruler, had a golden opportunity to revive the traditional republican institutions and resurrect the Empire in the

---

[72] The aged apostle John was eventually freed from his banishment in A.D.96, and he resumed his preaching of the Gospel until his death in the city of Ephesus at the close of the 1st Century A.D.(47)

tradition of Augustus, Trajan, or Hadrian. Instead, he established himself as an absolute ruler with a politically and economically unworkable bureaucracy, whose vines crept in to hobble the machinery of state, and to govern and restrict all aspects of the social and private functions of Roman life. The burgeoning bureaucracy infiltrated and impaired legitimate government functions. It crept into the highest levels of government with the formation of the Tetrarchy, a hierarchical system of government, unmanageable, bureaucratic, and autocratic, where officials spent more time dispensing and currying favors whilst looking over each other's shoulders. After restoring military order, alas, no attempt was made to restore the economic and political systems which had served Rome so well for so many centuries.

The rule of the Tetrarchy with the two Augusti (co-emperors) and two Caesars (sub-emperors) under the leadership of Diocletian performed its military function, which was the defense of the Empire, exceedingly well, but the economic policies were a catastrophic failure, an impeachment of central regimentation and overt totalitarianism. Ultimately, it served to place more nails in the coffin of the Empire. Christians were persecuted with the same fervor as in the time of Nero. Diocletian's absolute rule erased whatever semblance remained of republican government, as well as local self-government in the outlying provinces, a tradition which had been preserved for 300 years since the collapse of the Roman Republic.

The vestiges of republicanism were effectively nullified or obliterated under Diocletian's rule. Having abandoned its *raison d'être* – its philosophic tenets (i.e., natural rights of citizenship, Roman stoicism, self-reliance, honor, and justice), its political precepts (i.e., constitutional rule of law), and its economic ideologies (i.e., economic opportunity and social mobility) – the Empire was well on its way to a rendezvous with an apocalyptic destiny.

CHAPTER 14

HISTORIC PARALLELS

Injustice never rules forever.
> *Seneca the Younger*

When you have robbed a man of everything, he is no longer in your power. He is free again.
> *Aleksandr Solzhenitsyn (b.1918)*
> *Russian patriot, author, and Nobel Prize winner in Literature (1970)*

ARE THERE LESSONS TO BE LEARNED?

These lessons in Roman history should best be learned by our present leaders and technocrats in the self-procreating government bureaucracies, who are today attempting to micromanage America and give the country the same remedy that accelerated the economic and cultural declivity of the Roman Empire in its ailing years. These lessons should be particularly perused by those who continue to push and militate for further government control of the economy and by those eager to find excuses to rationalize government intervention as a vehicle to achieve their desired social, political, and economic objectives.

The bitter truth is that American taxpayers have found themselves, since the inauguration of Lyndon B. Johnson's (U.S. President,1963-1969) Great Society, more and more pillaged and plundered by the tax-and-spend policies of profligate Congresses and acquiescent Presidents who have been leading us down the same path as that taken by ancient Rome.

And health care has not been immune. Government intervention, not the free market, has caused skyrocketing health care costs which, in turn, has triggered the health care crisis in which we are immersed today. In fact, Dr. Robert Sade, Chief of Pediatric Cardiac Surgery at the Medical University of South Carolina, points out, that while in 1965 (the year of the inception of Medicare) 6.5% of the U.S. gross domestic product "went to pay for health care," by 1992, it had ballooned to a full 14%. Moreover, he elucidates, "beneficiaries had no incentive to control costs, but a great deal of incentive to demand more services. As a result, in its first 5 years, the cost overrun on Medicare was nearly 70%, and has become many times that in its first 25 years."(49)

And the story of government intervention in medical practice does not end there but has continued to evolve so as to restrain the free market in the health care delivery system. Meanwhile, the public believes that medicine in the U.S. is based on free market principles. Nothing is further from the truth. Sade correctly asserts: "The responses of the government to the inevitable huge cost overruns have included price controls (which failed for the same reason as placing a lid on a boiling kettle fails), encouraging the development of HMOs with the passage of the HMO Act in 1973, restricting hospital construction, as with the National Planning and Resources Development Act of 1974, regulating insurance, and in the 1980s, controlling the costs of Medicare with the DRG [Diagnosis Related Group] system."(49)

And to this list we should add the application of RBRVS (Resource-Based Relative Value Scale) – a government mandated system of payment for physicians, which both Robert Moffit, Ph.D., Deputy Director of Domestic Policy at The Heritage Foundation, and Jane Orient, M.D., Executive Director of the Association of American Physicians and Surgeons (AAPS), correctly assert is derived from the Marxist Labor Theory of Values.(50,51)

Sade unerringly holds: "Each of these reactions generated a new set of problems, requiring a new set of responses. The latest of these is the American Health Security Act of 1993."(49) This plan is President Bill Clinton's (and First Lady Hillary Rodham Clinton's) answer to the present state of health care woes. Why are health care costs out of control? Because of government intervention, as well as its corollary which Sade describes in one sentence: "When purchasing health care, people do not have the sense that they are spending their own money." Ninety-five percent of all costs incurred during hospitalizations and 81% of physician's fees are paid by someone (government or private insurance) other than the person seeking medical care.(49) As a result, patients do not have an incentive to reduce costs; market forces are lacking in the health care delivery system. The end result is that costs continue to escalate. More government and more bureaucracy is not the answer.

Time magazine has called this Presidential proposal, "the boldest most expensive social initiative since the New Deal, bigger than F.D.R.'s institution of Social Security half a century ago."(52) Likewise, *The Economist* proclaimed, "Not since Franklin Roosevelt's War Production Board has it been suggested that so large a part of the American economy should suddenly be brought under government control....Armed with his plans for reforming health care and waving his health security card, Mr. Clinton proposed nothing less than the government should seize the levers of an industry that accounts for one-seventh of the American economy."(53) And there is seemingly something in it for everyone – except, of course, physicians. Even California's Democratic Congressman Fortney "Pete" Stark, who is not a friend of Medicine, admitted upon studying the proposal that the plan will "destroy fee-for-service medicine as we know it."(54)

The economic brunt of the program will be borne almost solely by those already paying their fair share, the patient-consumer and the providers: hospitals and physicians. Thus, it is no wonder that the plan is touted as only costing a mere additional $480 annually per person for such an extravagant proposal and is boasted to insure all 37 million people who are presently uninsured.

We now know that of that number without insurance coverage, only 5-10 million are truly uninsurable or unable financially to obtain health care coverage.(55) The rest chose not to do so, either because they do not feel they need it, or had something else better to do with their money, like buying an automobile, or putting a down payment on a new home, etc. Besides, the present tax structure provides a disincentive for the self-employed and for the employees of small businesses that do not provide health care coverage to obtain their own coverage. Others in the rank of the uninsured are simply in transit from one job to the next and were uninsured because their policies provided by their employer and linked to their place of employment lacked portability. In the latter groups are where we find the other 25-30 million who "lack" insurance coverage.(55) Mind you, it is based on these false premises that we are getting ready to dismantle the best health care in the world without confronting the true underlying root causes of "the real crisis."(49,50,56-58)

The much touted Clinton plan promises to cost $700 billion dollars over a 5-year period, counting an expected $91 billion dollars left over, that ostensibly will be used to reduce the deficit!(59) So where does the rest of the money come from? Two of the enumerated sources are the "sin taxes," $105 billion, and Medicare/Medicaid savings, $238 billion. The numbers do not add up, so I suspect that an unenumerated (and largest) amount will come from the savings that will be realized supposedly from RBRVS implementation for all prospective payment plans and thence the reduction in "provider" reimbursement, as well as forthcoming unannounced taxation. In fact, a recent publication[73] notes that based on new proposals published in the *Federal Register* as of July 14, 1993: "HCFA plans in creating values (RVUs) for services not covered by Medicare because 'increasingly...private insurers base payment, in whole or in part, on the Medicare physician fee schedule.' In other words, the Medicare Fee Schedule (RVUs) may become the basis for all reimbursement." Amongst the insurers who have already adopted this fee structure (or plan to do so) are Blue Cross/Blue Shield plans, workers compensation, and many managed care entities (HMOs).

The various tiers of incredibly complex bureaucracy, amongst the redundant loops and bundles of red tape facing patient and doctors alike, would make President Clinton's health care proposal if passed by Congress, a bureaucratic nightmare. It would make overt, fully socialized medicine, as in Canada for example, comparatively attractive to American physicians. But it would be a disaster for patient-consumers, because overt and covert rationing of health care services and deterioration of the quality of health care would be the result.(60)

A new, mammoth, bureaucratic monstrosity, the National Health Board, would have unprecedented powers enforcing global budgets (price controls) and assuming control of 15% of the U.S. GNP. It would rival the IRS in centralization "prestige" and power.(59) As political commentator, P.J. O'Rourke writes: "The President has put a lawyer in charge of making doctors cheaper" (61) – and it shows. The medical liability (tort) reform package is weak and ineffective. The sky would still be the limit for the attorney-litigators.

If the Health Security Act of 1993 (or a look-alike managed competition plan) is implemented, there would be loss of the patients' freedom to choose their physicians, places of treatment, and health care plans. Patients would be discouraged from remaining with their long-time physicians, as the Act has strong financial incentives to encourage the dissolution of the previously sacrosanct patient-doctor relationship. The Act would provide financial incentives for patients to join HMOs chosen by the health alliances (another intervening layer of bureaucracy functioning as government cartels), and strong financial disincentives for the traditional "fee-for-service" plans, which would actually be quite limited. In essence, the concept of choice in health care would become moot.

Sade is indeed correct when he maintains: "The American health care system is in trouble, not because of failure of the marketplace, but because of the

---

[73] Southern Health Care Services Newsletter, Atlanta, Georgia, October 1993.

absence of a market. *The only lasting solution to the U.S. health care crisis is the creation of a true competitive market in health care* [his emphasis]."(49)

Needless to say, the timeless parallels between our present period and that of Diocletian's epoch are far too obvious – and the aftermath, too apocalyptic to be considered or even entertained by the statist health care gurus who want centralization at any price. These are indeed the times that try men's souls, and the times when the famous maxim of George Santayana (1863-1952) applies: "Those who cannot remember the past are condemned to repeat it."(11)

THE DOUBLE-EDGED SWORD OF CIVIL LITIGATION AND ADMINISTRATIVE LAW

Camarón que se duerme se lo lleva la corriente.
Old Cuban Proverb

Trouble will rain on those who are already wet.
Anonymous

From a fallen tree, all make kindling.
Spanish Proverb

The medical profession in the United States, because of its previous independence, the high status accorded to its members, and their relative prosperity, has been singled out of the judicial mainstream. For instance, physicians are practicing medicine under the constant threat of civil litigation, easy prey for unscrupulous attorney-litigators involved in a lottery system of medical liability that is eroding physicians' confidence in the judicial system. Contingency fee-driven litigation-on-demand; the absence of the necessary restraining English Rule in civil litigation, by which the loser pays all court costs; the lack of the necessary disclosure of collateral sources (which today allows plaintiffs to collect from multiple entities and defendants for the same alleged loss without this fact beknownst to the jury); the dismissal rule whereby plaintiffs can dismiss a claim (up to the time of trial) when they don't like the way the suit is going and refile it later – are all facets of the litigation juggernaut that is devastating America. For physicians who are frequently named in "malpractice" lawsuits, the injustice of long and arduous imposition of years of medical litigation can be demoralizing. Medical liability litigation may take many years for resolution of the claim, whilst a dark cloud looms over the integrity and competence of the defendant physician; it is also detrimental to the psychologic (and sometimes) physical well-being of patient-plaintiffs who have genuine grievances. In fact, because of these impositions and injustices, many physicians settle malpractice claims regardless of whether they have actually committed malpractice.(56,57,62)

Moreover, medical practice is controlled and regulated by draconian administrative decrees written and enforced by a myriad of government agencies and gargantuan bureaucracies which are unbound to the U.S. Constitution and literally out of control. In fact, 25% of all U.S. health care costs are consumed by administrative costs and a burgeoning bureaucracy. Physicians, frantic and sometimes in a state of outright panic, are doing everything they can to decipher and follow cryptic bureaucratic decrees and encoded regulations [74] to avoid the dreaded accusation of fraud or abuse. Indeed, the simplest accusation and mere allegation of wrongdoing could result in a formal investigation by any one of the government's watchdog agencies. Thus, physicians are doing all they can to educate themselves, train their office staffs, follow government regulations, in an attempt to deter potential prosecution for violating vague and arbitrary rules and sundry other decrees published in the *Federal Register*. [75] Thus, physicians have less time left to spend with patients and in the actual delivery of medical care.

In dealing with administrative law, e.g., fraud allegations, physicians have learned the hard way that they no longer have the benefit of constitutional safeguards such as "due process" and "equal protection before the law" as protection from the barrage of accusations and recriminations that follow the modish accusation of "fraud and abuse."

Yet, under the pretense of abiding by the 6th Amendment, medical and product liability litigation has been stretched to the breaking point, spawning a juggernaut of litigation that is tearing the fabric of our society.(56,57,62) For example, manufacturers are reluctant to invest money in the research and development of new medical products including much needed pharmaceuticals, medical appliances, and vaccines; doctors are closing or limiting their practices or retiring early because of a liability crisis. Despite popular belief to the contrary, it is the medical specialists who are trained to perform the most complex and highest-risk procedures, not the incompetent physicians (as the layman believes) who are most prone to be easy prey for the medical litigation industry.

The public in general and the medical profession in particular must realize that progress in the health care arena cannot take place until the monstrous medical and product liability crisis is brought under control. This fundamental fact must also be recognized by health care policymakers. The litigation juggernaut has been picking up steam inexorably in the last two decades and is now threatening the very foundation of our system of jurisprudence and constitutional government. The litigation juggernaut poses a threat to property and to progress because it thwarts innovation in the same manner as the expansion of administrative law presently poses an imminent threat to individual liberty. The circumvention of constitutional safeguards and their replacement with administrative mandates has effectively resulted in the demoralization of the medical profession and the erosion of the civil rights of a whole class of citizens, the American physicians, to the detriment of the traditions of this great nation.(65)

Authorized to impose mandates on physicians are a myriad of government agencies such as the Internal Revenue Service (IRS), the Department of Health and Human Services (HHS), the Health Care Financing Administration (HCFA), and the Occupational and Safety Hazard Administration (OSHA), to

---

[74] The cost of U.S. government regulation for the single year of 1990 has been estimated by the Joint Economic Committee, *Annual Report* (1992) at $461.4 billion.(63) In fact, based on the conservative estimate that for every $10 million incurred in regulatory costs to the economy, there is one premature death, the Competitive Enterprise Institute analyst, Jonathan J. Adler, computed that federal regulations result in 40,000 to 50,000 premature deaths each year.(37)
[75] According to Doug Bandow, Senior Fellow at the CATO Institute, during 1991 under President Bush, the *Federal Register* printed some 68,000 pages of rules and regulations, the third highest in history and the most ever, since President Jimmy Carter.(64)

mention but a few. [76] Although both civil litigation (litigation-on-demand) and the erosion of constitutional safeguards affect all, physicians have been disproportionately affected, as members of an unfavored minority in these egalitarian times. I have no doubt that to stem the tide, physicians, of necessity, will have to enter the gladiatorial arena to positively effect change in the political process. In fact, it is essential that the medical profession and its members become involved in the present political debate over health care policy and the future direction of medical practice, not only for the sake of their own survival but also to ascertain that physicians remain members of an independent profession that continues to render compassionate, ethical medical care, whilst still providing the highest quality medical care for their patients without having to resort to rationing or denial of medical care – a daunting task, no doubt, in these perilous and transitory times as we enter the 21st Century.

The attorney-litigators, with roughly 70% of their members in the United States and pushing through our court system 18,000,000 new lawsuits per year, remain directly involved in political issues, as well as legal matters.(56,57,62,67) Let me interject at this point that I believe that the majority of lawyers are conscientious and ethical professionals, many of whom also lament, just as we physicians do, the change in the ethical climate of the legal profession since the 1960s. Nevertheless, as the number of attorneys increase,[77] the government, which is already disproportionally composed of lawyers, has been able to expand the horizons of liability to immeasurable vistas. For it seems that as more attorneys pour out of law schools, almost reflexively, legislators pass more legislation that opens new avenues for liability litigation. They are supported by yet other newcomers, the self-styled consumer advocates, many of whom are attorneys themselves and who provide the raw material for what Walter Olson, Senior Fellow at The Manhattan Institute, has correctly pegged, "the sue-for-profit litigation industry."(62)

Unfortunately, these insidious and ingenious ways of opening new windows of opportunity for the attorney-litigators are simply grist for the litigation mill. [78] The fact remains that the creation of these myriad sources of legal disputes are accompanied by less jobs, less competitiveness, less productivity, less research, less development, and less innovation in the market place. They are also associated with more suffering in America's homes and more tension in the workplace. No matter which way you look at it: America loses.

---

[76] And as of this writing, if President Clinton's Health Care package passes, we would have a National Health Board (NHB) that would approach in power and bureaucracy that of the IRS. The IRS, incidentally, dwarfs the FBI in the number of employees and entrenched bureaucracy. The IRS, with 123,000 employees and an annual budget of approximately $280 million (1993), is five times larger than the FBI.(64) It is the largest government law enforcement agency, with vast and immense powers: it collects personal as well as financial information on all citizens (not just criminals), it imposes civil penalties at will without affording constitutional protection to defendants (not even the right to a day in court). Unlike other criminal proceedings, the IRS places the burden of proof on the accused taxpayer, who immediately upon the strain of an accusation becomes the hapless defendant.(66)

[77] New graduates continue to pour out of American law schools in record numbers, so that approximately 35,000 new attorneys are added each and every year to the nearly 800,000 U.S. attorneys already in practice.(67)

[78] Class action lawsuits, malpractice suits, product liability lawsuits, suits stemming from allegations of date rape and sexual harassment, not to mention, suits for environmental and regulatory violations, as well as suits stemming out of alleged violations of the Americans with Disabilities Act (ADA) of 1990 (compliance estimated to cost businesses $20 billion a year for at least the next 5 years), and although some of these violations may be serious, the vast majority are frivolous, fishing expeditions in search of deep-pocket defendants.(62) As if all of this were not enough, the renown economist, Dr. Paul Craig Roberts, has calculated that, "as much as 60% of the billions of dollars spent under the guise of the environmental clean-up Superfund program to detoxify allegedly contaminated sites by industrial wastes has been pocketed by lawyers for legal expenses." Yet, the Superfund program "is failing to clean up the environment, but is wiping out jobs and banks and is threatening our insurance companies."(64)

Up to this time, individual physicians have been relatively quiet relying on the leadership of the AMA to do their negotiating with government authorities. Yet they have been neither impervious nor immune to this litigation virus. They have been too busy taking care of their own patients, figuring that lawsuits and accusations of "fraud and abuse" just could not happen to them, not in America. A lawsuit, anyway, is something that happens to others, not to oneself. Vaguely aware of the danger, and unwilling to commit themselves to the task, physicians are now being made to suffer, being picked off efficiently by their tormentors with pinpoint accuracy, one by one, like doves flying over a hunting field.(65) It is time that physicians listen to the clarion of the political realities of our time. The medical profession must not remain dormant any longer and risk being swept away by the litigation juggernaut and the tsunami of government intervention.

In fact, the situation in which the medical profession finds itself today elicits in me vivid memories of my loving maternal grandmother who, whilst I was still a child sitting on her lap, told me didactic stories and recited old Cuban proverbs. And foremost amongst them: *Camarón que se duerme, se lo lleva la corriente*, "A shrimp that falls asleep would be taken away by the current."

In the opposite corner, the legal profession always controls the judiciary and they are forty-six times more likely than the average citizen to serve in Congress.(68) Therefore, they frequently control the legislative branch of both the state and federal governments; and not infrequently, as in the present, they also control the executive branch of government! [79] Perhaps this over-representation of the legal profession in government has something to do with the fact that the much needed legal reforms remain on the back burner of politics, protected, so it seems, by the conspiratorial silence of the media. Not infrequently the interest of the legal profession and the media coincide, and they coincide so thoroughly as to be virtually indistinguishable and as to constitute a profitable symbiosis: Publicity and sensationalism of alleged wrongdoings or injustices foster a climate conducive to litigation; whereas, media coverage of huge awards and other aspects of lottery-litigation beget publicity.

And this epiphany brings us up to the third great bastion, or rather current, of liberalism and egalitarianism (besides the media and the Hollywood cultural elites)(69,70) and that is, the entrenched liberal academia of the large American universities, the underwater volcanic explosions behind the tides of the tsunami: domestic socialism for wealth redistribution to placate the special interest groups and the seduced masses, litigation-on-demand to appease the attorney-litigator lobby (and effect yet more wealth redistribution), and global government to satiate the unquenchable thirst for maximizing profits by the corporate internationalists, who will be exempted from the misery that will be imposed on the rest of us.

So it should not be surprising that the fault for the alleged evils and shortcomings of the medical profession – charges of "fraud and abuse" (the shibboleth itself much hackneyed and abused) claiming an unsubstantiated 10% of the health care budget; overt failures to control escalating health care costs (due to public demand for unlimited medical care and access to the latest technology, etc.); and

---

[79] The president, Bill Clinton, is an attorney, as is the first lady, Hillary Rodham Clinton, who headed the Health Care Task Force that drafted the report, which U.S. physicians may have to follow to deliver medical care in the foreseeable future.

imputed failures (i.e., guaranteed clinical outcomes, not to mention the failure of the medical profession to find Ponce de Leon's fountain of youth that bestows immortality) – are all placed squarely on the shoulders of the medical providers. The fact is that as dedicated and exceedingly competent as physicians are, they are still men and women, and fallible human beings. Physicians, trained and competent as they are, are still subject to human error, and this is compounded by the fact that they practice an inexact science.(71)

Besides the obvious problem that physicians are not infallible human beings, there is also the problem of a public who refuses to accept the fact that, like used machinery, especially run-down, maltreated, and abused machinery, they are also subject to aging and decay. Defying conventional wisdom and self-evident truths, they expect everlasting youth and perfect health without, mind you, accepting the responsibilities of doing everything possible to stay healthy, or alternatively, accepting the consequences of leading unhealthy lifestyles and outright self-destructive behaviors, as many Americans are prone to do.(58,72)

Not even the President of the United States is as personally accountable to another single human being (except perhaps to the First Lady), as a physician is to each and every one of his/her patients. A case in point is that of the stereotypical surgeon who, alone in the middle of the night, undertakes the responsibility of operating on a sick or seriously-ill patient, a patient whose life is wavering between life and death, a life placed squarely on the surgeon's shoulder and the dexterity of his/her hands. Every second counts. Yet, despite all this drama, there are always limitations in what he or she can do. For, after all, the hand of Providence guides the surgeon's dextrous hands, or if you prefer, nature will run her course.

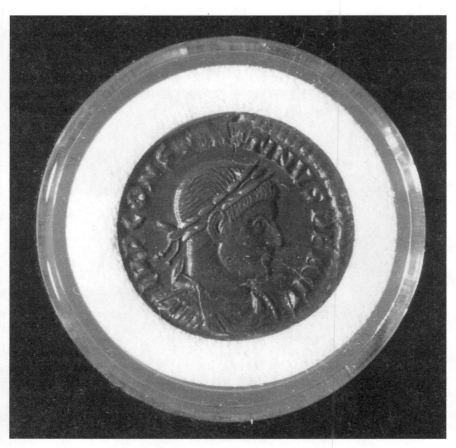

Plate 15 – Laureate head of Emperor Constantine the Great (A.D.306-337). Silvered bronze follis. Author's private collection.

CHAPTER 15

CONSTANTINE THE GREAT

Fortune favours the bold.
> *Terence (c.195-c.154 B.C.)*

To the victor belongs the spoils of the enemy.
> *William L. Marcy*

In A.D.312, Constantine I, "the Great" (reigned, A.D.306-337), mounted atop his horse and leading his armies of the Western Roman Empire, beheld a fiery vision on a cloud in the sky, a luminous cross inscribed with a divine message, "by this sign shalt thou conquer." This vision, appearing fortuitously just before a major and decisive engagement (the Battle of Milvian Bridge), meant, at least to Constantine, not only victory but victory with the acceptance of Christianity for the Empire. Moreover, the revelation was reminiscent of St. Paul's (4 B.C.-A.D.64) auspicious vision and subsequent conversion on the road to Damascus. For Constantine, the vision, his victory, and his change of heart would mean revolutionary changes for the Empire: Constantine attributed his crucial victory that day to the intervention of the Christian God. Constantine was so touched by this miracle that, thereafter, his Roman legionnaires always carried into battle shields inscribed with the Greek letters, Chi-Rho, the first two letters of Christ's name.

Indeed on that fateful afternoon, Constantine the Great was triumphant, defeating his rival, the co-emperor Maxentius (reigned, A.D.306-312). Maxentius, who had claimed the entire Western throne for himself, died on the battlefield. Constantine converted to Christianity, becoming the first Roman emperor to do so, [80] and quickly ended the persecution of Christians by introducing the concept of religious tolerance into the Empire with the Edict of Milan.(73) This imperial edict established Christianity as a legal and tolerated religion in the Roman Empire of the West. Constantine even established Sunday as the day of worship.

Constantine, nevertheless, still had battles to fight in order to consolidate his power, so next he moved decisively against the co-emperor Licinius (emperor of the East, A.D.308-324). In a series of battles, Constantine fought and finally, in a decisive engagement, defeated his Eastern rival. The decisive victory at Chrysopolis over the cruel Licinius resulted in the reunification of the Western and Eastern halves of t he Roman Empire. These victories consolidated the empire and fortified it. Yet, even more importantly and more enduring, was the fact that Christianity was suddenly transformed from a small persecuted religious sect [81] to a protected and established religion of a now reconsolidated and fortified Roman Empire, an empire that was still the supreme power in the Western world under the determined and powerful guidance of Constantine the Great.

---

[80] The emperor Galerius (joint emperor, A.D.305-311) who, along with Diocletian, had done his best to stamp out Christianity, converted to Christianity on his deathbed following an acutely debilitating and incapacitating illness. He even signed an edict ending religious persecution of Christians and asked Christians everywhere to pray for him, his relief from pain and suffering, and his recovery from the cruel illness to which he ultimately succumbed.

[81] Interestingly, Diocletian (d.A.D.313) who had perhaps carried out the worse persecutions of all, was still alive at the time of the fateful conversion of Constantine (A.D.312), although he was aged and retired at his castle near Salonae.

In A.D.325, Constantine convened the first world ecumenical council of the Christian church at Nicaea, which not only established the supremacy of Christianity throughout the Empire but also settled and ended several internal disputes which had arisen within the Christian church. Then in A.D.330, he moved his capital from Rome to the small town of Byzantium on the western side of the Dardanelles, and founded what later became the magnificent city of Constantinople (today: Istanbul, Turkey).

CONSTANTINE AND LEPROSY

Leprosy had been known to physicians since antiquity, but it was in the 4th Century A.D. that it became widely prevalent in Europe. [82] Leprosy was considered a disease of the soul, associated with sinfulness and immorality. Lepers were to be avoided and isolated from their communities. According to the church, doctors could treat lepers by dressing and cleaning their ulcerated wounds, and thus soothe their condition in this fashion, but it was felt that given the nature of this illness, a cure could not be effected. Religious authorities maintained that leprosy "was a manifestation of transgression against divine law, a sin"...that could only be "alleviated by moral regeneration."(74)

Be that as it may, legend has it that Emperor Constantine was struck with leprosy and to expiate his sins, his pagan priests advised that he bathe in the blood of 3,000 children. He rejected the barbarous advice, and in his stead, he was bathed by Pope Sylvester who "immersed him in the love of the church." By this atonement he was cured of the dreadful disease and gained divine misericordia.(74) Thankful, grateful, and so immersed in the love of the church, the story goes, he provided for the Donation of Constantine which gave the papacy mundane and earthly authority. In those days, this temporal authority was tantamount to geopolitical power and military authority.

THE DONATION OF CONSTANTINE

The story of Constantine the Great brings us to a remarkable document found during the very early Middle Ages, the *Donation of Constantine,* that bolstered the papal contention for the derivation of its temporal powers.

From the time of the collapse of Rome, the spiritual authority of the church was known to be derived from the Holy see of St. Peter, but whence derives the temporal powers of the church? The *Donation of Constantine* provided some answers. The document provided evidence that in exchange for Pope Sylvester I (St.Sylvester; pope, A.D.314-336) having once healed Emperor Constantine of leprosy and restoring him to good health, the emperor had, upon moving his capital to Constantinople, granted Pope Sylvester the title of "Temporal Successor in Rome." This power, in effect, established the worldly and earthly powers of the bishopric of

---

[82] Leprosy reached a peak in the 14th Century and then gradually declined, so that by the 16th Century it had run its course and was almost completely extinguished in most of Europe.

Rome, from the power of investiture to the authority of governing municipalities and even leading armies into battle. The *Donation of Constantine* enabled the papacy, as the bishopric of Rome was later called, to claim not only divine and spiritual powers leading to the salvation of the soul but also mundane and temporal powers, empowering the pope to govern kingdoms and municipalities as well as to crown kings and emperors here on Earth:

> *And inasmuch as our imperial power is earthly, we have decreed that it shall venerate and honor his most holy Roman Church and that the sacred see of blessed Peter shall be gloriously exalted above our empire and earthly throne. We attribute to him the power and glorious dignity and strength and honor of the empire, and we ordain and decree that he shall have rule as well over the four principal sees, Antioch, Alexandria, Constantinople, and Jerusalem, as also over all the churches of God in all the world. And the pontiff who for the time being presides over that most holy Roman Church shall be the highest and chief of all priests in the whole world, and according to his decision shall all matters be settled which shall be taken in hand for the service of God or the confirmation of the faith of Christians.(75)*

These temporal powers, in addition to the spiritual guidance that the pope already provided to his flock, gave the see of St. Peter tremendous power, unprecedented for any Christian ruler except perhaps the power later wielded by the Holy Roman Emperors, and even their power frequently rested upon the acceptance and approval of the Holy Church. The alleged *Donation of Constantine* also aided the power of the Christian church as it consolidated its authority as the official religion both in the surviving Roman Empire in the East and in the emergent nation-states of Europe in the West.

The *Donation* was considered authentic, and for centuries it was cited as the source of authority from which the Pope and the Church derived their power to involve themselves in earthly matters, erstwhile considered matters for the secular state. The document formed the riveting argument for the temporal power of the pope, and it remained so until the humanist scholar Lorenzo Valla (c.1407-1457) discovered in the midst of the Renaissance that this document was a masterful forgery, contrived by an artful and resourceful monk sometime in the years c.A.D.740.(1)

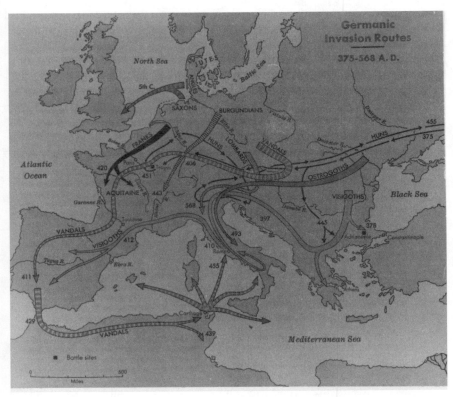

Plate 16 – Barbarians at the gates of the Roman Empire. Germanic invasion routes A.D.375-568. Brinton, Christopher, and Wolff, 1976.

CHAPTER 16

THE BEGINNING OF THE END IN THE WEST

This is the way the world ends, not with a bang but a whimper.
T.S. Eliot (1888-1965)

VALENS AND ADRIANOPLE

As we have noted, the 3rd Century A.D. brought civil war and chaos. We will not dwell on this point. Then, in A.D.378, the Roman war machine, a semblance of its former self, suffered a spectacular military defeat, a major disaster that presaged the collapse of the Western Roman Empire. In that fateful year at the Battle of Adrianople, the Visigoths, pressured by the Huns, fought and inflicted a decisive defeat upon the Roman legions led by the Emperor Flavius Julius Valens (emperor in the East, A.D.364-378). Emperor Valens was killed in battle, and the Roman lines were breached.(1,10,24,45) The penetration of the previously impervious Roman defenses by the Germanic hordes portended the beginning of the end.

Nevertheless, from the disastrous occasion in A.D. 7 at the time of the rule of the first Roman Emperor Augustus up until the Battle of Adrianople, it is fair to say that despite the period of anarchy that ensued in the 3rd Century, the imperial Roman legions had, for the most part, held the line and kept the barbarians at bay.

Emperor Valens' debacle in the 4th Century A.D. was almost without parallel. A trend was becoming evident. Moreover, by the 5th Century A.D., substantial numbers of Teutonic barbarian warriors were literally within the Empire, and as the year A.D.410 approached, it was clear that they were amassing outside the city's walls, surrounding the seven hills, preparing for the final onslaught upon the gates of Rome.

ALARIC AND THE VISIGOTHS

In A.D. 410, Alaric (c. A.D.370-410), who had been a general of an auxiliary Gothic regiment in the Roman army, ascended the throne as King of the Visigoths and almost immediately turned against Rome. He knew from first hand experience that he held moribund Rome within his grasp, and towards this end, he set out to conquer the Western portion of the Roman Empire by ravaging southern Greece and wreaking havoc amongst the hapless population. He was then poised to strike and when the opportunity presented itself, Alaric struck at Rome herself. After two savage but unsuccessful sieges, he finally penetrated Roman defenses and sacked Rome in A.D.410. Alaric became the first barbarian in 800 years to sack and capture Rome.

It should be understood that by this time the Roman army was not only composed of large numbers of Germanic tribesmen but was also even commanded in the field by some Teutonic generals. One such general was the capable Stilicho, a member of a Vandal tribe to which Rome had previously opened her gates. Unfortunately, however, by the time his kinsmen struck at Rome, he was no longer there to prevent the ravaging and pillaging of the once glorious mistress of the Mediterranean. Stilicho, who had triumphantly led Rome's army and who had previously defeated Alaric and his Visigoths in the Balkans, had been accused of high treason and executed in A.D. 408. [83]

By now, the Eternal City was only a semblance of her former self. She was only a vestige, the remaining symbol of a once formidable empire. The young Emperor Honorius by this time had moved his court to Ravenna, and Rome, lacking the necessary leadership and manpower, was incapable both politically and militarily of halting the barbarians. Moreover, Stilicho's less capable successors were betrayed, and the garrison guarding Rome, overwhelmed.

It was said that Rome was sacked continuously for three horrible days, unable to defend herself from the massive looting and plundering. One can sense the strong feelings of uncertainty, helplessness, anguish, and despair that must have seized the Roman citizenry during those barbarous and horrific times. Yet more years of trials and tribulations were in store for the citizens of the Western Roman Empire, for more anarchy and chaos would be forthcoming.

For example, from North Africa, a territory nominally under the Romans but now under the ravages of the Vandals, we have the story of the woman scholar, Hypatia (c.A.D.370-415). Hypatia, a mathematician and member of the Neoplatonic school of philosophy, was head of the school of Alexandria during this apocalyptic time, a time when the light of culture and learning not just in Alexandria, but all over the Western world, was twinkling dimly and fading fast. She was the last star of the Alexandrian school and library.(76) One day in A.D.415 on her way to the library, her carriage was attacked by an angry mob. Hypatia was dragged from the carriage and murdered in the street. The light of the last remaining star of Alexandria, alas, had been extinguished.

And as if this unspeakable situation was not enough, after the looting and pillaging of Rome, the seemingly most barbaric of the barbarian hordes, the Huns, were fast approaching Rome. In fact, it had been the Hunnish onslaught which had forced the Germanic warriors across the Danube and the Rhine to invade Roman territory with a fury. Now the fierce tribesmen of Central Asia and Eastern Europe were themselves threatening to strike at the weak but still symbolic heart of the empire, Rome.

ATTILA AND THE HUNS

Attila, King of the Huns (A.D. 434-453), had not only been extorting tribute from the Eastern and Western Roman emperors but was now ready and confident to challenge the Western half of the realm, for he had never been defeated on the field of battle. Then, at the Battle of Châlons on the Catalaunian plains in A.D. 451, the hand of Providence finally appeared to intercede for Rome. Attila and his

---

[83] Stilicho had been the chief military officer for the powerful Emperor Theodosius, and after Theodosius' death in A.D. 395, Stilicho served as regent for the 11-year-old Honorius (A.D.393-423). But the inexperienced young emperor had him executed for high treason on the ill-advised urging of his older brother Arcadius (A.D.377-408), emperor of the Eastern Roman Empire.

Huns were defeated by the combined forces of the Roman General Aëtius (d.A.D.454) and the Visigothic King Theodoric I (d.A.D.451). Theodoric, who planned the battle strategy with Aëtius and was none other than Alaric's son, had allied himself to Rome in the face of the Hunnish advances in Europe. In a fierce clash and tempestuous battle, Attila was defeated and forced to withdraw. King Theodoric himself was killed in the ferocious battle.(26)

Châlons was the first and only military defeat of Attila's career.(10,24) Yet the battle is considered by military historian Edward Creasy to have been one of the world's fifteen most decisive battles of antiquity. Creasy points out that this defeat prevented the Western Roman Empire from falling to the pagan Hunnish hordes; instead, it would hold out for a quarter of a century more, to fall to the Christianized Germanic barbarians.(26)

Nevertheless, despite this major defeat, Attila the Hun rearmed, regrouped, and refurbished his fierce, multi-ethnic, heterogenous forces. Rather than being discouraged, Attila carefully prepared to launch a final massive attack against the feeble but still beating heart of Rome. And within a year, he was ready to strike. And so it was that in the year A.D. 452, Attila and his Hunnish hordes were again preparing for total war and massing at the outskirts of Italy.

On the Roman side, the persistent and pervasive sense of doom lingered within the gates as the citizens braced for the worst. Remembrances of A.D.410 must have been evident in their collective memory. The Western Roman Empire had by now been effectively reduced to the Italian peninsula. The torch of the Empire had passed to Byzantium and the Eastern Roman Empire, but Rome, nevertheless, remained emblematic of Roman power.

At this time, the Western Roman emperor was Valentinian III (reigned, A.D.425-455) who although considered a mediocre and at times irascible ruler who took little interest in the affairs of government, had nevertheless provided some degree of stability to the Western Empire during his nearly 30-year rule.(10) So as Attila the Hun approached Rome in preparation for the final onslaught, Valentinian waited impassively for the apocalypse. To make matters even worse for Rome, this testy ruler ignored the counsel of Aëtius, the hero of the Battle of Châlons, who had fallen from favor with the emperor because of suspected disloyalties, palatial intrigues, and petty jealousies. Valentinian himself judged the Roman army incapable of defeating Attila's reorganized armies (1,10,77), and was preparing to sue for peace when the semi-legendary Pope Leo I, "The Great" (pope, A.D.440-461) interceded and miraculously dissuaded Attila from attacking Rome.

The private meeting between the old pope and the "Scourge of God" took place on the outskirts of the Italian frontier. The saintly Pope Leo is said to have approached Attila's camp leading a procession of priests and monks. The venerable old man, with his white beard and dressed in white ecclesiastical garments, rode a white horse. Upon seeing this curious procession, Attila mounted his black charger, Villam, and surrounded by his royal retainers is said to have inquired of the strangers the exact nature of their unexpected arrival.(77) He then called to a halt his advancing warriors, and on the banks of the river questioned the saintly old man dressed in white who led the procession. His name was Pope Leo. Attila crossed the river and on the other side of the stream, the "Scourge of God" and his counterpart, the pious Pope Leo, held the famous secret counsel, so secret that the contents of their conversation were never divulged.(77)

How Pope Leo I was able to convince Attila not to descend upon Rome, or why Attila was so dissuaded, remains to this day one of those great puzzling secrets of history. Perhaps, as leadership expert Wess Roberts asserts, "it was the destiny of Rome to be spared."(77) In any event, Attila and his retinue followed by his mighty heterogeneous horde of Hunnish warriors turned northward and back to the Valley of the Danube, whence they had originated.(1,7,10,12,24,45,77)

GAISERIC AND THE VANDALS

As we have seen, several serious wounds had already been inflicted upon Rome, but at least for the time being, Rome managed to survive. Still, more diffi-cult times were yet to come to haunt the moribund city before the final cataclysm. In A.D.455, for instance, the Vandals under King Gaiseric responded to the appeals of the queen of the newly assassinated emperor, Valentinian III. [84] Valentinian, iras-cible and impudent, had made many enemies for having ordered the assassination of Aëtius, Rome's last great general and the victor at Châlons. Valentinian's wid-owed queen was now being forced to marry the new emperor, Petronius Maximus (emperor in the West, March 17 to May 31, A.D.455). According to historian Michael Grant, she had nothing but contempt and animosity for the new emperor, whom she held responsible for Valentinian's murder.(10)

Petronius ruled for only 70 days. During the Vandals fierce assault upon Rome, he was killed in a cowardly attempt to flee the besieged city. The Vandal attack was successful; Rome's defenses collapsed, and Gaiseric and his warriors sacked Rome. Again the city was pillaged and plundered by Germanic barbarians, and this time the Roman gentry and clergymen were persecuted by the brutal raiders.(10,24) Gaiseric and his Vandals then resumed their locust-like invasion, subduing North Africa and the islands of Sicily, Sardinia, Corsica, as well as the Balearic Islands, where they finally settled to enjoy their loot and plun-der.(1,7,10,24) The city on the Palatine Hill now lay mortally wounded, and the end was in sight.

ODOACER AND THE GERMANS

The final blow struck the Eternal City and her western half in A.D. 476 during the ill-fated rule of the hapless, teenage emperor, Romulus Augustulus (emperor in the West, October A.D.475-September A.D.476). The young emperor, who was ironically named after both the legendary founder of Rome, Romulus, and the first Roman emperor, Augustus, was dethroned by the Germanic general, Odoacer (c.A.D.433-493). The Germanic chieftain formally and finally ended the Western Roman Empire in that unfortuitous year, and from that day onward

---

[84] Perhaps a sign of the times, Attila the Hun was likewise enticed to Rome by a woman of high and regal rank, none other than Honoria, Emperor Valentinian's sister, who proposed an alliance of marriage and then bequeathed herself to Attila who, so encouraged, not only claimed her hand but also demanded half of the Western Roman Empire as dowry. To claim these prizes he had marched his warriors upon Rome in A.D.451-452.

historians consider the event concomitantly to mark the fall of Rome, and the inception of the Dark Ages in Europe. Although one must keep in mind that the Eastern Roman Empire, the Byzantine Empire with its majestic capital at Constantinople, survived and endured for another millennium. But for the Western territories, it was the beginning of a painful period of social unrest, economic ruin, civil strife, rampant warfare, chaos, and the collapse of many erstwhile institutions of the preceding centuries.

THEODORIC THE GREAT AND THE OSTROGOTHS

Odoacer, the conqueror of Rome, was in turn defeated in A.D. 493 by another Germanic chieftain, Theodoric (c.A.D.454-526) King of the Ostrogoths, who had been appointed and sent as Consul to Italy by the Byzantine emperor, Zeno. Odoacer surrendered to Theodoric near Ravenna and was executed. So unceremoniously ended the life of the man who gave the *coup de grace* to the Roman Empire of the West.

King Theodoric then severed his ties with the Eastern Roman emperor, Zeno (reigned, A.D.474-491), and went out on his own to conquer Italy, becoming known in history as Theodoric the Great. His long rule was relatively beneficent, aided perhaps by the fact that he respected the vestiges of the erstwhile Roman institutions and restored law and order in Italy.(10,24) Yet, he allowed Boethius (c.A.D.475-525), the Roman philosopher and statesman, to be falsely accused of treason and executed in A.D.525. Boethius' *Consolation of Philosophy*, a treatise on ancient music, was written whilst he was imprisoned and awaiting execution. Boethius' work was considered "the unquestioned authority on Western music for many centuries."(7)

Eventually, a *novus ordo* emerged out of the chaos. The birth of a feudal society with the reimposition of law and order, the rise of monasticism, the strengthening of Christianity and spirituality, which were to be the new order and guiding principles of Europe during the ensuing Dark Ages. Yes, in time we would witness the resumption of an orderly Christian and spiritual tradition, the seeds of which had been sown in the fertile minds of the Germanic invaders during the decline of Rome. Many of the Germanic conquerors, in fact, had embraced Christianity before their final onslaught.[85]

Of singular importance to us during this time was the growth of monasticism and the birth of monastic medicine, which saved and preserved, albeit in rudimentary form, some of the medical knowledge of the Græco-Roman world, medical knowledge which, as we shall see later in our narrative, would in time blossom to fruition during the Medieval period and Renaissance.

[85] Although many of the Germanic barbarians followed the creed of the Arian heresy at this time, many later embraced Roman Catholicism. *Arianism* was the Christian heresy expounded by the Alexandrian priest, Arius (c.A.D.256-336), which maintained that Jesus was neither divine nor human, but a supernatural being. The heresy was condemned both by the Council of Nicaea in A.D.325 and the First Council of Constantinople in A.D.381.(7)

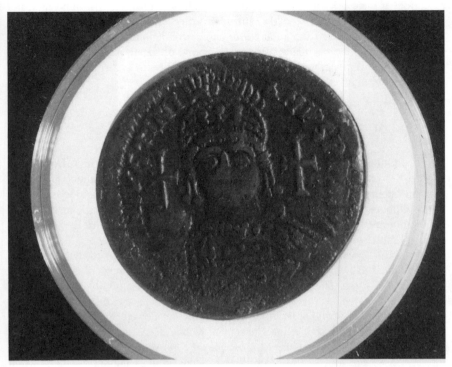

Plate 17 – Justinian I, "the Great" (A.D.527-565) in full military regalia. He holds a shield in his left hand and a globe surmounted with a cross in his right hand. Large bronze follis. Author's private collection.

CHAPTER 17

JUSTINIAN AND THE BYZANTINE EMPIRE

Although Constantine the Great was not strictly a Byzantine ruler, for he ruled over both Western and Eastern Roman Empires, he nevertheless founded and moved his capital to Constantinople, at the site of the ancient and sleepy village of Byzantium in Thrace, which later lent its name to the remaining Eastern Empire: the Byzantine Empire.

The Roman Empire of the East, referred to as the Byzantine Empire (or the Eastern Roman Empire) with its capital centered in Constantinople, survived and continued the tradition of the Roman Empire in a different form and in a different direction. For one thing, as time passed, the Eastern Roman Empire became more and more Greek and less and less Roman. It also became more of a grandiose citadel than a vast empire. Even so, the Eastern Roman Empire would last another thousand years (until 1453), and would remain the bastion of Orthodox religion, a guardian of sorts for European civilization, as it presented a formidable obstacle to potential military incursions into Europe by ambitious Eastern potentates.

Of all the Byzantine rulers, in my estimation[86] Justinian towers head and shoulders above the others, despite the fact that his reign spanned one of the most difficult and calamitous periods in the known world, the inauspicious 6th Century A.D.

THE REIGN OF JUSTINIAN

Character is a long-standing habit.
> Plutarch (c.A.D.46-c.120)

In A.D. 525, Justinian (emperor of the Eastern Roman Empire, A.D.527-565) assumed the title of *Caesar* (under Diocletian's Tetrarchy, a "sub-emperor"). His reign began two years later with his ascension to the rank of *Augustus*. But even before that, the clever and young Justinian had frequently advised his uncle, Byzantine Emperor Justin I (reigned,A.D.518-527), regarding matters of state.

Justinian's reign was seemingly destined for glory as he assumed the appellation of Emperor of the Eastern (Byzantine) Roman Empire. Beside him, at his coronation, was his wife, Theodora, a former actress and daughter of the animal-keeper of the imperial menagerie. Accounts to the effect that "she used a number of beastly men as stepping stones between her father's animals and the throne"(78) was likely slander spread by the Byzantine court historian, Procopius (d.A.D.565), who wrote scandalous histories about the imperial family and held extreme animosity toward the empress.(79)

Theodora not only married Justinian, but was crowned *Augusta* in her own right. In her own time, she was reputed not only to have been brave, intelligent, and beautiful but also to have been the great power behind the throne, at least

[86] Constantine the Great is not included in this estimation.

in the early years of Justinian's rule. As Panati declares, "it should have been a reign of imperial splendor, and it began that way. Justinian erected magnificent buildings, fortified his territories with chains of castles, recruited excellent armies of skilled pikemen and bowmen, and his code of laws, which embodied those of ancient Rome, would be the basis of European justice."(80)

Theodora was Justinian's principal adviser, and together, they mastered the ways of the slow-moving bureaucratic government of Byzantium and dealt with the courtly intrigue of their stately palaces and royal domain.(81) Throughout her life, Theodora remained active in social, political, and civic Byzantine affairs, exerting considerable influence in legislative reforms such as those dealing with the status of women and their civil rights.(22)

Justinian, energetic and always calculating, soon became a formidable and outstanding emperor, and his greatest achievements were accomplished in the earlier portion of his reign (for reasons that, as we shall discuss, were beyond his control). Public-minded, he gained a reputation for his hard work employed in domestic projects and his indefatigable energy given to building and construction within the empire. In or near his capital at Constantinople, Justinian built impressive monuments attesting to his building passion: fortresses, monasteries, and churches including the awe-inspiring Cathedral of Hagia Sophia in Constantinople, still standing, majestic and resplendescent, in Istanbul today. He also stamped out corruption in the bureaucratic government and stimulated commerce throughout the empire.(80)

Concerned with the security of the empire first and with the expansion of Byzantine rule second, Justinian's armies, under his two capable generals Belisarius (c.A.D.505-565) and Narses (c.A.D. 548-559), relentlessly castigated the horde of Germanic barbarians who had congregated on the outskirts of Byzantium, or those who were descendants of the tribesmen who had overrun Rome and settled in the erstwhile territories of the then defunct Western Empire. Justinian then set to the daunting task of reconquering the old empire and punishing the barbarians. What is even more amazing is that he was largely successful. He reconquered major portions of the old empire including regions of North Africa where, as you would remember, the Vandals under King Gaiseric had settled decades earlier (after their urge for sacking, pillaging, and plundering had been satiated). The Vandals were crushed in A.D.534 by Justinian's forces led by Belisarius, and North Africa was expeditiously reconquered.

Likewise in Italy, Justinian's armies also fought and defeated the Ostrogoths (East Goths) who had settled throughout the Italian peninsula after their largely successful earlier years of conquest under their capable king, Theodoric the Great. Belisarius defeated the Ostrogoth armies in several battles, reconquering Naples, then Rome (A.D.536), then Milan, and finally Ravenna in A.D.540, the Ostrogoths' seat of government. Then Narses squelched an Ostrogoth revolt led by their last king, Totila (reigned, A.D.541-552), and subdued the rest of Italy.(7) Not only had the Italian peninsula been reconquered, but the Ostrogoth kingdom had been effectively erased off the maps of Europe. Justinian pursued the barbarians up to Spain and even recaptured parts of the Iberian peninsula from them.

Of the Germanic tribesmen who had penetrated Roman defenses and sacked Rome during the preceding century, only the Visigoths (West Goths) seemed to have escaped the wrath of Justinian's armies. They settled far beyond the

Pyrenees, became Christians, and merged with the native Spanish population restricting themselves to the Iberian peninsula. The Visigothic kingdom survived until the spectacular Islamic conquests by Moorish troops in A.D.711.(1,7,45,80,82)

Despite these glorious and spectacular conquests, Justinian's greatest and most lasting achievement was the codification of Roman laws into his *Code of Justinian*. Recognizing that for justice to prevail law must not only be written but also clear to both the judges who interpret them and the people who must obey them, he set himself the task of compiling the Roman laws which had been evolving for over 15 centuries since the time of the great Republic and the revered *Twelve Tablets*. This was certainly no small task, considering that these laws included not only the venerable laws of the Roman Republic but also imperial decrees, senatorial statues, magisterial and judicial edicts, and even the added commentaries to the laws by the various Roman jurists of the ages.(1,7,12,22,78,81)

For this arduous, tedious, and scholarly legal task, he appointed the jurist, Tribonian, perhaps the greatest and most illustrious legal scholar of his day, and a committee of 10 jurists to study and assimilate this legacy of laws. The work was then assembled into a *codex*, which appeared in A.D.529 and was later called the *Code of Justinian* (or the *Justinian Code*).

The first part of the code, the *Codex*, also became the first part of the *Corpus Juris Civilis*. The second part of the *Corpus Juris Civilis* was the *Digest,* or *Pandects*, an edited summary of the collection of commentaries on the laws compiled up to that time. This second part was assembled by a committee of 17 who also worked under the direction of Tribonian. The third part, the *Institutes*, became a textbook for legal students and lawyers. This comprehensive *Corpus Juris Civilis* was revised and enacted into statute in A.D. 534. Finally, those laws enacted after the codex, and the legal supplements providing information about the new laws, were compiled as the *Novellae* and published after Justinian's death.(1,12,22,78,81)

This comprehensive body of Roman laws was centuries later available to medieval Europe and served as the legal foundation for European law. As early as A.D. 1100, the study of Roman law had been revived in Italian universities and served as a blueprint for the developing legal systems of continental Europe, whose countries are said to have civil-law systems, as opposed to the common-law system that is generally followed in English-speaking countries.

The *Corpus Juris Civilis* provided the raw material for the *Code Napoleon* which was proposed by Napoleon (1769-1821) in 1804 as the Civil Code of the French People. Nevertheless, the Napoleonic code, like the Justinian code, originated with the collection of existing laws. Moreover, the Napoleonic code was also influenced by the Enlightenment's concept of the laws of nature, as well as some of the principles and ideals of the French Revolution. The Napoleonic code, like Justinian's code, survived its creator to the extent that even as Napoleon's army withdrew from the faraway countries of Europe after being defeated on the battlefield or expelled from formerly occupied countries, the provisions of the code were retained, and formed the basis for the modern European legal systems.(1,7,22,78,80)

At the peak of his reign in A.D.540, after accomplishing major political, judicial, and military successes, Justinian's empire was struck by the old enemy of mankind, one that not even Justinian could conquer: pestilential disease. The bubonic plague, which struck with a vengeance in A.D.540, is justifiably the worst recorded pandemic to ever afflict humanity. Records regarding the dimensions of the devastation, suffering, and death were carefully kept by Justinian's chief archivist and secretary (none other than the court historian, Procopius), [87] whom we have already mentioned.

At the time that the horrible plague struck, Justinian was engaged in a war that was being waged fiercely on two fronts. We have already described the military feats of his armies as they battled the remnants of the Germanic tribes in the West. But during the years A.D.541 and 542, Justinian was also engaged in the East fighting the recalcitrant Parthians led by the Persian king, Khosru I (reigned, A.D.531-579).

If we think of the dimensions of the devastation of the bubonic plague of the 6th Century in the midst of the Dark Ages – the savage imperial wars waged against the barbarian hordes, the terrible famines, the ubiquity of death and destruction, and finally the full unleashing of the cataclysmic pandemic, the worst pestilence the world has ever seen – it should not be difficult to find within man's psyche invocations against the full horror and conjurations in the face of the surrealistic visitations of the dreaded Four Horsemen of the Apocalypse, as described in the biblical book of *Revelation.*

Justinian, defeated by the cataclysm, realized that the bubonic plague was a new and unconquerable enemy, an enemy that was demolishing his once invincible armies and killing his generals faster than the wounds inflicted on the battlefield by his mortal enemies. Demoralized and disheartened, he returned to his capital, Constantinople, only to find that there too the terrifying pestilence was relentlessly killing his people, rich and poor, regardless of kinship or station in life. The mortality in the city at this time was approaching 5,000 deaths a day and would eventually reach an all-time high of 10,000 deaths daily.(80) In despair and in need to fill the void, Justinian sought solitude, and the comfort and solace of religion.

THE BUBONIC PLAGUE OF THE 6TH CENTURY

And I looked, and behold, a pale horse; and his name that sat on him was Death.
Revelation 6:8

The bubonic plague is caused by the virulent, pathogenic bacterium, *Pasteurella pestis,* transmitted generally by the black rat, *Rattus rattus.* The plague is passed from rat to rat by fleas. Man becomes infected when he unwittingly interrupts the infectious cycle by being bitten by an infected flea.(80,83,84)

Since the fall of the Western Roman Empire, there have been three major bubonic plague pandemics which decimated large segments of the population in the continuous Eurasian landmass, and usually North Africa as well, not just because of its geographic proximity and geopolitical continuity via the Middle East cultural bridge but also because of its close commercial ties with Europe. [88]

---

[87] Procopius' scurrilous chronicles, *Secret History of Procopius,* should be considered in a different light than his more sober histories and scholarly firsthand accounts contained in his masterpiece, *Procopius' History of His Own Time.* The latter contains priceless information about the plague that assailed mankind during his time, the Plague of Justinian.
[88] For the record, the epidemic that lashed at most of the known world in A.D.166 during the reign of Marcus Aurelius was probably not the bubonic plague, but more likely smallpox.(85,86)

The death toll from these three devastating pandemics is today, for most of us, incomprehensible. These pandemics were: the Plague of Justinian (6th Century A.D.), the Black Death (14th Century A.D.), and the Bubonic Plague (1665-1666; also known as the Great Plague of London) which coincided with another catastrophe, the Great Fire of London. Although these three pandemics have been estimated to have resulted in approximately 137 million dead, Panati reminds us that these cataclysmic pestilences took place in a world that was much more sparsely populated than it is today.(80)

To make matters even worse, one must also remember that these pestilences assailed and ravaged mankind at a time when the average life-span was short – less than two decades during the Middle Ages.(85) Humanity deemed pregnancy itself with great trepidation, because the natural act of childbirth carried a frighteningly high mortality for both mother and baby, a mortality comparable to a serious illness. Survival to age 5 was a miracle not only because of endemic disease, dirt and filth, concomitant poor hygiene and sanitation, but also because of the primitive state of medical knowledge. Pestilential disease thrived under such conditions and inauspicious environments. Moreover, during the Middle Ages, bathing and cleanliness, even in the upper classes, was a rarity because of ignorance. These salutary activities were believed to be unhealthy, as well as irreverent – acts of vanity in the face of God.(85)

But let us now return to the pathophysiology of the bubonic plague: Once the infection takes place, *Pasteurella pestis* causes the Black Death by septicemia (blood poisoning), or death may be caused by the pneumonic form of the plague, another ominous presentation of the disease. In the highly contagious pneumonic form, the disease is transmitted directly from person to person via the pulmonary (aerosol) route.

The predominant form of the disease, though, was the bubonic form, characterized by severe involvement of the lymphatic system with the formation of *buboes*, from which the disease takes its name. The buboes are swollen, infected lymph nodes most commonly involving the inguinal and/or the axillary lymph node chains. The buboes may grow to a significant size to erode through the skin and spontaneously burst, draining infectious purulent material. In pneumonic cases of the plague, it was said that one day a person would cough-up phlegm and then be dead by the fifth day. With the predominant (more subacute) bubonic form of the plague, the disease resulted in buboes, and the clinical course was characterized by painful, swollen, purulent, and draining lymph nodes, and a slower and more agonizing death. Very few so afflicted lived beyond 10 days with this pestilence, which carried a mortality of 90 percent.

The pandemics of bubonic plague were veritably history's greatest scourges. In the case of the first (and worst) pandemic, which occurred during the reign of Byzantine Emperor Justinian and Empress Theodora, the epidemic furiously ravaged the population for five decades between A.D.540 and 590, and caused an incomprehensible fatality rate estimated at 100 million deaths.(80) The Black Death of 1346 to 1361, which inflicted morbid devastation and rampant desolation along with pestilential disease and death in medieval Europe, exacted a death toll of perhaps 27 million lives and lasted 15 to 20 years; whilst the Great Plague of London, which assailed England from 1665 to 1666, at its peak killed 2000 Londoners a week and mercifully only lasted several months.(80,85)

Therefore, the worse epidemic was certainly the one which occurred during the reign of Justinian. That epidemic lasted longer, killed the most people, and caused the most destruction, giving a new, unintended meaning to the term Dark Ages. At the height of the Plague of Justinian, the mortality from the disease reached such high proportions that the traditional and religious practice of "individual graves had to be abandoned" in favor of mass graves which, in any event, "could not be dug fast enough."(80) Thus writes Procopius as recorded in Panati's book, *Extraordinary Endings*: "To accumulate the corpses, Justinian ordered that roofs be removed from the towers and forts and that the towers high columns be stacked with bodies. When no more corpses could be crammed in, lye was poured down the shaft and the roof replaced. Once all fort towers were filled, ships were loaded with the mounting dead, rowed out to sea, and abandoned or set ablaze."(80)

During the Plague of Justinian, entire villages and towns were obliterated and the apocalyptic visitation was considered divine retribution from God as punishment for worldly sins. Justinian himself withdrew from public affairs and in solitude immersed himself in the study of theology.

The plague of the 6th Century marred the otherwise glorious reign of Justinian. It was the bubonic plague that prevented Justinian, the scourge of the barbarians, from consolidating the military gains of his foreign policy. As you would remember, he had eradicated the Vandal's kingdoms in North Africa (their remnants were absorbed by the native populations), and the Ostrogoths were driven into historic oblivion after he forced them beyond the Alps.

Even Justinian's judicial reforms were interrupted by the horrible plague, which, incidently, was believed to have started in Egypt, then to have spread via merchants to Palestine. Ultimately, it reached Byzantium via itinerant scholars who likely came to Constantinople from Alexandria or Antioch. Nevertheless, despite the plague, Justinian was able to complete his most important and durable project: He was able to compile his code of laws dating back to the Roman Republic which centuries later would form, in part, the basis for European civil law.

It is ironic that the learned physicians of Justinian's day, who at the time followed the precepts of Græco-Roman medicine, were discredited "since their notions and nostrums proved useless at a time when they were most needed."(80) Instead, the people turned for consolation, mercy, and even healing to monastic medicine and the teachings of Christianity. The Christian church did rush in, and as best it could, tried to fill in the medical void. The monks in the monasteries quickly became the spiritual, as well as corporeal, healers by tending both to the needs of the soul and the requirements of the body. With the failure of Græco-Roman medicine, they used prayer and only the rudiments of physical or herbal medicine. This new episode in medical history, appropriately referred to as monastic medicine, will be discussed in great detail in Part Six.

Unfortunately, medicine regressed, and disease in general was again equated with vice and sin, rather than with filth, poor hygiene, and natural causes. In some cases, natural causes did correspond to vices from a medical standpoint (as we very well know today), and perhaps even to sin (if examined from a purely theologic perspective), but further moralizing is, nevertheless, beyond the scope of this discussion.

Of one thing we can be sure, and that is that the humbling of the medical profession, as a result of its impotence to control or to do anything that could medically control or eradicate the apocalyptic pestilence of the 6th Century, essentially halted the advancement of medical knowledge for centuries.

But in the ensuing centuries, medicine would not be alone in its abeyance. It along with the other previously advanced professions such as law, engineering, and the natural sciences, not to mention the liberal arts contained in the Greek and Roman classics, were all but forgotten, erased, so to speak, from the collective memory of humanity. All areas of human endeavor were doomed to intellectual dormancy. Progress stopped. The turning wheels of Western culture and civilization had ground to a shrilling halt.

Humanity was now fully immersed in the midst of the Dark Ages. New hordes of barbarians were marauding and ravaging the West, whilst the plague was humbling the East. With the Plague of Justinian, the Dark Ages had now, in effect, once and for all closed the curtains of human progress upon the stage of Western civilization.

PART FOUR: GRÆCO-ROMAN MEDICINE

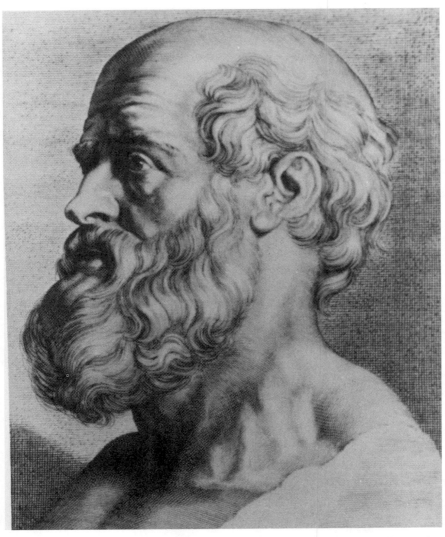

Plate 18 - Hippocrates (460-370 B.C.), as envisioned in an engraving by Paulus Pontius (1603-1658). National Library of Medicine, Bethesda.

CHAPTER 18

THE LEGACY OF HIPPOCRATES

The art and science of medicine in Græco-Roman times – from the Golden Age of Greece through the golden ages of Rome and up to the period of a hint of decline of the Western Roman Empire (the late 2nd Century A.D.) – was exemplified by two renown and illustrious Greek physicians, Hippocrates of Cos and Galen of Pergamon, and two Roman *medici,* Celsus and Scribonius Largus.

We have discussed Celsus in the context of the Hellenistic to Roman transition, and Scribonius Largus will be discussed at length in the section on Græco-Roman medical ethics. That leaves us with two ancient and venerable physicians that will be discussed at length in this section: Hippocrates (Classical Greece) and Galen (Roman Empire).

HIPPOCRATES – THE MAN AND THE FOUR HUMOURS

Primum non nocere (first do not harm).
        Hippocrates

Hippocrates of Cos (460-370 B.C.), the "Father of Medicine," is credited not only with the famous code of medical ethics but also with the judicious and novel concept of combining judgment and experience in medical practice.(1) According to Greek legend, he was a descendant of Æsculapius, the god of medicine, and Hercules, the mythologic hero.

In his Hippocratic collection, the *Corpus Hippocraticum*, composed of over 60 books, Hippocrates and his followers described the etiology of diseases, signs as well as symptoms of illnesses, and thoroughly documented clinical observations and pathologic processes affecting their patients.(2) Hippocrates also discussed the Humoural Theory of diseases in which he propounded the concept that the body consisted of Four Elements: blood, phlegm, black bile, and yellow bile. These elements allegedly caused disease when the normal mixtures and arrangements became unbalanced in the human body. This imbalance in diseased states, for example, resulted in fever and prostration.

Hippocratic physicians also stressed the importance of the examination of the human body, body fluids, and secretions. They recognized that immobility was a prognostic indicator of the severity of an illness. Hippocrates himself paid considerable attention to the symptoms described by the patient and to the physical signs obtained from the medical examination.

According to Hippocrates, nature has medicative and healing powers. A good physician, therefore, assisted nature in restoring health. Hippocrates was a proponent of the Critical Day doctrine, which maintained that on certain numerically-assigned days from the onset of an illness, the role of the physician was supportive only. Yet in actual clinical practice, Hippocratic theory went further, asserting that the introduction of a morbid agent into the human body affected one or more humours, thus causing health imbalance and precipitating disease. To expel this morbid agent from the body, the physician needed to treat throughout "the period of crisis," assisting nature only when needed.

Hippocrates also proposed the doctrine of *Contraria-Contrariis-Curantur*.(3) This doctrine stated that a physician should do to the body the opposite of that which the disease itself causes or creates. For example, in dermatology, it meant the application of cold to hot areas and moist to dry areas to heal skin lesions. Perhaps Hippocrates' second most recognized and accepted principle, after his code of medical ethics, was the axiom that the human body has the inherent power to preserve and heal itself as well as to combat disease and its detrimental effects.

Arguably, his most important and notable contribution, as we have previously stated, may have been that of assigning to diseases natural rather than supernatural causes. The corollary was that the treatment of disease involved the appropriate natural remedy rather than the use of magic or the invocation of supernatural beings, which was the case in previous civilizations up to the time of the Ionian Greek philosophers and classical-age physicians.

Hippocrates is also credited for his conservative treatment of abdominal diseases by observation first, and when the course of the illness warranted it, by interventional methods such as surgery. Nevertheless, he believed that serious intestinal wounds were uniformly fatal. He described the clinical sign known today as the Hippocratic sound, "audible splashing noise with a bouncing palpation over the distended abdominal area secondary to intestinal obstruction."(4)

According to the medical historian Harry Bloch, Hippocrates taught "that water and sunshine blended together in the human body to produce the most healthy of conditions."(5) He was therefore one of the first to believe in the beneficial effects of the solar rays. Perhaps as a result of his teachings, the later Romans "indulged in sunbaths in their solaria (Heliosis) which was followed by cold sponging," to preserve and improve their health. According to Bloch, the Roman physician, Caelius Aurelianus (fl. 5th Century A.D.), "prescribed sunbaths for a wide range of diseases. Romans named the spring water in Bath, England, *Aquae Sulis*, for the water brought health to those who drank it. Both Greeks and Romans linked mountain streams to aqueducts that extended over long distances to assure contact of the water with the sun and air before the water reached their cities."(5)

THE CORPUS HIPPOCRATICUM

The collective works of Hippocrates, the *Corpus Hippocraticum,*[89] was compiled in Alexandria around 300 B.C. and, as previously mentioned, it is characterized by the epochal proposition, the novel idea, of disease causation as the result of ascertainable natural phenomena, not abstruse supernatural forces – a giant step forward in medical history, indeed. Moreover, it followed by logical inference, that the conquest of disease was within man's reach by the judicious use of natural remedies and treatments, rather than by the invocation and intervention of a myriad of deities residing on Mount Olympus and environs, not to mention the

---

[89] The Hippocratic collection includes such treatises as the *Hippocratic Oath, Law, Decorum, Precepts, Prognostic, Epidemics* – all of which have extraordinary passages still relevant today.

Underworld, whence they brought about unpredictable supernatural phenomena.

Yet despite all of his accomplishments, Hippocrates is best known for his code of medical ethics. Indeed, even the layman knows that the Hippocratic Oath remains the bedrock of medical ethics – 2,500 years after its proclamation by Hippocrates and his followers during the 4th and 5th Centuries B.C. Here is the celebrated Oath:

> *I swear by Apollo, the physician, and Æsculapius and Hygeia and Panacea and all the gods and goddesses that, according to my ability and judgment, I will keep this oath and stipulation: To reckon him who taught me this art equally dear to me as my parents, to share my substance with him and relieve his necessities if required: to regard his offspring as on the same footing with my own brothers, and to teach them this art if they should wish to learn it, without fee or stipulation, and that by precept, lecture, and every other mode of instruction, I will impart a knowledge of the art to my own sons and to those of my teachers, and to disciples bound by a stipulation and oath, according to the law of medicine, but to none others.*

> *I will follow that method of treatment which, according to my ability and judgment, I consider for the benefit of my patients, and abstain from whatever is deleterious and mischievous. I will give no deadly medicine to anyone if asked, nor suggest any such counsel; furthermore, I will not give to a woman an instrument to produce abortion.*

> *With purity and holiness I will pass my life and practice my art. I will not cut a person who is suffering with a stone, but will leave this to be done by practitioners of this work. Into whatever houses I enter I will go into them for the benefit of the sick and will abstain from every voluntary act of mischief and corruption: and further from the seduction of females and males, bond or free.*

> *Whatever, in connection with my professional practice, or not in connection with it, I may see or hear in the lives of men which ought not to be spoken abroad I will not divulge, as reckoning that all such should be kept secret.*

> *While I continue to keep this oath unviolated, may it be granted to me to enjoy life and the practice of the art, respected by all men at all times, but should I trespass and violate this oath, may the reverse be my lot.*

As noted from the text, the first part of the Oath provides for the self-perpetuating apprenticeship system of learning, medical education and training, that characterized medicine as a learned profession, a profession that restricts its knowledge to the initiates and reserves its wisdom for the distinguished members of the sect. Unfortunately, secrecy led to suspicion of physicians through the ages by the lay public, an attitude that was reserved not just for physicians but for other professionals possessed of special knowledge; generally though, this suspicion was greatest towards physicians.

Those who currently support unrestricted abortion and many recent biomedical ethicists who militate for the so-called proper allocation of resources and the subtle rationing of health care (usually beginning with the elderly) by quoting classical writings in support of their liberal agenda should perhaps pay heed to the Hippocratic

Oath. Hippocratic physicians, as required by the Oath, generally repudiated abortion (except when the life of the mother was in danger or other extenuating circumstances, for the life of the mother was apprised above that of the unborn baby) and generally deemed abortion unacceptable medical practice. Needless to say, active euthanasia was strictly proscribed by Hippocratic teachings; otherwise the physician was only bound by this Oath to consider what was to the benefit of his patient. Although today one hears and reads a lot of mainstream media references (mostly inaccurate) about physician obligations to society, I have yet to hear or read a serious mainstream media piece ever reporting the Hippocratic Oath's stance on abortion, euthanasia, or the fact that physicians' obligations were restricted to their individual patients, not to society at large.

So, true to its Pythagorean influence, the Hippocratic Oath forbids abortion and euthanasia, but does not proscribe surgery. The Oath reflects the attitude of those Asklepiads who became followers of Hippocrates and who believed in specialization – an attitude which was also assimilated by the *physiks* and *medici* of Hellenistic and Roman times,[90] and later by the physicians of the Middle Ages – that Hippocratic physicians should not perform surgery which they were not trained to do and which required the skills of a specialized surgeon. The same situation held true and applied to cases of nephrolithiasis (urinary stones) which required treatment. Here again, the rationale was that since those cases required special expertise and since the doctor had the duty to advise what was best for his patient, he would turn over or refer those cases of urinary stones to surgical specialists who possessed the necessary ability and skills, as well as the versatility required, for the treatment of that specific malady.

So what at *prima facie* may seem inconsistent is clearly not.(6) The reference to the practice of surgery and urology was the recognition for the need and the creation of two surgical specialties that were not yet considered part of the House of Medicine. The proper interpretation of the Oath, therefore, requires Hippocratic physicians to refer their surgical cases to the surgical specialists adept in the surgical arts who were, only later, during the Renaissance (although their close relationship was noted during the Middle Ages), to join the physician's ranks.

The Asklepiads, followers of Hippocrates, maintained that "a physician should recognize the limitation of his knowledge and should have the courage to admit that he is ignorant of certain parts of the art." This formulation is consistent with other passages from the collection of Hippocratic writing, the *Corpus Hippocraticum*, which reads in part: "When a physician is uncertain as to the condition of a patient and is disturbed by the novelty of an affliction that he has never seen before, he should never be ashamed to call in other physicians to examine the patient with him...."(2)

Thus, as early as 2,500 years ago, Hippocratic physicians recognized that as medical science progressed, it would be difficult, if not impossible, to master all the accumulated knowledge, and therefore, unrealistic and unfeasible for a physician to be versed in all branches of the profession. Therefore, both explicitly and implicitly in their writings were the concepts of specialization, consultations, and appropriate referrals for the benefit of the patient, first; and for the advancement of the art, and science of medicine, second.

---

[90] The term doctor is derived from the Latin, *docere, doct*, which meant "to teach" – and it came to mean "learned," and thus, was given to physicians as the title for their degree in the medieval universities.

The term physician is derived from the Greek *physike*, which meant "knowledge of nature" and hence, *physiks* which later connoted the meaning of a medical doctor with philosophic rather than technical inclinations.

The term *medicus* is the Latin for "healer" and is derived from *medicina* and *mederi* which signified "to heal." The Roman *medicus*, on the other hand, later connoted a doctor with technical skills.

The Oath of Hippocrates is not the first document to propose a set of precepts of expected medical behavior and conduct. The Edwin Smith Papyrus was not only the first surgical text but also the first treatise to give specific advice with respect to both medical treatment and specific moral judgment, at least with regard to the treatment of traumatic injuries. Nevertheless, the Hippocratic Oath comprises the first set of precepts to formulate systematically a voluntary, self-imposed code of ethics – an edification of professional morality – unsurpassed in history.

As a guide to highly ethical and venerated professional conduct, the Oath also prohibits sexual relations between doctors and their patients – a situation perhaps even more applicable to psychiatrists and other psychotherapists. Failure to abide by this proscription has resulted in a plethora of ethical and legal problems in the modern age. The Oath also provides for ethical conduct in treating the ill and vulnerable, as well as protects patient confidentiality – noble concepts heretofore unknown in any other profession, except the clergy.

The medical historian Dr. Ilza Veith, who studied the *Corpus Hippocraticum* at length, reminds us of the importance of honor and the need for a physician in Græco-Roman times to remain above reproach. This ideal was not an abstraction but a truism for a member of a respected and learned profession, which at the time was "entirely free of legal supervision." For instance, in the Hippocratic tract, *Law*, it is stated, "Medicine alone in our states has been made subject to no penalty, except dishonour, and dishonour does not wound those who are compacted of it."(7)

The treatises *Decorum* and *Precepts* deals almost exclusively with physicians' behavior, etiquette, and expected medical conduct in and out of the patient-doctor relationship. For instance, in *Decorum*, we find the following advice:

> *As all I have said is true, the physician must have at his command a certain ready wit, as dourness is repulsive both to the healthy and to the sick. He must also keep a most careful watch over himself, and neither expose much of his person nor gossip to laymen, but say only what is absolutely necessary. For he realizes that gossip may cause criticism of his treatment. He will do none at all of these things in a way that savours of fuss or of show. Let all these things be thought out, so that they may be ready beforehand for use as required.(2)*

As Veith points out in *Precepts*, Hippocratic teaching gives prudent advice to physicians:

> *I urge you not to be too unkind, but to consider carefully your patient's superabundance or means. Sometimes give your services for nothing, calling to mind a previous benefaction or present satisfaction. And if there be an opportunity of serving one who is a stranger in financial straits, give full assistance to all such. For where there is love of man, there is also love of the art. For some patients, though conscious that their condition is perilous, recover their health simply through their contentment with the goodness of the physician. And it is well to superintend the sick to make them well, to care for the healthy to keep them well, but also to care for one's own self, so as to observe what is seemly.(7)*

In *Precepts*, Hippocrates discusses fees; this discussion is still relevant in today's ongoing debate regarding physician fees and health care costs. At least two major conservative think tanks, the Dallas-based National Center for Policy Analysis and the Washington-based Cato Institute, and in my own state, the smaller Atlanta-based Georgia Public Policy Foundation, all envision an ingenious and common sense approach to health care delivery: what I have called the *patient-oriented, free-market* approach which requires the doctor to fully discuss fees with his/her patients prior to rendering non-emergent care (i.e., before undergoing surgery or initiating drug therapy).(8) With this approach, physicians and their patients would discuss fees much in the same manner that physicians now discuss informed consent information prior to initiating any type of medical treatment. This practice is underscored by the fact that more than 90% of care rendered today by physicians is not emergent.(9)

This issue of medical fees and health care costs is a tremendously important and transcendental issue reaching to these modern times from antiquity. Today, everyone knows we are afflicted with spiraling health care costs. The way to control escalating medical costs is through the time-honored methods of free-market incentives which appeal to the sense of self-interest and personal responsibility inherent to the human species. Human nature is such that when individuals (including patients) act based on self-interest in the consumption of goods and services (e.g. medical marketplace), they act as prudent consumers, conserving resources of their own volition, and this behavior in the marketplace results in tangible benefits to the community as a whole.

Discussion of fees, then, between patients and their physicians must rely on age-old incentives, competition, personal responsibility, and free-market forces for the patient-consumer, tempered by the enlightened self-interest, virtue-based ethics, and civility of modern-day Renaissance physicians.(1) Only by instituting these historically-tested principles can we rein in health care costs whilst providing equitable access to health care without sacrificing quality and/or instituting overt or surreptitious involuntary rationing.(8,9,10)

According to the treatise, *Precepts*, fee discussions naturally will not be appropriate in those cases dealing with the very sick or critically ill – the 10% or so who enter the patient-doctor relationship on an urgent basis. This is the specific commentary regarding fee discussions with critically ill patients: "For should you begin by discussing fees, you will suggest to the patient either that you will go away and leave him if no agreement be reached, or that you will neglect him and not prescribe any immediate treatment. So one must not be anxious about fixing a fee. For I consider such a worry to be harmful to a troubled patient, particularly if the disease be acute....Therefore it is better to reproach a patient you have saved than to extort money from those who are at death's door."(7)

In *Prognostic*, Hippocrates discusses proper bedside conduct and gives physicians advice as to the proper way of discussing disease processes, diagnoses, and prognoses with patients, even to preserving one's own medical reputation in the face of treatment failures:

> For it is impossible to make all sick people well – that would be still better than foretelling the course of their illness. But men do, as a matter of fact, die; some through the severity of their disease, before the doctor is called in – some immediately, some living on a few days, others a little longer, before the physician can bring his art to bear on the illness in question. Hence we must show the nature of these diseases, how far they are superior to the bodily powers. In this way one will

justly gain a reputation and will be a good physician; one will indeed be better able to save those capable of cure if he has made up his mind long beforehand in each case, and no blame will attach to him if he has already foreseen and announced who is to die and who is to be preserved.(7)

In *Epidemics*, Hippocratic dictum declares that "the patient must cooperate with the physician in combating disease."(2) This is a harbinger for today's emphasis on patients taking charge and responsibility for their own medical care as consumers of health care – with the information and advice provided by their own physicians.

After careful analysis of the Hippocratic Oath and the other treatises of the *Corpus Hippocraticum* dealing with professional ethical behavior, Veith has deduced that "the picture of the ideal doctor that is given in these writings does not show him as saint or as a philanthropist but as a person who works for a living with dignity but without impulse to charity."(7)

The profession provided the Greek physician prestige, as well as a good life and an honorary status in his community. He worked hard for his patients and bore great responsibilities – namely, decisions regarding the life and death and well-being of his patients – but he was remunerated appropriately for his knowledge, efforts, and for the responsibilities he assumed. His services were handsomely remunerated both financially and emotionally, for the simple reason that his services were recognized and highly valued by an appreciative public.

Whether in pursuit of fame and fortune in a dignified profession or imbued with altruism to help their fellowmen in need, the fact is that the physicians' services were appreciated by a grateful community. Most physicians performed then, and do today, individual acts of personal charity [91] and self-sacrifice that were not (and are not yet) mandated by the state. Rather, these dignified acts were then, and still are today, humane acts inspired by true charity and compassion, a compassion that comes from the heart of a devoted professional and from professional fulfillment.

Special qualities were (and still are) inherent to physicians – viz, enlightened self-interest and virtue-based professional ethics which are imbued with the ideals of compassion and philanthropy, charity and humanitarianism. Physicians, of necessity, possess these qualities as unwritten prerequisites for performing the duties and obligations of a truly demanding, noble, and ancient profession.

[91] On this point, I differ slightly from Veith's view.

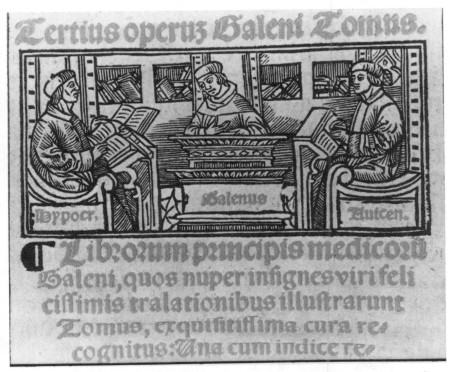

Plate 19 – Manuscript illustration showing Hippocrates, Galen and Avicenna, from an edition of Galen's works published in Lyons in 1528. National Library of Medicine, Bethesda.

CHAPTER 19

GALEN: PHYSICIAN PAR EXCELLENCE

[Regarding Galen] I have but one physician and he is a gentleman.
> *Marcus Aurelius (Roman emperor, A.D.161-180) after being treated successfully for a stomach ailment*

The most famous doctor was named Galenus (Galen). If one juggles the letters, one gets angelus, meaning an angel – and that is what every doctor ought to be.
> *Abraham of Santa Clara (1644-1709) a Viennese monk who extolled Galen's virtues as a physician in the care of the sick.(4)*

GALEN – THE MAN AND THE LEGEND

Claudius Galenus (Galen, A.D.130-200), a veritable medical giant of the 2nd Century A.D., devised a medical system which remained in effect, with very little modifications, for 1,300 years. About him it would be fair to say, that in the same vein as Aristotle who was considered "the Philosopher" during the Middle Ages, Galen should be considered "the Physician."(1)

As a young man, Galen studied in Alexandria which was still a center of learning, although by this time, the city on the Nile delta had lost much of its luster to the grandeur of Rome. After completing his studies, Galen returned to his home in the Ionian city of Pergamon, where, as a young physician, he was given an official post as physician to the gladiators – a job in which he excelled.(3)

Galen's success in Pergamon helped him to seek brighter horizons in Rome, the still shining city on the Palatine Hill, where he ultimately settled to practice medicine as a *medici*. By the age of 30, Galen had set up office in Rome, and learned and confident of his knowledge and intellect, he practiced ethical medicine at its best. In his spare time, he mingled with scholars, philosophers, other *medici*, and well-placed patricians, thereby establishing lasting friendships as well as creating some envious and jealous enemies, mostly within his own fraternity of physicians.(1,3,11,12)

An eclectic by nature, Galen led medicine back to the precepts of Hippocrates and away from the cults, sects, and political influences in which medicine had become enmeshed in those pivotal days of the Roman Empire. All told, he practiced medicine for over 40 years, encompassing the reigns of Antonius Pius (emperor, A.D.138-161), Marcus Aurelius (emperor, A.D.161-180), Lucius Verus (co-emperor, A.D.161-169), Commodus (emperor, A.D.180-192; Galen's office in Rome burned during the great conflagration of his brutal reign), and Pertinax (emperor, January-March A.D.193). Galen returned to Pergamon and died there during the reign of the great ruler Septimius Severus (emperor, A.D.193-211).(3)

Galen's anatomic knowledge is said to have surpassed that of the Alexandrian scholars Erasistratus (fl.c.250 B.C.) and Herophilus (335-280 B.C.), the noted physiologist and anatomist, respectively. Roman law, however, did not permit dissections of the human body. Though Erasistratus and Herophilus have been credited with performing the first systematic human dissections and associated physiologic work, [92] it is also well known that after 150 B.C., human dissection was prohibited even in Alexandria, and the law was strictly enforced by Rome.(13)

Although Galen had ample opportunity to study the human body as physician to the injured gladiators during his sojourn in his native city of Pergamon, his experience with human cadaveric dissections was quite limited. Galen did mention in his writings one occasion in which he had an opportunity to dissect a human body – that of a corpse of a robber that he found lying alongside a highway. For the rest of his anatomic works, Galen relied on animal dissections, primarily apes and pigs. Because of this shortcoming, the paucity of cadaveric human dissection, it was inevitable that anatomic errors occurred and erroneous observations were made. These errors crept into his voluminous written works. The application of animal anatomy to human anatomy and physiology was to result, indeed, in great errors in medical knowledge that would unfortunately go uncorrected for 13 centuries.

Galen followed the natural philosophy of Aristotle. He believed in the hypothesis of the all-encompassing existence of the Four Elements: fire, water, earth, and air – which had been proposed by the philosopher Empedocles (c.490-430 B.C.) and accepted by Aristotle. These elements were associated with the all-pervasive Four Qualities: heat, moisture, dryness, and coldness. Galen also subscribed to the medical theory of the Four Humoural Principles of Hippocrates, with blood being the fluid *par excellence*. Each humour was associated with a principal quality, for example, blood is hot and moist. Lymph (phlegm in the Hippocratic tradition) is cold and moist. Yellow bile is hot and dry, and black bile is cold and dry. He also predicated that the majority of diseases resulted from an excess, deficiency, or alteration in the relative concentrations of these four fundamental humours and their qualities within the body.(1,3,11,13)

Like his medical and philosophic mentors of old, Hippocrates and Aristotle, Galen asserted that preservation of health depended on the harmony of the four humours and their four qualities. Perfect health was associated with a perfect equilibrium of these humours. But Galen went a step further, devising his Four Principles of Temperaments, namely the sanguine, the phlegmatic, the vilious, and the melancholic. These temperaments or "idiosyncrasies" supposedly predisposed individuals to specific conditions or diseases. Moreover, for Galen, each disease required different treatment modalities, and specific remedies were given to purify the vitiated humours; purgatives were given to remove superfluous humours. In addition, the humours were subject to plethora. General plethora occurred when all four humours were in excess; local plethora occurred when there was excess of a single humour.(3)

Galen expanded further on symptoms of diseases and prognostic signs and developed the concept of *pathognomonic* signs of diseases. He was a strong proponent of the examination of the pulse for diagnostic as well as prognostic

---

[92] Nevertheless, the first human dissection is credited to the physician Alcmaeon of Crotona (fl.500 B.C.) who followed the philosophic teachings of Pythagoras and Empedocles.

purposes. He expanded on "the seat of the affection" concept, and thus, like Hippocrates, he stressed the importance of localization of diseases to the organs involved. He emphasized that the correlation of function and disease was imperative in medical practice. For example, micturition was a problem traceable to the bladder; abdominal distension, a problem of the bowels.

In clinical practice, Galen upheld the Hippocratic doctrines of crisis and critical days and the axiom of *Contraria-Contrariis-Curantur*.(3) In fact, in reviewing Galen's writing, most authorities agree that the majority of therapies formulated for specific diseases as well as for the preservation of health were in line with Hippocratic therapeutics.(1,3,11,13) Both Galen and Hippocrates stressed special diets, exercise, bathing and hygiene, massage, moderation in eating and drinking, and the promotion of excretion. Only as a last resort did Galen resort to blood letting. He was an advocate of blood letting only in moderation and only after carefully considering all the indications and contraindications. For example, he bled in cases of plethora, and the amount bled was always proportionate to the patient's constitution, temperament, and strength. He never bled children under the age of fifteen. He believed it was better to err on the side of insufficient blood letting than on the side of excess.[93]

Galen prescribed opium for sleep, pain relief, and diarrhea; otherwise, he prescribed few internal medications. He occasionally prescribed *Theriaca* (3), an interesting pharmacologic concoction whose origin deserves retelling here. According to our earliest information, Theriaca (also Theriac or Theriacum) originated as an antidote for poison developed by none other than King Mithridates VI of Pontus, who was, you will remember, Rome's recalcitrant arch enemy. Legend tells us that the belligerent King Mithridates led a precarious existence because of his many enemies. He therefore sought personal protection against potential assassination attempts by frequently consuming small amounts of poison so as to develop bodily resistance. And so it was, that after he was defeated by Pompey the Great and threatened by his own rebellious troops, his attempt to commit suicide by ingesting poison proved unsuccessful. He had developed immunity to the venom, and the poison was therefore ineffective. In imminent peril of capture, he finally ordered a trusted soldier to dispatch him with a sword.

After his death, Mithridates' antidote was "rediscovered" and used as Theriaca. The word itself is derived from the Greek for "wild beast"; it was coined by Nero's physician, Andromachus (fl.1st Century A.D.), after he added viper's flesh to the preparation. The recipe for this concoction varied from a mixture of several ingredients to what has been called a "pharmacologic monstrosity" that contained 50 to eventually 100s of ingredients.(15) The concoction was used as a panacea for a variety of illnesses over the succeeding centuries, up to the mid-1700s.(16)

It should not be left unsaid that Galen was not only a prolific writer who left the most voluminous body of writing in antiquity, but he was also a trained observer of nature and a compiler of knowledge. As Osler himself pointed out, "It was he who corrected the error of Praxagoras and Erasistratus – that the arteries

---

[93]The age of overzealous blood letting was yet to come, in the 17th Century. One final interesting observation speaking to the manifest resilience of Galenic medicine, in particular bloodletting and the careful examination of the pulse as expounded in the ancient writings of Galen, is the fact that these medical practices are still used today in the remote mountainous country of Bhutan in the Himalayas as reported in *National Geographic*.(14)

contained air and hence their name on that account." By experimentation, Galen showed that the arteries contained blood, not air.(17)

Not unexpectedly, Galen was also a successful and prosperous physician who was well compensated for his services (and thus disliked by some of his envious colleagues). He is supposed to have received 400 gold aurei (about $2,000) for a fortnight's attendance upon the wife of a wealthy man named Boethus.(17) For the "sin" of being prosperous in his medical practice and having wealthy patients as patrons, Galen has been maligned through the centuries, and for his teachings, labeled a dogmatist.

As if these charges were not harmful enough, Galen, who one would have expected to have been protected by the uncertainty of evidence and the profundity of time, has also been accused and inculpated for allegedly "fleeing the epidemic" of A.D.166. Nevertheless, before I address this contentious issue, I would like to discuss two related items which I have previously mentioned in passing, but are worth recounting at this time.

First, is the influence of contemporary philosophy on the judgment that we render writers of antiquity. It seems that, more and more, we tend to judge ancient writers by the standards of our own age. For instance, such physicians as Paracelsus (1493-1541) – whose philosophy of non-conformism and contumacy is today modish with the prevailing zeitgeist of liberal ideology – have been judged quite favorably by current standards; whereas, others such as Galen – who embodied the spirit of what was best of the predominant ideas and institutions of his time – is today labeled a dogmatist, whilst being judged unfairly and harshly by current standards.

Second, is the issue of physicians' behavior during epidemics. Though it is true that many physicians throughout the ages have been accused of running away from epidemics, fearing contracting pestilential disease both as acts of self-interest and naked self-preservation, it should be emphasized that the vast majority of physicians (notwithstanding the wearing of elaborate protective masks and robes to ward off disease) did participate with perseverance and courage in the treatment of the afflicted.(18-20) Nostradamus, Chauliac, Chekhov, and Copernicus, to mention but a few, all participated courageously in the treatment of the sick whilst risking their own lives during the dreadful epidemics of their times.

Moreover, during epidemics there have been physicians readily available to take care of the sick, except in those instances where there were no physicians left alive to treat survivors, as was the case of Greek physicians during the Peloponnesian Wars (431-421 B.C.).(21)

Regarding the old assertion that Galen "is notorious for having fled the plague in Rome in A.D.166," a recent writer quotes Galen: "having sojourned three years in Rome, the great pest beginning, I hastily set out from the city going eagerly to my native country."(22) With this alleged admission, understandably to some extent, his critics believed that he had been caught *flagrante delicto*. And this quotation, no doubt highly incriminating at first glance, nevertheless, should be closely analyzed. As it turns out, one of the main sources from which this quote has been extracted and recently popularized, is the scholarly article by medical historian Dr. Joseph Walsh written in 1931 entitled, "Refutation of the Charges of Cowardice Made Against Galen." This well-known work by Dr. Walsh as the title implies, vigorously defended and, in my view, justly exonerated Galen of the infamous charges.(12,18)

With sound scholarship, Walsh showed that Galen actually left Rome *before* the epidemic had become manifest there and argued that even if he had known of the coming epidemic, there was as much of a chance of the epidemic reaching Pergamon, his native city (already in the path of the epidemic) and to which he [Galen] allegedly "fled," as of it reaching Rome. According to Walsh, this widely quoted statement was taken from a catalogue of Galen's work at the request of a favorite pupil, Bassus, two years before Galen's death, and has been wrongly interpreted despite all the known facts of the case.(12)

Walsh explicated why Galen left Rome: He was exhausted from fighting the many rivalrous sects of physicians (including the troublesome Thessalian methodists) whose enmity he had aroused for many reasons but predominantly because of *professional jealousy*, that timeless malady which has afflicted the House of Medicine throughout the ages. Also, Galen's call for the return to Hippocratic medicine, higher ethics, and higher standards of learning was detested by the quacks he wanted to weed out of the practice of medicine in Rome.(1,3,11,12)

Instead of the aforementioned and widely quoted statement, Walsh explains: "He [Galen] left Rome where the epidemic had not yet begun and no one expected it, and actually went into the regions where it was already a menace." Walsh's authority is a work written 13 years after the pestilence assailed Rome, Kühn's *Galeni Opera Omnia* (Liepzig, 1821). And in Galen's own words, "When I understood the war was ended I set out immediately from Rome....Not long after Lucius Verus returned."(12)

The great pest of A.D.166-167 was brought back to Rome by the victorious armies of co-emperor Lucius Verus upon their return from the Parthian campaigns. The pestilence was probably smallpox. It decimated 25 million people near the acme of the Roman Empire, which at the time had an estimated population of 100 million inhabitants and an army of 375,000.(23)

Another author, the medical historian H.W. Haggard, in *The Doctor in History*, speculated that Galen went to Pergamon to help his native city, which would have been more in need of physicians than Rome at the time.(11) Moreover, there were probably more physicians to attend the potential victims of the plague in Rome than there were in any other city. And, I might add, two years later when Emperor Marcus Aurelius, who was battling the Germanic hordes, ordered Galen to join the army at Aquileia where a plague was decimating the Roman army more effectively than the Germanic tribes, Galen left immediately and joined the army to treat those afflicted. The pious Emperor Marcus Aurelius later fled to Rome with his adopted brother, the co-emperor Lucius Verus (who died of the pestilence on his way to Rome)(24), whilst Galen stayed with the army at Aquileia. Walsh correctly opines that this act is "hardly the act of a deserter."(12)

Galen also served under Commodus, Pertinax, and Septimius Severus (during whose reign he died in A.D.200). I seriously doubt that a coward physician (which is what Galen would have been if he had "fled") would have survived the political intrigues of the time or the wrath of those tough and resilient Roman emperors!(18)

ST. LUKE AND DIOSCORIDES – TWO CONTRASTING PHYSICIANS OF THE 1ST CENTURY A.D.

Not all physicians have been properly recognized for their meaningful contributions to medical practice; others have been noted for their achievements in related areas of endeavor. The following two physicians, one a Christian saint, the other a pagan military surgeon, exemplify divergent views of physicians during the transitional period of the 1st Century A.D.

St. Luke (fl.1st Century A.D.) is by theologic tradition a physician as declared by St. Paul, "the beloved physician." [94] St. Luke is better known as one of the apostles, as a devout Christian leader, and as a biblical evangelist who was canonized by the early Christian church for his pious acts. He was born in Turkey and lived during the 1st Century A.D. at the time of Christ.

St. Luke was one of the 12 original disciples as well as the author of the third synoptic gospel of the New Testament [95] and the book of *Acts of the Apostles*, which relates to the early history of the Christian church and deals with the works of St. Paul and St. Peter.(26) He is considered the most literary of the New Testament writers. His account of Christ's ascension is believed to be based on contemporary eyewitness accounts.(27) St. Luke's works are thought to have been written between A.D. 80 and 100.

His famous admonition, *medici, cura te ipsum*, "physician, heal thyself" (Luke 4:23), has become an article of faith within the medical profession, as well as an admonition to return to the Christian ideals of morality. It is also an important nexus between the ideals of simple Christianity and the precepts of medical ethics, and a reminder of the limitations and vulnerability of physicians throughout the ages.

St. Luke, a gentile, accompanied St. Paul, the Apostle to the Gentiles, on his second evangelical journey to Rome. It is, therefore, not surprising that St. Luke's teachings were adopted by the early Christian church and accepted on faith.(26,27) Moreover, St. Luke's teachings of the Christian faith were augmented and fortified by the persuasive teachings and logical analysis of St. Augustine. St. Luke's teachings were also, incorporated into the logical arguments of the greatest of medieval theologians, St. Thomas Aquinas. In due time, the teachings of "the beloved physician" would become part of the New Testament, one of the four synoptic gospels of holy scripture, to help guide man in his eternal quest for salvation.

Pedacious Dioscorides (A.D.40-90) was a surgeon in Nero's army c.A.D.60.(16,28) He wrote and illustrated his magnum opus, *De Materia Medica*, the standard botanical illustrated reference which held grip on medical illustrations for 15 centuries.

In *De Materia Medica*, Dioscorides described 519 species of plants and herbs and their medical and pharmacologic usages. It was the product of years of diligent work compiling medicinal plants (as well as animal products and even minerals believed to have medicinal value), whilst serving the highly mobile Roman army in three continents during the expansive 1st Century A.D. Dioscorides' monumental work should have stimulated others to perform their own observations, data collection, and investigations in nature; instead it was merely copied and

---

[94] St. Paul, the Apostle to the Gentiles, has been said to be the most influential person in the development of the Christian church after Jesus.(25) A Jew, he was born in Asia Minor as Saul of Tarsus, the son of a Roman citizen. A zealous nationalist educated in Jerusalem, he approved of the martyrdom of St. Stephen. Called to suppress Christianity in Damascus in A.D.33, he was blinded by a powerful heavenly light and heard Jesus querying: "Why persecutest thou me?" Later, he regained his sight, was baptized in the Christian church, and became an arduous proselytizer for the new faith.(26) He would later be the most ardent proponent of Christianity and the most influential theologian in church doctrine.(25)

[95] This book also contains a unique account of the birth and boyhood of Jesus.

recopied. Because the book was copied so many times through the centuries, the illustrations were rendered useless for the practice of herbal medicine or as a source of information for botanical studies. The illustrations lost their informative and teaching value, and later assumed a more decorative function, appropriately used to adorn texts of botany or medical history.(1,16,28)

Dioscorides' botanical medical illustrations, which have been reproduced time and again, were accepted by succeeding scholars as uncontested facts and incontrovertible knowledge rather than verified by direct observation of nature or experimentation. His botanical and pharmacologic tenets were accepted as dogma despite the shortcomings of the later reproductions.(28) It is ironic that some of these aspects of secular medicine such as the pharmacopoeia of Dioscorides and Galenic medicine remained virtually unchallenged until the Renaissance, despite their failure to alleviate the ill and the suffering, either during the Plague of Justinian or during the recurrent pestilences of the Middle Ages, particularly the Black Death of 1346-1361. In both of these direful pandemics, medical remedies and herbal potions prescribed by Græco-Roman physicians failed to mollify suffering and death, and as we shall see, both had significant impacts on the course of history and the parlous fate of humanity.

CHAPTER **20**

THE CHAMPIONS OF CHRISTIAN THEOLOGY

Faith is the substance of things hoped for, the evidence of things not seen.
St. Paul

THE PHILOSOPHIC BASIS FOR MEDICAL KNOWLEDGE

A brief review of the major religions and moral philosophies of the East, insofar as their influence on medical practice, Western thought, and Judeo-Christian values, was given in Part I. Let us now touch upon the remarkable Christian theologians, those responsible for melding and reconciling Græco-Roman thought with Christian theology, from the time of the harrowing experience of the fall of Rome to the chaos of the Dark Ages and the doldrums of the Medieval period.

It is beyond the scope of this book to discuss the individual contributions of Jesus and St. Paul, the founders of Christianity, or Abraham and Moses, the founders of Judaism. But we will take this opportunity to discuss the leaders who had a pivotal role directly on our story, and whose importance will become clear henceforth.

Amongst the champions of Christianity stand tall the figures of St. Augustine and St. Thomas Aquinas. By sheer force of intellect and logical argument, they were able to integrate Christian thought into the evolving Western intellectual tradition as well as weave the Græco-Roman inheritance into the fabric of Judeo-Christian morality and the mores of the common people. Moreover, they were able to reconcile Christian dogma with the prevailing philosophies of their times, thereby militating, not only for the survival of Christianity, but assuring its ascendancy as the major religion of the West.

The strong moral arguments and commonality of the arguments of Christian ideas assured not only compatibility with the mores of the working classes but also with the upper classes. They included the very few intellectual elites (those few in the nobility who were l iterate and the clergy) who lived in the epoch just before the onset of (and during) the Dark Ages and extending through the years up to the end of the Medieval period.[96]

ST. AUGUSTINE

St. Augustine of Hippo (A.D.354-430) was the most influential theologian in the eclipsing years of the Western Roman Empire. In his philosophic and theologic writings, he effected a profound impact on the direction that Christianity

---

[96] The Dark Ages roughly incorporate the period from A.D.476 to A.D.1000, whilst the Medieval period can be categorized as the era beginning roughly in A.D.1000 to A.D.1400. This entire epoch comprises the Middle Ages.

would take in the closing days of the Roman Empire. Survival and consolidation of his ideas were ensured by the fact that 500 of his sermons, over 200 of his letters, and several of his books amazingly survived through the tumultuous fall of Rome and the throes of the Dark Ages up to the present day.

In what is perhaps his most famous book, *The City of God*, St. Augustine refuted the charge by some authorities that the Roman Empire's decline and presaged eventual collapse was a result of divine retribution against the Romans for the abandonment of Roman pagan religion and the formal adoption of Christianity by the Empire.(29)

In religious matters, the thrust of his arguments were on the importance of spiritual progress and the attainment of salvation via the infinite grace of God through the instrument of the Christian church on Earth. He reaffirmed the idea of original sin, the precept of predestination, the perversity of sex – all of these ideas coming from a man who had earlier led a worldly life and existence. It was St. Augustine who purportedly exclaimed, "Lord, make me chaste – but not yet," and wrote, "Love, and do what you like."(30) Obviously, he repudiated the indiscretions of his youth, repented, and converted to Christianity. St. Augustine later wrote about his former hedonistic life, including its trials and tribulations, in another theologic and literary masterpiece, *Confessions*.(31)

St. Augustine believed in the supremacy of spiritual power and the church over temporal matters and the state. As if to make sure that this belief would prevail, and perhaps even anticipating the chaos that was to come, he took pains to set the church on solid footing prior to his death before the gathering storm, the onset of the Dark Ages. St. Augustine accomplished this very difficult task by reconciling religious dogma with many of Plato's ideas and philosophy, thereby becoming one of the founders of Neoplatonism. Most importantly, his work provided a conduit for many worthwhile Græco-Roman theo-philosophic ideas which survived and later took root in medieval Europe.

St. Augustine's theologic ideas, together with the moral philosophies of Neoplatonism, provided the post-Roman, Western world an oasis of philosophic and theologic thought that would give people comfort, solace, and the much needed pabulum to help them survive in the desert of incertitude, turmoil, and chaos that befell the Western world during the Dark Ages, particularly in the 5th and 6th Centuries A.D.

At the time of St. Augustine's death at age 76, the Vandals were besieging his hometown of Hippo in North Africa. Within a few weeks of his death, the marauding Vandals finally overran the defending garrisons and captured the city. Hippo was pillaged and plundered, but miraculously, St. Augustine's library and cathedral were left intact.(25) St. Augustine's influence over medieval theologians, such as St. Anselm (1033-1109), St. Thomas Aquinas (1225-1274), and John Wyclif (c.1328-1384), and later such Renaissance protestant leaders as John Huss (1369-1415), Ulrich Zwingli (1484-1531), and John Calvin (1509-1564), was as enormous and powerful as it was self-evident and pervasive, in the writings of these eminent theologians.

St. Anselm

St. Anselm (A.D.1033-1109) also played an important role as a philosopher-theologian, bridging the gap of time between St. Augustine's Christian dogma and Neoplatonism, and St. Thomas Aquinas' scholasticism. St. Anselm, an Italian-born Benedictine monk, developed an ontologic argument in support of the existence of God, which no doubt later influenced St. Thomas Aquinas' theology. St. Anselm's ontologic proof deduced God's existence from man's conception of a perfect being possessed of all faculties, omniscient and omnipotent. He helped pave the way for St. Thomas Aquinas' teleologic approach to logic and the development of scholasticism.

Scholasticism, as you may well know, became the predominant philosophy of the late Middle Ages, and remained so at least until 1879 when Pope Leo XIII (pope, 1878-1903) enunciated that the system of scholasticism forged by St. Augustine, St. Anselm, and St. Thomas Aquinas was official Catholic philosophic dogma.(26)

St. Anselm became the Archbishop of Canterbury in 1093 and was canonized in 1494. His writings even influenced a leader of the Enlightenment, René Descartes (1596-1650), who used a similar logic and ontologic argument to prove the existence of God during the 17th Century, the "Century of Genius" that followed on the heels of the Renaissance.

ST. THOMAS AQUINAS

St. Thomas Aquinas (1225-1274) was, without a doubt, the greatest of medieval theologians. A Dominican friar, he was the most erudite scholar and prodigious writer of his age. In the controversy between the Realists and the Nominalists which raged in the Middle Ages, he was a moderate Realist who used orderly logic and common sense to solve abstruse philosophic problems. [97] He reconciled the conflict between the medieval Nominalist and Realists using the same teleologic approach that he had used to prove the existence of God. Similarly, he reconciled the teachings of Aristotle to medieval Christian faith.(33,34) Aquinas' synthesizing of Aristotle's natural philosophy and Christian dogma, along with his development of scholasticism, has been hailed as the greatest achievement of medieval philosophy.(26)

As we have seen, St. Augustine had already welded Christian scriptures to Neoplatonic thought at the dawn of the Dark Ages, and had helped pave the way for the Christianization of the denizens of the crumbling Roman Empire. St. Thomas Aquinas, always rational in his logic and scrupulous in his accounts, was also careful to cite the scriptures of St. Augustine in his monumental works, *Summa Theologica* and *Summa Contra Gentales*.(33,34) These works were veritable encyclopedias of medieval learning, thought, philosophy, and logic, all scholarly compiled. Aquinas believed that through faith, truths were directly revealed from God. He also asserted that when thinking is rightly and rigorously pursued, it confirms the truths revealed by faith. Therefore, if man arrives at a different conclusion from that of Christian orthodoxy, he must have used faulty logic. This was the main axiom of the tenets of the scholasticism of the Middle Ages. This teleologic concept of logic, also referred to as the Doctrine of Final Cause embodied in scholasticism, influenced Christian thought

---

[97] The Nominalists argued that concepts have no objective reality outside the mind and that only things and events exist objectively outside the mind. The Realists, on the other hand, asserted that universal ideas and concepts have an independent existence outside the human mind.(26,32)

through the late Middle Ages to the present age.(1,16,32,33)

St. Thomas Aquinas also forged the concept of the human body made up of a spiritual mind and a material body. The spiritual principle was an emanation from God, a ray of divine intelligence. Although he adapted Aristotelian philosophy to Christian dogma, as a moderate Realist he was always careful to distinguish faith from reason, not making one exclusive of the other.(1,16,32-35)

Despite the strength of scholasticism during the Middle Ages, there was no complete unanimity of thought even during the late Medieval period. As we have already mentioned, the controversy between the Nominalists and Realists seethed during this epoch. In the early Medieval period, a precursor to St. Thomas Aquinas, the French philosopher, theologian, and moderate Nominalist, Peter Abelard (1079-1142), who is also considered the founder of the University of Paris, held that the dialectic system of logic of Aristotle could be utilized to achieve truths of faith and universal truths, thus anticipating the theologic concepts and logical arguments of St. Thomas Aquinas.(26,32)

Abelard was the subject of one of the most tragic love stories and one of the most famous and poignant romances in the Middle Ages. Abelard, the most renown dialectician-philosopher of his age and teacher at the University of Paris, began a torrid love affair with a student, Heloïse. Their love was consummated in a secret marriage. Upon learning of this, Heloïse's uncle had Abelard emasculated by common thugs. Abelard, in profound despair, became a monk and secluded himself in the monastery of St. Denys. Heloïse became an abbess.(26,32) Abelard's writings were later considered heretical. In his final years, he retired to the monastery of Cluny, and "allowing no moment to escape unoccupied by prayer, reading and writing or dictation...in 1142, he died at the age of sixty-three."(32)

Then in the late Medieval period, the English reformer John Wyclif, an extreme Realist and follower of St. Augustine, attacked orthodox church doctrine and championed the people against the church. He was especially opposed to the liturgy of transubstantiation and maintained that the writings of holy scripture were paramount over church doctrine.(26,32)

And before the dissenter Wyclif, there was John Duns Scotus (1265-1308), a Scottish Franciscan theo-philosopher who rejected the doctrines of St. Thomas Aquinas (Thomism), asserting that faith was irreconcilable from reason (Scotism).(35) He believed that will, not reason or faith, was the ruling philosophic principle. He modified St. Anselm's ontologic arguments to predicate that the existence of God must be evinced from the experience of the senses.(26) In time, these divergent theologies would lead to an irreparable schism in Catholic church dogma and indirectly influence the events that set in motion the cascade that eventually resulted in the explosion of the Renaissance and the leviathan conflict of the Reformation.(1)

It was St. Thomas Aquinas' scholasticism, which reconciled faith and reason and explained observed natural phenomena, that led to a relatively smooth, philosophic transition to the early Italian Renaissance.(1,16) The same scholasticism that taught that observed natural phenomena could be explicated by known or assumed truths, also reconciled successfully the theory of the Four Humours with Christian theology, and provided needed stability during the transition.

THE CULT OF CHRIST THE HEALER

Before concluding this chapter on the Champions of Christian Theology, allow me to digress briefly to bring forth and discuss the cult of Christ the healer.

The Jewish communities, created after the diaspora c.A.D. 66-70, increased along the seashores of the Mediterranean and were well known for their moral and religious way of life. They were renown as well for their principles of charity in the care of the sick and the poor, and their belief in the ideals of the Good Samaritan in dealing with fellow human beings (Luke 10:30-35). Moreover, the fact that the Jews would not associate with pagan cults made their communities ideal for proselytizing Christians. Thus, it was amongst these God-fearing Jewish people that Christianity found many of its early converts during the 1st and 2nd centuries.(36)

The synoptic gospels of Matthew, Mark, and Luke contain a number of "miracles" performed by Christ; of these, in at least 13 of them, either sickness is cured, disability is healed, or the dead are restored to life. These medical miracles, as well as the affirmation by St. Luke, the physician, transferred the miraculous and divine healing power of Christ to his disciples: "He called the twelve together and gave them power and authority over all devils, and to cure disease." According to the medical writers Frederick F. Cartwright and Michael D. Biddiss, this power was later extended to the 70 disciples and followers of Christ, expanding the role of Christian leaders in the cult of Christ the Healer.(36)

To the citizens of the Roman Empire in the 2nd Century A.D., assailed by so many deadly pestilences (we have already discussed the pestilence of A.D.166-167, which continued endemically until A.D.180), Christianity offered the hope and comfort that could not be found in other exhausted creeds or cults, of which there were many within the Empire and its border states. In Christianity, there was the belief in miracles that could restore health to those with mortal illnesses, that could conquer death via spiritual and physical resurrection, and that could even promise ultimate bliss in a heavenly paradise for those sinners who earnestly repented.(36)

As the underground Christian church consolidated itself during the 3rd Century A.D., another horrendous epidemic broke out in A.D. 250, the Plague of Cyprian. St. Cyprian was the bishop of Carthage who presided over the mass conversions that took place at the height of that horrible epidemic, a true pandemic, which assailed the known world for 16 years. The Roman Empire was so shaken by this plague that the legions withdrew behind the natural frontiers of the Empire, the Rhine and the Danube, and Rome itself was fortified. It was said that the good Bishop and his North African priests were baptizing 200 to 300 people a day into the Christian faith during those ominous times. Thus was the growth of the Christian faith – unlike the secular Græco-Roman medicine practiced by the physicians of the time – accelerated by such natural disasters.(36)

As we have seen, with the inability of the Roman Emperors Decius (reigned, A.D. 249-251) and Diocletian (reigned, A.D.284-305) to eradicate Christianity, or Julian the Apostate (reigned, A.D.361-363) to reverse its ascendancy, Christianity grew deep roots within the Empire. Its message of hope and salvation became firmly entrenched, inveterate amongst the wistful and enduring population. Constantine the Great established Christianity as the state religion and

Theodosius the Great fortified its status by enacting laws against paganism, making the epochal permutations wrought by Christianity virtually irreversible within the Western world.

CONSEQUENCES OF THE CATACLYSMIC BUBONIC PLAGUES

We have already noted some aspects of the Black Death in earlier chapters (and it will be discussed in more detail in a later chapter), but I think it is appropriate to draw at this time a parallel between the consequences of the Plague of Justinian of the 6th Century A.D. and the Black Death of the 14th Century.

Just as the Plague of Justinian changed the population irreversibly, such that it in effect sealed the fate of the Western Roman Empire to extinction and rendered Græco-Roman medicine dormant for several centuries, the Black Death of 1346-1361 changed the English, and later, the rest of the Western European landscape. According to Cartwright and Biddiss, the feudal economic system disintegrated as indentured servants, serfs, and previously impoverished peasants became tenant farmers and land owners because of sheer depopulation of landed estates and farmlands.(36)

Moreover, the Christian church's inability to deal with the Black Death exerted a negative influence on the authority of the church; Cartwright and Biddiss note: "The remarkable grasp of the church upon Europe enabled Christianity to weather the storm, but the authority of the church did not survive the Black Death unscathed."(36)

Indeed, disenchantment and opposition to the church developed in the years after the horrible pestilence. Taking advantage of the different schisms and dissension already existing within the Christian church, John Wyclif, the noted English theologian, his pupil, John Huss of Bohemia, and later during the upheaval of the Renaissance, the priest Martin Luther (1483-1546) all questioned the "Holy Church's hitherto unchallenged power."(36) Whilst the Plague of Justinian reinforced Christianity (Græco-Roman medicine's nostrums had failed), the reverse occurred with the Black Death of the 14th Century (the church failed, and Græco-Roman medicine would later be rediscovered and revitalized, incarnated in the Renaissance physicians). The failure of religion to provide adequate physical or spiritual comfort during the Black Death pandemic may have provided the seeds that germinated into the Protestant Reformation. These rifts within the church, the unholy pestilences terrorizing humanity, and the advent of the rediscovery of the Greek and Roman classics all contributed to the cultivation of the soil that reaped the abundant intellectual harvest of the approaching Renaissance.

PART FIVE: GRÆCO-ROMAN MEDICAL ETHICS AND INTIMATIONS FOR THE PRESENT

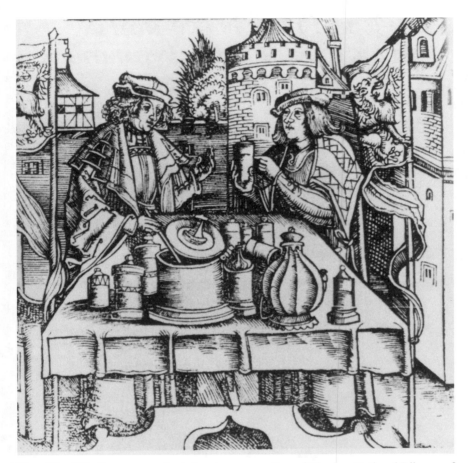

Plate 20 - 16th Century woodcut showing preparation of Theriac. National Library of Medicine, Bethesda.

CHAPTER 21

TRANSCENDENTAL QUESTIONS OF ETHICS

The little foxes that spoil the vines.
Song of Solomon 2:15

What is morality in any given time or place? It is what the majority then and there happen to like and immorality is what they dislike.
Alfred North Whitehead

THE EARLY GREEK STATE PHYSICIANS

During the 6th Century B.C., two generations before Hippocrates, Herodotus, the Father of History, described the well-organized public medical service already in existence in some of the Greek city-states. Plato also discussed the role of state physicians and their method of election by public assembly: "when the assembly meets to elect a physician...he was to serve for one year and when the year of office has expired...the physician has to come before a court of review...before he could serve another year."(1) To my knowledge, this process appears to be the first attempt in medical history by which competent physicians were elected to serve as public health officers in a process reminiscent of our present-day peer review. Elections of medical officers therefore appeared to be based on merit and competence. The existence of a selection process for state-physicians in the Greek city-states evolved and survived into Roman times. These state-physicians who served the public apparently were independent of the temples of the Asklepiads. They were well paid, secular, and held in high esteem in the communities in which they served. It is apparent from both the writings of Plato and Herodotus that there was keen but meritorious competition between distinguished physicians who wanted to serve in these public posts.(1)

Early Greek physicians of necessity were also philosophers, *physiks*; others were more prone to study the natural sciences and were more akin to the later day Roman *medici*. Greek physicians performed dissections early in their training to procure knowledge in anatomy and physiology, like the medical scientists in Alexandria of later ages. Yet as philosophers, Greek physicians sought basic truths and pursued arguments to reach logical conclusions about the nature of health and disease. So in this light, it is not surprising to find that the Greek physician Alcmaeon of Crotona (fl. 500 B.C.), credited with performing the first human dissection, and his colleague, Diogenes of Apollonia (who also performed elaborate human dissections) were not only esteemed anatomists and physicians – but also genuine philosophers who strove to find answers to the great questions of their day (i.e., the laws of nature and the nature of disease).(2)

The Greek philosophers, Socrates, Plato, and Aristotle all denied divination and asserted, just as Hippocrates had predicated, the view that rational explanations should be sought for the causes of diseases. They supported a rational explanation for the basis of Greek medicine and for the formulation of secular ethical principles. Yet, it must be noted that these great men of antiquity and their Stoic successors, as is implicit in their writings, all believed in a transcendental Higher Being.

In the case of Roman society, Pliny the Elder tells us that the Romans did not have professional physicians until approximately 220 B.C. when Greek physicians, many of whom were slaves, began streaming into Rome. For one thing, as we stated previously, Roman citizens considered medicine beneath their dignity, and thus they shunned medicine as a vocation. So until the time that medical practice became commonplace and generally accepted, the head of the family – the *Pater familias* –treated his family with folk remedies and sacrificial rites to specific deities, praising those associated with health and appeasing those responsible for disease.(3)

EARLY GREEK MEDICAL ETHICS

One of the earliest ethical accounts with regard to Greek medicine may be found in Homer's *The Iliad* (8th Century B.C.) which recounts the great courage displayed by the physician-brothers Podalirios and Machaon during the Trojan War. We also encounter questions of medical ethics in Herodotus' accounts of the Persian Wars (490-480 B.C.)(4), as well as in the unembellished historic accounts of the Greek historian Thucydides in his *History of the Peloponnesian War.*(5) It is in this last source that the reliable Thucydides describes the great epidemic that broke out in Athens in 429 B.C. in which the Athenian statesman Pericles (c.495-429 B.C.) perished. Thucydides writes, "so great a plague and mortality of men was never remembered to have happened in any place before. For at first neither were the physicians able to cure it, through ignorance of what it was, but died faster themselves, as being the men that most approached the sick."(5)

So here we have a profession which from the earliest of times had been pursued by virtuous men thirsting for knowledge and striving to heal the sick, which had been guided by enlightened self-interest, a profession which was now involved in the process of setting for itself ethical standards to be followed by its members. This was a remarkable, voluntary, and unselfish act by any profession in antiquity and unprecedented in history. These standards were set without coercion or intimidation from any government entity and were guided only on the basis of what was right and what was wrong, accepting both the "good" (the advantages) with the "bad" (the sacrifices). The "good" was the esteem and prestige conferred on Greek physicians, and more importantly, the value of the services provided by virtue of being a healer, possessed of the knowledge to alleviate pain and suffering, and postpone death, and yes, the financial rewards. Greek physicians were paid handsomely for their travails and responsibilities.

The "bad" part was not really bad at all, at least for those who had answered "a calling." From time immemorial, the ethics of Greek medicine required that when treating patients, the obligation of physicians was to place the patients' interests above their own, and for them to do their utmost to maintain and enhance the standards of the profession, to keep abreast of new philosophic arguments and new medical theories (and medical treatments) so as to be able to provide the best medical care and procure the most benefit for their patients. Even under the worst of circumstances, physicians were expected to maintain equanimity, uphold benevolence, and radiate compassion.

Historically, it has also been the inclination of physicians, even when poorly organized, to provide voluntary services to communities in direful times, in periods of crisis – such as in wars, pestilences, and other catastrophes – and to provide and deliver care to those in need, including charity care for the indigent and the dispossessed. But no where in Græco-Roman medicine was it obligatory for physicians to provide care without compensation or be so regimented as to become *de facto* servants at the disposal of the state. In Græco-Roman tradition, financial rewards and personal prestige went hand in hand with successful medical practices. A successful medical practice was expected to be associated with material success and personal prestige which, in turn, was commensurate with the degree of hard work, dedication, perseverance, and other qualities associated with compassionate and devoted physicians – as we have seen from the examples of Hippocrates and Galen.

As we shall see, it will not be until the rise of Christian asceticism in the Dark Ages and the advent of monastic medicine that the overlapping of the duties of the monastic monk and the Græco-Roman secular physician redirected the basis of medicine from an enlightened virtue-based paternalistic ethic of a learned and independent profession to an altruistic public-service directed deontologic ethic. Later, the medical profession would be further redefined as the roles of both physician-priests and lay physicians passed through evolutionary stages in the Middle Ages. Ultimately, medicine would separate from the priesthood and become a learned trade, initially as an apprenticeship in the guild system, and later with scholarship within the rubric of the medieval university. To the patient-doctor relationship, the Judeo-Christian tradition added the ideals of the Good Samaritan and charitable public service. During the phase of monastic medicine, the new ingredients of asceticism, austerity, submission, total self-effacement, and charity – all qualities expected of a Christian saint – were added to the already present components of individualism, philanthropy, humanitarianism, benevolence, and the compassion of ordinary human beings who happened to be endowed with these extraordinary qualities as well as possessed of special knowledge.

Despite the great demands imposed on physicians, they have managed to survive as members of a dedicated profession throughout the ages, because people recognized two important facts: First, that physicians, for the most part, have been devoted and compassionate human beings; and second, that the art and science of medicine has limits, limits perhaps set by nature, by the Creator, or by the limitations of ordinary human beings. It is time for the public to recognize these limitations as basic, simple, and eternal.

AN OBLIGATION TO TREAT?

In his monumental review of historic evidence on the question of whether there is a historic basis for the obligation of physicians to treat patients during pestilential diseases, Dr. Walter Friedlander, the renown medical historian and ethicist, found that historic evidence pointed to the fact that physicians have in general behaved properly and acted appropriately throughout the ages, for the most part acting as individuals, not as a monolithic group of self-entrenched, self-serving professionals.(6) Furthermore, he found evidence that physicians based their individual behavior and actions on their own ethical behavior, based on their own virtues, their own moralities and convictions, as well as their own self-interest. In his estimation, judged as a whole, the profession always has had its heroes and its villains (or cowards), but by in large, the virtues of the physicians succeeded in providing appropriate care during times of crisis, such as wars and plagues, for the rich and poor, for remote villages and urban areas, without the need for government intervention.(6)

Others have also found that care of the sick during times of plagues and pestilences has taken place by physicians, for the most part, by relying on the support and infrastructure provided by the business community. To solve the problems of medical care shortages even during times of plagues and pestilences, towns and communities relied, not just on professional "duties," but also on the proper free-market incentives to obtain the required medical services, as was the case with the town-guilds of the Middle Ages.(2,6-8)

In his scholarly treatise, Friedlander concludes, "this history of what physicians have done when faced with mortal risks and the care of patients goes back at least to the time of Hippocrates....Some physicians have avoided and others have accepted the risks...[of treating patients during deadly epidemics]....There are insufficient grounds for an assertion that physicians are obligated to treat patients with AIDS because of what the vast majority of physicians have done in the past...,a conflict of principles makes it difficult to site an obligation to act in a particular manner." He goes on to say that some other standards [other than historical precedents] should be considered such as a "contractual or moral basis" in the obligation for physicians to treat patients with AIDS.(6)

Yet, for AIDS, the AMA unfortunately has created an unnecessary contradiction between the AMA's own Code of Ethics, Principle VI, which says, "a physician shall, in the provision of appropriate patient care except in emergencies, be free to choose whom to serve, with whom to associate, and the environment in which to provide medical services"; and subsequent proclamations that addressed the issue of the obligation of physicians to treat patients with AIDS. In 1988, for instance, the AMA Council of Judicial and Ethical Affairs stated, "it is the view of the Council that Principle VI does not permit categorical discrimination against a patient based solely on his or her sera positivity."(9) It goes without saying that physicians should treat patients with whom they have an established patient-doctor relationship (except in emergencies), and who have illnesses within the physicians' realm of competence and expertise. And in this light, I ask who is better qualified than the individual physician to judge his/her own degree of expertise in a particular area? Moreover, the above statement by the Council is in itself a moot point for contention in our increasingly adversarial society. It only adds fuel to the already controversial and potentially explosive issues of physicians' need of referral, acceptance of patients for treatment, and patient confidentiality.

Historic precedents, supported by Græco-Roman ethics and the Judeo-Christian tradition, clearly establish that the patient-doctor relationship should be preserved, along with physician and patient autonomy. Moreover, economic incentives should be used to solve whatever potential manpower-related problems occur, whether it be AIDS today, or any other epidemic in the future. (7,8)

If anything, the behavior of physicians reflected during peace times and even during most epidemics, wars, and other historic calamities, reinforces the need for applying voluntary free-market incentives to solve the problems in the health care delivery system, along with the revivification of compassion, charity, and trust – not the government takeover of a prosperous health care industry and the coercive compassion of government bureaucrats. This point should be kept in mind in our own age as we grapple with the increasing problems of infinite demand brought about partially by the perception of free care coupled with finite and dwindling resources – both problems created by government intervention in the health care field.

The proper allocation of health care resources should be entrusted to free-market incentives, with the government providing the means to health care access via the private sector. This must occur if we are to remain a free society, free of oppressive and stifling government regulations, and a society that respects individual liberties, freedom of association, and the sanctity of contracts. It is also imperative if we expect to move medical ethics and high-technology medicine unhindered through the corridor of time into the 21st Century.

ON CRITICIZING COLLEAGUES

From the outset let me say that unethical physicians do exist and need to be weeded out of the profession via the proper channels (by reporting to state medical societies or to the state medical boards.[98] Physicians have an ethical obligation to report unethical or incompetent colleagues to disciplining bodies, but many times this is not done. One reason for this is government antitrust regulations which in effect allow errant physicians to file lawsuits against those participating in the disciplining process. The medical profession should be empowered to enforce ethical and clinical standards and allowed to police itself – but as we shall see, this is only one side of the story.

Another problem is that of inappropriate, critical remarks uttered about fellow colleagues. Perhaps animated by professional jealousy or petty rivalries, some physicians have been known to openly criticize colleagues in hospital corridors or even deride colleagues in patients' rooms as acts of petty self-aggrandizement, thereby casting into the wind the proverbial seeds of unfounded accusations and medical lawsuits. Unfortunately, some of these land on fertile soil.

As difficult and painful as it is to admit, Walt Kelly's famous cartoon character, Pogo, a witty Georgia opossum inhabitant of the Okeefeenokee swamp, once said, "we have met the enemy and it is us." Yes, the medical profession is notorious for self-inflicted wounds. According to the AMA, as well as most specialty codes of ethics (including my own specialty code of ethics as written by the American Association of Neurological Surgeons (AANS), colleagues who practice unethical medicine or who are deemed incompetent should be exposed by their

[98] The state medical boards are the statewide body polity authorized with disciplining health care professionals.

peers to the proper authorities. By in large these individuals who have gone through long and rigorous education and training to become physicians should be amenable to re-education and re-training. Those truly incorrigible should be weeded out of the profession, to protect the public and maintain professional standards. Therefore, to a significant degree, physicians themselves are responsible for their colleagues' standard of practice. Yet if and when physicians make the judgment of exposing a colleague who is allegedly incompetent or suspected of unbecoming conduct, then I think the exposers also have a responsibility to stand by their convictions in the disciplining process. Truth and justice, one way or the other, should prevail – the ethics of our profession demand it.

As with any other accused citizen, physicians subjected to peer review investigations and the disciplining process deserve the same just and fair treatment as those put through the rigors of court proceedings. Accused physicians should be given due process and equal protection before the law. Physicians should be accorded the benefits of the central tenets of American justice, that he/she is innocent until proven guilty, that his/her confidentiality is protected during the investigation process and/or disciplinary proceedings, and he/she should be judged impartially by the weight of credible evidence and convicted only when evidence establishes guilt beyond a reasonable doubt.

In civil cases, it is my conviction that lawsuits should not be allowed to go forward unless a pre-trial screening panel, after reviewing the body of credible evidence, finds that the physician has likely performed negligently. That is, that he/she has performed below an established minimum standard, as demonstrated by the preponderance of scientific evidence. In criminal cases, pre-trial publicity should be avoided and kept to a minimum to protect the accused, who may after all, be innocent. As Thomas Fuller (1608-1661), the English clergyman and author, once asserted, "even doubtful accusations leave a stain behind them."

The AMA Code of Ethics (Principle II) states, "a physician shall deal honestly with patients and colleagues and strive to expose those physicians deficient in character or competence, or who engage in fraud or deception"(10), and the AANS Code of Ethics (Section III-H) states, "neurological surgeons should be responsible for helping their medical colleagues maintain a high level of performance and integrity in the practice of medicine, and should refrain from repeating false charges about another health care professional."(11) Both statements are remarkable for their brevity, clarity, and sincerity.

From the foregoing, it is clear that slandering colleagues on the basis of unfounded accusations, insinuations, gossip, or hearsay is unethical. By the same token, participating in a conspiracy of silence to protect colleagues who are known to be incompetent or who engage in professional misconduct is likewise unethical and should be deplored. When in doubt, one should perhaps consult Aristotle who counselled moderation, the Golden Mean, "virtue...the mean between extremes." And above all, I think most importantly, whether in criminal proceedings or civil litigation, physicians should always remember one of the Ten Commandments, at least the one most pertinent to our discussion, "thou shall not bear false witness" (Exodus 20:1-17).

EVOLUTION OF MEDICAL ETHICS

As we return to our discussion of early Greek medical ethics, we should also expound on the evolution of those ethics. In this vein, let us note that by the

2nd Century A.D., the Neoplatonists had established Galen as the unchallenged authority in medicine. Galen believed in the virtue-based ethics of the ancient Greek physicians. It was his concept of ethics that predominated until the rooting of Christianity and the integration of Judeo-Christian ethos throughout the territories of the old Roman Empire. Physicians eventually became a privileged class, but these privileges were accompanied by required services and responsibilities. In fact, as early as the 1st Century A.D., the philosopher Seneca the Younger (5 B.C.-A.D.65) had asserted that "the physician had become the friend of the patient," and that "it was generally recognized that the work of physicians and their responsibility went beyond monetary remuneration."(12)

Thus, recognizing the value of services rendered, imperial decrees did much to improve the lot of physicians in Roman times. Those privileges which were conferred upon physicians were bestowed by rulers not because physicians were of royal or noble blood – indeed, many of the physicians of the early Empire were Greek slaves rather than Roman citizens – but because of their hard-earned status and reputation as compassionate healers, and for the valuable services that they provided to Roman society. Physicians had already proven themselves by rendering services in the treatment of the afflicted during plagues and pestilences and ministering care to the wounded during the many Roman wars and campaigns fought throughout the Empire.

The Edict of Vespasian, for example, granted all physicians exemption from taxation and from "the burden of having soldiers billeted in their houses." This edict was later curtailed by Antoninus Pius (Roman emperor, A.D.138-161) because it was abused by other itinerant practitioners and charlatans who were not qualified physicians, but who claimed the status only to gain exemption from taxation and other special privileges.(12)

Only seldom were established Greek or Roman physicians (who belonged to specified sects) censured for misbehavior or unethical conduct. On the other hand, itinerant quacks and charlatans who belonged to no philosophic school and who had received no training (apprenticeship) in medicine abounded. To avoid being censured, these peripatetic practitioners seldom stayed in one place for long and were nearly always on the move. Later during Byzantine times (6th-15th Centuries), privileges likewise would be granted to physicians based on competency, knowledge, and professional merit, as well as their purported moral character.

In the Western world during most of antiquity (especially during Græco-Roman times), medical practitioners were independent and free to practice as they pleased. Physicians generally subscribed to and followed one of the many philosophic sects or schools of thought into which medicine in those days was splintered. Later, laws were written to deal with specific medical issues such as fee disputes, contractual contentions, or death alleged to be the result of physician treatment.(12) The fact that government recognized that physicians were valued members of a learned profession whose purpose and function benefitted the state was also a major impetus for the government to leave physicians alone to practice their trade or profession, as well as the fundamental reason for the bestowal of special privileges. Moreover, emperors and government officials were also keenly aware that even though morality and ethics could be enforced and transgressions severely prosecuted, the state could not of itself legislate an individual's innate ability, intelligence, and acquired knowledge. These were qualities recognizably more akin to the individual and his temperament than to the nurture and purview of the state.

In those antiquated times, it was expected that the patients themselves had a responsibility for seeking and obtaining care from "the right physician" as affirmed by the Roman physician and ethicist, Scribonius Largus in the 1st Century A.D., who very succinctly observed: "Rarely does anyone make an evaluation of the doctor before putting himself and his family under his care. And yet, if people have their portrait painted, they will first try to make sure of the artist's qualities on the basis of that which experience can tell, and then select and hire him."(12)

And no where is this observation more relevant than in today's debate over health system reform, not only from a quality perspective, but also from a fiscal viewpoint. Thus, for modern patients who pay their premiums and their deductibles (or co-payments), but not the larger portion of their doctor's or hospital's bills, there are no fiscal restraints. Despite the *prima facie* impression of fee-for-service capitalism in the medical market place, the fact is that those much talked about free-market incentives are illusory. Moreover, doctors for the most part have not been encouraged to discuss fees with their patients. That practice nevertheless could give impetus to the much needed implementation of true free-market incentives. Generally, patients have not focused on the fiscal aspects of health care and have not made serious attempts at cost containment. The truth is that when Americans seek medical care for themselves or their families, health care costs are deemed largely irrelevant, immaterial – even impertinent.

In today's health care environment, patients, as consumers of health care, have no real vested financial interest in controlling health care costs since nearly 80-90% of their medical expenses, as we have noted, are paid either by the government or by other third-party payers. [99] This has created a widespread myth that health care is free and its supply infinite, rather than a commodity which, one way or another, has to be paid for by the patient-consumer. Moreover, when this commodity is used unwisely, it must be paid with higher premiums, higher deductibles, and higher co-payments. Those who have closely studied the puzzling questions inherent in the health care costs dilemma recognize that true incentives for cost containment are conspicuously absent. The bottom line: Patients should be empowered to make their own informed health care decisions, a responsibility rooted in and called for since Græco-Roman times.

Once this simple concept stemming from individual responsibility is grasped, only the most statist of elites, whose ideology precludes them from embracing the concept, and government bureaucrats, who have a stake (their jobs) in preserving the status quo of government intervention and dependency, would oppose this rational concept of patient empowerment. They base their opposition on the false assumption that patients "would not know how to find the 'right' doctor, or that patients would not be capable of making the correct health care decisions for themselves, therefore those decisions are best left to government."

Today more than ever, physicians should take the initiative to advise their

<hr />

[99] Statistics from 1990, the last year for which comprehensive statistics have been made available as of this writing, show that 42% of total health care expenditures are already funded by state or federal government agencies; 33% are funded by private health insurance, and 10-20% are "out-of-pocket" expenses.(13)

patients about health care matters within the purview of the patient-doctor relationship. This in fact had been the case until the U.S. government invaded the health care field in the 1960s, consolidated its hold on medicine in the 1970s and 1980s, and prepared for the complete takeover of the health care system in the 1990s.(14-17)

Today, government interference in the practice of medicine permeates all of the professional activities of the physician. Whenever government deems it appropriate, it violates what was previously considered the sacrosanct patient-doctor relationship. Today, the leadership of many national organizations such as the AMA seem headed in the wrong direction, for they are too eager to please the government and too quick to capitulate to its demands. Thus, some observers, with good reason, question whether those organizations can continue to truly represent the wishes of their rank and file members. They suspect that they have become instruments of government coercion by which physicians are made to conform to cryptic, vague, and cumbersome government regulations,[100] and in this fashion, taking the easy way out of the struggle through appeasement of the entrenched government bureaucracy. Consequently so emboldened, this ever-growing bureaucracy prints yearly tens of thousands of pages of rules and regulations for health care providers which strangle the medical profession and take time away from patients. And this bureaucracy today will cling tenaciously to its position of power and control at any cost.

In closing this chapter, we should invoke the late professor of ethics and medical history, Ludwig Edelstein (1902-1965), who wrote, "Among the ideals conceived by the ancients, none was loftier than that which envisages love of humanity as the professional virtue of the physician...."(12) And ponder his belief that "Osler extolled the idea of ancient medical humanism and held it up as the idea to be followed in the future." (I wonder if humanitarianism, rather than humanism, would have been a more descriptive and appropriate term.[12,19,20])

Physicians should be wary of the realistic possibility of the abject surrender and total capitulation of the medical profession by an overly pragmatic leadership devoid of vision and ideals who in time may even come to justify the planned government takeover of medicine by its arrogated authority. Moreover, physicians should also be careful about embracing a medical philosophy based solely on humanistic principles, that could be interpreted as justifying the government takeover and the incorporation of medicine as an appendage to the parasitic body of government, spiritually void, and forever afflicted with the pervasive anguish and despair that permeates the present age.(21-30)

---

[100] It is perhaps worth repeating the words of journalist Alan Stang who once noted, "One of the hallmarks of a dictatorship is that its laws are deliberately vague. A dictator wants vague laws in order to make obedience difficult so that he may call you guilty whenever he likes."(18)

CHAPTER 22

THE ORIGIN OF MEDICAL PHILANTHROPY AND MEDICAL HUMANISM

All strangers and beggars are from Zeus, and a gift, though small, is precious.
Homer (c.8th Century B.C.)

PHYSICIANS OR CHARLATANS

In the early Græco-Roman tradition, medical practitioners were physician-philosophers, because they wanted to understand not only the etiology of illnesses and their proper treatment but also the meaning of human existence. They believed in the validity of the eternal quest for truth. To the Greek physician, love for his fellow man, his patients, and his profession were not only necessary attributes but also intricately interwoven entities and interrelationships that needed to be understood to carry on a successful medical practice.

Osler once said, "where there is love of man, there is also love of the art." Philanthropy, as Prof. Edelstein pointed out, involves the ideal that "...the love of humanity of the ancient physician was associated with the love of his craft."(12)

These ideals were established in Greek civilization by the time of the classical age of Athenian Democracy, which not surprisingly coincided with the Golden Age of art and philosophy.(31) It was in this milieu, in the flourishing atmosphere of Greek politics and arts, that the lofty ideals and the moral ethical principles of the profession were established. For instance, physicians were willing to accommodate fees to the financial circumstances of their patients, and were willing to treat those who were not able to pay – since professional ethics gave physicians leeway to charge patients according to their ability to pay.

Within this context of beneficent paternalism and enlightened self-interest and the respect accorded a dignified profession, the noble ideals of the Greek physicians were "totally adequate to serve the public interest well."(12) Today, unfortunately for the public, the situation is quite different. In the government-created atmosphere that physicians cannot be trusted in monetary matters because of their purported rapacity, physicians today have neither the leeway to decide what they can bill their own patients nor the option to charge according to the patient's ability to pay. By law, physicians today must collect from Medicare patients any amount applied to their deductible and/or co-payment.[101]

In antiquity, the enlightened self-interest ethics of the virtuous Græco-Roman physicians required the attainment of high standards of medical practice.

---

[101] Today, cost shifting takes place largely in the hospital setting where insured patients end up paying more to subsidize the care of the indigent, the uninsured, and Medicare patients.

Such high standards were set up to distinguish legitimate practitioners from travel-ling charlatans. It must be remembered that in those days most physicians were peripatetic or itinerant *iatros* who practiced without formal schooling. They were primarily bound by the ethical precepts of the philosophic sects to which they belonged. It was not only by its manifest knowledge but also by adherence to its own ethics that the nascent medical profession recognized and distinguished charla-tans from the *iatros*, the true physician-philosophers, for it was essential that the profession recognize its authentic members for its own benefit, as well as for the benefit of society.

Prof. Edelstein asserts, "abuses by quacks and charlatans...could be pre-vented only in the individual's decision to make himself responsible before the bar of his own conscience, the conscience of a good craftsman, and this responsibility he assumed by the adoption of a strict etiquette. A great achievement indeed! *For not only did the physician voluntary establish a set of values concerning sound treatment* [my emphasis], but he also gave, so to speak, a personal pledge of safety to his patients, badly needed in a world that knew no other protection for them."(12) Thus, it was no coincidence that the Greek word for being an "expert and good" sets the physician apart from itinerant quacks and mountebanks.

The ethics of the Greek physicians as ascertained from the early books of the *Corpus Hippocraticum*, including the books *Precepts* and *On The Physician*, entailed discussions of the proper behavior of physicians toward those with whom they came in contact with during treatment. Other books, as we have already noted in the section on Hippocrates, discussed medical etiquette, bedside manners, the setting of a doctor's office, his *iatreion*. In discussing these books, Prof. Edelstein brings forth the fact that once treatment is started, it should be completed and "that the physician should not withdraw his help from the sick so as to avoid blame or other unwelcome consequences."(12)

Prof. Edelstein also affirms another important precedent which was set in the books *Epidemics* and *Problemata* of the *Corpus Hippocraticum*, and that was, that the physician was to do his art and craft to the best of his ability as an "ethic of outward achievement rather than inner intention." By this statement of affirmation, it was also understood, "...the physician's motives in practicing medicine, he was engaged in order to make a living. Nor was there any conflict between his pecu-niary interest and the exigencies of craftsmanship as long as he remembered that love of money, of easy success, should not induce him to act without regard for the benefit of the patient...." Moreover, "if he learned to forget personal advantage for the sake of doing the right thing, he had...done all that was necessary."(12)

I think that today, despite what one reads or hears in the mass media, most physicians would agree with the great philosophers Socrates, Plato, and Aristotle who proclaimed that the primary function of medicine is to treat and heal the sick. Socrates, for example, asserted that "the physician is not a money maker or an earner of fees, but a healer of the sick," and Prof. Edelstein quoting Plato's *Republic*, writes that, "when Socrates is asked rather mockingly: 'is this true of the shepherd also? Does he too have the good of his flock in mind?' He answers emphatically in the affirmative. So that the same response is true for all the arts and trades that rely on public service, that they were invented not for the sake of per-sonal advantage, but rather for the purpose of performing a service...."(12)

In discussing physicians and wealth, Prof. Edelstein sheds light onto the issue from the perspective of historic precedents. We learn that even though Aristotle also predicated the belief that the purpose of medicine is "that of causing health not of producing wealth," from the point of economic theory, he nevertheless also maintained that medicine belongs to the art of acquisition which deals with exchange and "labor for hire."(12,32) Plato in his *Eryxias*, in discussing the relation of wealth and virtue in the crafts, classifies the latter not under "limited servitude," but on the "acquisition of wealth," and therefore more noble. Moreover, it is in this context that he cites the example of the "expert pilot" and the "skilled physician."(12,33)

Prof. Edelstein also reminds us of several crucial points stemming from the judicious thinking of the Greek classical age. One was that all manual labor was judged by the standards of performance and not morality. Morality was reserved for man's private life, so that even medicine was "impervious to moral consideration"; second, that work was considered "a dire necessity not an ennobling activity"; third, that the classical age did not recognize the concept of "profession," and artists, physicians, and others were classified with common craftsmen.(12,31) It was Aristotle, perhaps nature's most astute observer, who maintained that unlike the slaves who were subject to "unlimited servitude," artisans and craftsmen were subject only to "limited servitude." By this he meant that with regard to a man's job, he was obligated to do his task well; his personal morality was his own affair.(12,32)

THE CONCEPT OF WORK

If a man will not work, he shall not eat.
                    2 Thessalonians 3:10

There is dignity in work only when it is work freely accepted.
                    Albert Camus

Faith without works is dead.
                    James 2:20

The concept of work evolved from classical times and since physicians initially were considered craftsmen and subject to "limited servitude," it is worth cataloguing the significance of the concept of work during this time. The Pythagoreans insisted on the moral implications of work and considered it "a noble toil." This concept was amplified by Aristotle during classical times; his interpretation and amplification became widespread during Hellenistic times, when men were asked to be both morally upright and to perform their work with pride. Aristotle distinguished "the happy life" presuming independent means and "the good life" presupposing an occupation.(12)

The Stoics subscribed to the idea that the acquisition of wealth through organized toil was compatible with morality and taught that "whatever station in life one may find oneself," one must live to the rules of morality and ethics.

Socrates, whose teachings were subsequently paramount to the formation of professional ethics, maintained that for the poor to remain idle, rather than working, was shameful. Hesiod, the Greek poet of the 8th Century B.C., proclaimed, "The gods rank work above virtue." Lucius Seneca, "the Elder," (c.54 B.C.-c.A.D.39) believed that "love of bustle is not industry." Cicero wittily quoted a contemporary adage, "accomplished labours are pleasant." And Galen himself pronounced that, "employment is nature's physician, and is essential to human happiness."(34)

According to Prof. Edelstein, Greek tradition recognized virtue not in inner subjective feeling and content, but rather in objective human action. Moreover, because of his work, a physician who had the right kind of philosophy and all the virtues of a gentleman was considered "equal to a god" in traditional stoic philosophy. It was also believed that a true physician was the peer of the sage. Conversely, the Greek philosopher Epicurus (341-270 B.C.) held that all forms of activity that did not result in happiness were merely vulgar and mundane activities. Prof. Edelstein notes that "none of the Hippocratic treatises considered the obligation of the physician inherent in his medical task." Thus, medical etiquette, ethical principles, and the responsibilities of a professional medical practice were accepted voluntarily. The *Corpus Hippocraticum* then served the purpose of adapting seemingly abstract philosophic ethics to the apparently more concrete and practical clinical practice of medicine.(12)

THE PHYSICIAN AS THE TRUE PATIENT ADVOCATE

The writers of antiquity wrote and discussed ethics merely as individuals trying to find out the best way and the right way to conduct themselves in their dual functions as philosophers and medical practitioners. They did not intend to impose on others their own ethical code or their own morality. The same should be true today, and to enforce good medical practice and medical ethics we should re-invigorate our own ethics, looking not only to history but also to the reality of changing times. Ethics should reflect the authentic feelings of the members of the profession about what is right and what is wrong, not the echoes of what is politically expedient, or the subtle braggadocio of leaders merely seeking publicity, self-aggrandizement, and the opportunity to climb the ladder of medical organizations, or the imposition of the exigencies of sworn enemies of the profession for the purpose of appeasing its detractors (and tormentors). Physicians' survival will depend on their ability to articulate eloquently to the public the fact that they have been and remain their patients' best advocates. If physicians are not successful in conveying this message, the medical profession will become an enslaved government trade union rather than remaining an independent and honorable profession. That is, in short, what is at stake for the House of Medicine!

As if to corroborate this fact from history, Prof. Edelstein with great clairvoyance points out that in the Hippocratic book, *Oath*, the Pythagorean concept of the physician as the patients' advocate is clearly expressed. Moreover, it is also in this book, composed during classical times, that the concept of trust – as a virtuous quality and state of mind that the physician must engender in his patients who are ill and vulnerable—is clearly promulgated within the patient-doctor relationship. The development of patients' trust in their own physicians is asserted as of paramount importance, because illness is a time of vulnerability, a time when patients must put themselves in the hands of their healers. They do this solely on the basis of trust in their physicians' knowledge, honor, and virtue, and I might add, friendship.(12)

According to Prof. Edelstein, the origin of scientific medicine took place in ancient Greece when ordinary medical practitioners immersed themselves not in the study of science *per se*, but in the study of philosophy. Philosophic schools proliferated during the classical period; later, during Hellenistic times, philosophic schools further fragmented into various medical sects. Predictably, individual physicians then embraced the particular ethics of the sects to which they belonged.(31) For example, it was specifically the sect of the Empiricists, who were not only practicing physicians but also skeptic philosophers, who during Hellenistic times exerted great influence in the realm of medical ethics. Their motto explaining the goal and aim of a physician was: "to practice medicine for the sake of reputation or of money, of neither of which he desires to have too much or too little, but just as much as is adequate and guarantees peace of mind."(12) Erasistratus, the renowned anatomist and physiologist of Alexandria, who epitomized the Hellenistic period, was also interested in medical ethics. Prof. Edelstein quotes him thus, "...the physician is both, perfect in his heart and most excellent in his moral conduct. But if one of the two should happen to be missing, then it is better to be a good man devoid of learning than to be a perfect practitioner of bad moral conduct, and an untrustworthy man...good morals compensate for what is missing in art, while bad morals can corrupt and confound even perfect art."(12)

Both the philosophers of the Peripatetic sect and the school of Stoicism founded by Zeno of Citium (c.300 B.C.) have been given credit for the important synthesis of medicine and philanthropy. Others have asserted that philanthropy was mankind's natural inclination to help his fellow man in dire need.

Physicians, men and women, listen to their calling and follow a career in medicine instinctively cognizant of this truth. Physicians have an ardent desire to help their fellowmen in times of dire need – particularly times of serious illnesses and unrelenting suffering – those moments of intimations with death. Only the most cynical of individuals would go into this profession primarily for the monetary rewards. Students of medicine, the cream of the academic crop, could have easily gone into any other field of endeavor, such as business or law, in which they would have the potential for even greater remuneration with certainly less toil, without having to deal with the unpleasant subject of pain and suffering and the prospect of being confronted *vis-à-vis* death with the constant remainder of their own mortality. This, physicians do day in and day out whilst consoling aggrieved relatives, never knowing when they will be hit with a lawsuit in spite of all their labors.

Self-interest does not necessarily negate altruism, as has been amply demonstrated by most physicians and many other professionals in the clergy and even the legal profession at various points throughout the ages. There was one other reason, besides desperation, that drove patients to physicians in remote times, despite the fact that it was not until the turn of the 20th Century that a patient seeking the professional help of an ordinary physician actually benefited from that visit. That was, the public sought the thoughtful advice of physicians. Suffice it to say that despite the rudimentary state of medical knowledge during much of recorded history and civilization, patients flocked to consult compassionate physicians.[102] They knew that physicians had answered a calling of caring and benevolence, and generally displayed a devotion rarely seen in other occupations (excepting perhaps the clergy).

In the formulation of the Græco-Roman deontologic ethics, the Peripatetic school of medical philosophy stressed "the Hellenistic concept of the unity of man," whilst the Stoics emphasized the concept of obligations inherent in the patient-doctor relationship, and an idealistic "love of mankind" that flourished in the upper circles of Roman society in the 1st Century A.D.(12,19)

Prof. Edelstein sums up this stage in the development of medical ethics with Galen, the sage of Pergamon, who asserted that "the physician should be contemptuous of money, interested in his work, self controlled, and just. *Once he is in possession of these basic virtues, he will have all the others at his command as well* [my emphasis]." Moreover, Galen subscribed to the idea that "philosophy is indispensable for medical practice just as it is for medical theory and...the physician must take up not just logic and physics but must also take the third part of philosophy, namely ethics." Thus, in effect, "the morality of outward performance characteristic of the classical era was now supplemented by a morality of inner intention."(12,31)

From his voluminous and magnificent body of writings, it would seem that Prof. Edelstein agreed with Galen who believed that medicine was philanthropic, in and of itself, because it intended to relieve suffering and treat the sick. Moreover, Galen's writings are permeated with the paramount idea that the motives of scientific inclination, glory, monetary reward, or philanthropy are not only matters of personal conviction but also necessities, and that when a physician does his/her job well, such motives have no overt bearing on the practice of compassionate ethical medicine. Thus, the great physician himself, Galen, was devoid of the sanctimonious moral overtones, the sense of self-righteousness, and moral pseudo-crusading that is so prevalent today amongst those non-physicians professing to be patient advocates. Instead, he clearly established what should be expected of physicians: competency and adherence to the tenets of the ethical code of the philosophic school to which they personally adhere.

Today, with the politicization of many aspects of medical practice and the tendency for knee-jerk ethical pronouncements by some medical organizations, physicians more than ever must be above reproach by strict adherence to professional integrity and his/her chosen moral code of professional ethics. Physicians must be ever careful of the ethical pronouncements of the professional organizations in which they belong, as they will be expected to abide by the ethical code of that organization.(35) Thus, today, it is imperative that he/she knows what the various medical organizations stand for and join those to which he/she can most clearly identify – politically, morally, and ethically.

Though Galen may not be considered "politically correct" by today's liberal standards, he stated his opinions clearly and precisely, taking into account human nature as well as the fact that physicians of necessity must place their

---

[102] Admittedly, the profession in general was ridiculed and sometimes distrusted in the post-Renaissance epoch (particularly the 17th and 18th Centuries) when acquisition of medical knowledge palpably slowed in the wake of the upheaval of the Renaissance.

patients' interest above their own in the patient-doctor relationship. Thus, he implicitly accepted the notion that physicians were virtuous human beings; and for him, underlying motives were irrelevant, in view of the fact that physicians pursued a medical career that not only demanded rigorous studies and arduous training voluntarily but also that was, of itself, thoroughly philanthropic. For Galen, therefore, explaining the underlying motives of competent, compassionate individuals who adhered strictly to the ethics of their particular philosophic sect was irrelevant for under those conditions it did not appear to affect clinical practice.(12,31)

THE ETHICS OF THE ROMAN PHYSICIAN SCRIBONIUS LARGUS

The man who is anybody and who does anything is surely going to be criticized, vilified, and misunderstood. This is part of the penalty for greatness...
> Elbert Hubbard (1856-1915), American author who
> promoted the ideal of America's rugged individualism.

Just as the term *philanthropy* derived from the Greek term *philanthropia* which connotes one's goodwill to his fellowman, so the term *humanitarianism* conveyed an analogous and similar meaning to the Romans.[103] As we direct our attention to the ethics of the Romans – the empire builders, and ultimately, the assimilators of Greek culture – we find the word philanthropy transformed into humanitarianism and humanistic ethics. With this perspective in mind, let us discuss the humanistic ethics of Scribonius Largus (fl. A.D. 40) who, in the glorious 1st Century A.D., warned physicians of the evil of professional jealousy. In his book On *Remedies*, in which he discusses the use of drugs and herbs in medical treatment: "Why is it," he inquires, "that my colleagues refrain from the application of drugs? Are they unfamiliar with them? This would be just reason for accusing them of negligence. Or are they aware of the usefulness of drugs, yet they deny their use to others? If so, they are even more culpable, because they burn with envy, an evil that must be despised by all men, and especially by the physician who is himself despised by gods and men if his heart is not full of sympathy (*misericordiae*) and humaneness (*humanitatis*) in accordance with the will (*voluntatem*) of medicine itself."(37)

As Prof. Edelstein points out, Scribonius Largus goes much further embodying the ethics of the new age: the physician "is not allowed to harm anybody, not even the enemies of the state (*hostibus*). He may fight against them with every means as a soldier (*miles*) or as a good citizen (*virbonus*) should this be demanded of him. [As a physician though, he must not harm anyone] since medicine does not judge men by their circumstances in life (*fortuna*), nor by their character (*personis*). Rather medicine promises (*pollicetur*) her succor in equal measure to all who implore her help and she professes (*profitetur*) never to be injurious to anyone."(37)

It was Scribonius who called medicine not merely an art or a science or a

---

[103] For its part, the term *humanism* relates a devotion to the humanities and the revival of classical letters as during the Renaissance. Today, humanism embodies a doctrine or way of life centered on human interests or values.(36)

trade, but "a profession," *professio*. [A] profession, according to Prof. Edelstein, is a Latin word that refers to trade or workmanship "that emphasizes an ethical connotation of work and an obligation to duty in the part of those engaged in the arts and crafts." Moreover, "it approximates most closely the Christian concept of 'vocation' or 'calling,' except of course that for him who has been 'called' to do a job, his obligations are ordained by God, while for the member of an ancient profession his duties resulted from his own understanding of the nature of his profession."(12)

Toward the end of the Roman Republic in the 1st Century B.C., the great statesman, politician, orator, and writer, Marcus Tulius Cicero (106-43 B.C.), explicitly mentioned architecture, education, and medicine (besides, of course, rhetoric and law) as the socially acceptable professions because of their requirement for human insight and contributions to human life; thus he considered them "the proper" (*honestae*) occupations for those for whose station in life it is fitting.(37) As an aristocrat and as a product of his time, Cicero considered only political and public activities which he himself engaged in, as the proper professions for "a member of the Roman nobility," [104] the nobles (*nobiles*), the successful entrepreneurs, now the elite class of the late Roman Republic.(31)

But it was Panaetius of Rhodes (185-110 B.C.) of the Stoic sect who underscored the importance of the virtues of all professions in civilization. For example, "a judge must adhere to truth while the lawyer may sometimes defend the probable even if this may not quite coincide with truth. Obviously here man's particular task imposes upon him certain obligations; each one has its own morality, from which there is no exception." So it follows that, "the judge is not permitted to indulge in bias or favoritism out of friendship."(37)

The foundation for the duties and obligations of medicine and the other major professions, such as architecture and education, appeared to have been laid down from the 1st Century B.C. to the 1st Century A.D. Thus, Scribonius may have been influenced by his predecessor, Panaetius, and his stoicism may have been transmitted via Cicero in the formulation of professional conduct.

In my estimation, it is very likely that Cicero, a noted legal scholar, orator, and leading statesman of his age, was most likely responsible for the formulation of professional ethics – by incorporating features of both the philanthropy of the Greeks and the humanism and humanitarianism of the Latin scholars – ultimately adopted by the evolving legal and medical professions. Cicero has also been credited with suffusing the profession of law and general jurisprudence with what is (or should be) their distinct virtue, namely, *truth*. In Cicero's view, each profession or career has its own ethos to which it must adhere *ipso facto* as a matter of ethical principle.(31) Both in the views of Cicero, who lived during the late Roman Republic, and Lucius Seneca "the Younger," the great Roman philosopher who lived in the early years of the Empire, the work of a craftsman, although considered an *officium*, also conveyed a moral obligation in the tradition of Socrates.

In the 2nd Century A.D., Galen refuted the assertions of those who, like Menodotus and Pliny the Elder (A.D.23-79), excoriated the medical profession for allegedly holding nefarious inner motives and intentions. The philosopher Menodotus predicated, for example, that the physician's objective was the

---

[104] This concept is expounded by Cicero in his book *On Duties*.(12)

accumulation of wealth and the accretion of honor. Pliny the Elder's criticism of the medical profession was more a diatribe against the physician's alleged deviation from the ethos of medical philanthropy than a specific complaint supported by logical arguments.

Seneca the Younger, on the other hand, defended the physicians and contended that men owe much more to physicians than financial remuneration.(12) And Pliny the Elder, despite his noted skepticism and sometimes open criticism of physicians, correctly stressed the importance of individual accountability and responsibility. Furthermore, he asserted that "all the crimes committed by physicians should be attributed to the individual and not the medical art."(12)

From the foregoing, it is evident that although many scholars, including physicians, have ascribed medicine's ethics of universal brotherhood to Christian medical ethics, much of this legacy actually originated with the Greek and Roman secular, medical humanism. Yet this notation does not detract from the benefits accorded by the additional ethics in later centuries derived from the Judeo-Christian heritage. This augmentation and further refining in medical ethics will become evident in later chapters.

We have already noted that Prof. Edelstein attributed philanthropy to the Greek tradition via the Pythagoreans and the followers of the School of Cos. To Scribonius, the Roman physician and early humanist, we can credit the infusion of humanism into medicine; and to Cicero, the Roman orator, we can ascribe credit for the setting of professional standards. Philanthropy and humanitarianism influenced the noble antediluvian concepts of caring and compassion as affected by the vicissitudes of the ages from the times of the medicine man of Neolithic times, through the era of the Greek philosopher-physician, and finally culminating in the professional physician of Roman times. Later, the key element of charity would be added to the mix, becoming a fundamental ingredient in the formulation of evolving medical ethics in the Christian era, beginning with the onset of the barbaric Dark Ages and winding through the slumberous evolution of the Medieval period.

This seminal formulation of medical ethics remains refreshing in the words of an early Greek Stoic philosopher-physician who thus advises:

> *You desire to be one of the healers (of sickness), you had the benefit of having (good) teachers. Now, practice your art faithfully. Be reliable; cultivate love of man; if you are called to your patient, hastingly go; when you enter into the sick room, apply all your mental ability to the case at hand; sharing the pain of those who suffer; rejoice with those who have found relief; consider yourself a partner in the disease; muster all enough for the fight to be fought; consider yourself to be of your contemporaries the brother, of those who are your elders the son, of those who are younger the father. And if anyone of them neglects his own affairs, remember that this is not permissible for yourself, and that it is your duty to be to the sick what the Dioscuri are to the sailors (in distress).(12)*

The medical writer I. Galdston does make a distinction between the "pagan *Græco-Roman individualism-humanism and Christian altruism* [my emphasis] which is confluent with the 19th Century secular-humanist ideology which asserts that Græco-Roman ethics lack any recognition of social responsibilities on the part of the physician."(38) Moreover, this writer correctly asserts that even when diseases were linked to social conditions, "the gospel of brotherly love took account only of the relationship between the individual doctor and his patient."(38) Moreover, medicine, as Scribonius has written, "does not judge individual men by their circumstances, station, or personality."(37)

This pronouncement is very significant and still relevant today when, in our own century, totalitarian systems have used the phraseology "brotherly love" or "for the good of society" as utilitarian pretexts to abrogate individual rights. That was not the case with the virtuous Græco-Roman physicians, when enlightened self-interest on the part of physicians – in association with a voluntary philanthropic and humanitarian ethic – was the rule of the day without state intervention, compulsion, or oppression. In the same light, the admission of the existence of the inherently human qualities of self-preservation and self-interest in virtuous physicians enlightened not only by their acquired knowledge but also by the fact that they are sworn to put the interests of their patients above their own, would tremendously enhance the modern evolving ethics of medicine – as we rapidly approach the 21st Century. It would then be self-evident that the new collectivists' philosophy of coercive compassion and forced egalitarian ethics afflicting us today would no longer be needed, for those false ethics only serve to distribute suffering equally to all citizens.

But let us again return to history. Another interpretation of Scribonius' humanism was recently provided by the medical ethicists, Dr. Edmund D. Pellegrino and Alice A. Pellegrino in an interesting and informative essay. According to these authors, Scribonius may have been one of Emperor Claudius' physicians who participated in the highly successful expedition and invasion of Britain in A.D.43. In the tradition of the Roman encyclopedists, Pliny the Elder, Marcus Vitruvius, and Pedacius Dioscorides, Scribonius wrote a popular catalogue of medical remedies which may have been used by the *Pater familias* for treating his family, for the Romans were indeed both self-sufficient and health-conscious.

Scribonius' *Compositiones Medicamentorum* is believed to have been written between A.D. 44 and 48, sometime after the return of Emperor Claudius from his famed expedition in the British Isles "and before the death of Empress Messalina"(39) who was executed for her reputed concupiscence and infidelity to Claudius.(40) According to these writers, the Roman physician, Aulus Cornelius Celsus, may have been Scribonius' teacher and "his guiding light"(39); some authorities believe that their works may have been compiled together in some editions.

The authors Pellegrino ascertain that an important translation of the text *Compositiones* begins with a salutation to Scribonius' patron, Gaius Julius Callistus, who, as Emperor Claudius' secretary, commissioned Scribonius' book. According to these authors, Scribonius' *Compositiones* shows a humanistic philosophy of medicine and medical ethics unprecedented in earlier Greek works. Accordingly, Scribonius' uses the word *humanitas* and *misericordia*, respectively, connoting the feelings of "humaneness" and "compassion" in similar usage to that of many other authors of the Augustan Golden Age. Yet these authors point out that Seneca the Younger [105] equates the word *misericordia* "with pity, a mental defect that blunts the mind, interfering with discernment of facts, good judgment, justice, and prudence."(39) So that the meaning of the word was by no means accepted universally.

[105] The original source here is Seneca's *De Clementia*.(39)

We also learn that *dignitas* was the most prized possession of the Roman citizen because it embodied all the ideals of worth, honor, glory, and reputation. Therefore to preserve *dignitas*, a Roman would make "any sacrifice." Thus, in the opinion of the authors Pellegrino, "it was in defense of his *dignitas* that Julius Caesar crossed the Rubicon river in 49 B.C. and began the civil war with Pompey the Great."(39) Because of his *dignitas*, Caesar defied the Senate and fulfilled his ambitious destiny. Perhaps even more precisely, by crossing the Rubicon, Caesar wrought the death knell of the Roman Republic. This act alone would seem to support Scribonius who seems to suggest to both Prof. Edelstein and the authors Pellegrino that, "at least for the physician when practicing medicine, even dignitas must take second place to humanitas."(12,31,39)

It is ironic that many ethical principles and humanistic tendencies were expressed by Scribonius at the time of the premier golden age of the Roman Empire, irrespective of the ethics of the reigning emperors, for Scribonius wrote his ethics during a period encompassing both the reigns of the depraved and infamous Caligula as well as the efficient and studious Claudius. Such are the ironies of history.

The most influential of the stoic philosophers from the Roman perspective may have been Panaetius of Rhodes, as we have intimated, for he introduced stoicism made more adaptable to the old Roman virtues of courage, temperance, honesty, justice, benevolence, and family; this was definitely stoicism with a more humane touch yet molded as to befit the practical Romans. The authors Pellegrino also point out the strong influence of Cicero, whose name today is nearly synonymous with "great oratorical and rhetorical skills." They remind us that Cicero himself attended stoic philosophy lectures given by disciples of Panaetius in Rhodes in 78 B.C. This early experience may have been of paramount importance in the formation of his attitudes and ideals which he, in turn, projected into Roman society.(39) They note that in his *De Officiis*, written between 46-43 B.C., Cicero expounded on his ideas of morals, duties, and obligations, and at least in the views of these authors, he ultimately resolved the long-standing conflict of duty and civic obligations.(41).

Cicero, the quintessential rhetorician, was also the ultimate Roman jurist, lawyer, and philosopher whose Latin treatises were inspired by the classical Greek philosophers, particularly Plato and Aristotle. Cicero, along with Seneca the Younger and the stoic philosophers, notably Panaetius of Rhodes, was largely responsible for the introduction of Greek philosophy, culture, and aesthetics to ancient Rome. Seneca the Younger, a connoisseur of rhetoric and history, albeit not a physician, should also be given credit for the formation of practical Roman humanism, based in part on the Roman legacy of natural laws and the Greek ideals of philanthropy.

According to the Pellegrinos, Cicero, in discussing the professions in general, and Scribonius, in discussing medicine in particular, fostered the Roman ethics underlying the Hippocratic Oath as a professional contract – a *sacred trust*. Cicero, for example, discussed the "sacredness of good faith, trust, morality over financial gain," whilst Scribonius Largus propounded on the humanity, *humanitas*, and compassion, *misericordia*, of the medical profession as sacred oaths. Many other features of Cicero's stoic philosophy, such as choosing virtue and duty, particularly morality over expediency and financial gain, characterize a good person. Thence, we can all surmise that Cicero may have been the primary source of information and knowledge to have influenced the physician Scribonius Largus' humanistic and secular medical ethics.(39)

The medical historians, Profs. Darrel W. Amundsen and Gary B. Ferngren, as well as the authors Pellegrino affirm that Cicero's and Scribonius' idea of *humanitas* and *misericordia* exceeded the Hippocratic notion of *philanthropia*.(39,42) In fact, E.D. Pellegrino goes a step further to assert that the sense of humanitarianism and compassion displayed by Scribonius (and Galen) "was only exceeded in beneficence by the Christian notions of *Agapés and Caritas*.[106] (43)

Medical bioethical imperatives derived from the old stoic philosophy and Scribonius' writings are virtue-based, which is the oldest ethical theory. Virtue-based ethics emphasizes the professional integrity of the physician, rather than the requirement of resolution of every complex medical ethical dilemma. In this vein, the authors Pellegrino point out: "Scribonius' ethics...is based on the humanity of both the physician and the patient, and on the special kind of human relationship that binds physician and patient to one another. It places the source of the obligation on the dependent and afflicted humanity of the person who is ill."(39) They conclude their excellent essay on Scribonius' humanism and ethics with a peroration that deserves quoting: "The ethical principles we find in Scribonius are based in an evolution of Greek *philanthropia*, as exemplified in the Hippocratic ethic, and Roman *humanitas*, as exemplified in Cicero. These two concepts provide a solid basis for a humanistic ethic – one that sees the essence of the physician-patient relationship and a promise that the physician will serve beyond self-interest. It is a sacred promise that embodies trust and, therefore, imposes a sacred obligation of fulfillment. It is, in fact, a covenantal promise – not a contract." And they conclude: "To opt for a virtue-based ethics is not to deny the utility or importance of ethical analysis and clarification that dominates Anglo-American medical ethics. But, when all is said and done, the patient is dependent upon the character, the trustworthiness, the moral sensitivity, and the resources of the physician. This is understandably difficult to accept in an egalitarian and democratic age, but is ultimately inescapable."(39)

The text of Scribonius Largus also gives insight into Roman medicine. For example, he mentions opium extracts and the use of beneficial herbs and effective drugs, whilst rejecting superstition and the use of magical remedies. As a high-society Roman and Latin scholar, he continued the Greek Hippocratic tradition of natural (scientific) medicine. Yet Scribonius was no conformist. He criticized the main Græco-Roman sect of physicians, the Asklepiads, the followers of Asklepius, the legendary physician-priest who venerated the healer god Æsculapius. Scribonius criticized the Asklepiads because of their inclination to use diets, baths, and exercises whilst at the same time they capriciously rejected the use of drugs and medicinal herbs in their treatment, for as we now know, Scribonius used medicinal herbs and drugs frequently in his practice and encouraged others to do likewise.(37,39)

The era encompassing the times of Cicero and Scribonius was an ebullient period in the history of medical and legal ethics, although it was not recognized as such at that time. Even though the Greeks had established the medical art of the *Iatros* as an ethical profession, it was left up to the Romans to bestow upon the

---

[106] *Caritas* refers to charity. Agapé refers to one of the three types of love referred to by the ancient Greek philosophers and later assimilated by Christianity; *Philos* refers to brotherly love; *Eros* to sexual love. *Agapé* refers to the overflowing, spontaneous, unmotivated, unrequited kind of love given to others regardless of their personal foibles.

physicians, the *medici*, the legal recognition that the Greek physicians never attained. And in this regard, it should be noted that although Emperor Augustus recognized the physicians as an important class of citizens in society, it was not until the reign of Emperor Septimius Severus (reigned, A.D.193-211) that medical practice was legally and judicially ordained as a distinct (and privileged) profession.

CHAPTER 23

MODERN PERSPECTIVES

We shall return to proven ways – not because they are old, but because they are true.
Barry Goldwater, Former U.S. Senator (R-Az)

Humanism has been recently defined by medical historian, Dr. C. Rollins Hanlon, as "a devotion to human interest from an individual standpoint, as contrasted with a view of the human race in general." He added, "it has a second meaning of devotion to studies of human culture, such as those carried on by the humanists after the Renaissance...especially with the cultures of Rome and Greece as determined from the literary traditions."(44)

Humanism comes from the Latin word *humanus*, which is derived from the word *homo* for man. Yet, it seems that the terms humaneness (which we have previously discussed) and *humanitarianism* may be more in tune with the underlying meaning of the word *humanism* as used in the context intended by the Roman physician and scholar, Scribonius Largus. These terms connote sympathy (or even empathy), love of fellowman and consideration for the welfare of mankind—terms more akin to the Greek word, *philanthropia* that denotes beneficence and fraternal love, than to humanism as a "devotion to human interest from an individual standpoint."

Humanism, as opposed to humanitarianism, is then a more individualistic term that conveys interest of people, as individuals, and fondness for certain disciplines of human endeavor, such as history, philosophy, literature, language, art, and music – that are loved purely for their own sake.

In his erudite essay, "Surgery and the Humanities," Hanlon relates that the National Foundation for the Humanities also adds to these definitions of humanism the theoretical study of linguistics and jurisprudence, as well as comparative religion and ethics. As Hanlon notes, today a controversy rages between the comparative importance of secular humanism and orthodox religion to the development and evolution of medical ethics. Yet, it should be obvious that they both exert considerable influence, not only on the evolution of medical ethics, but also on medical practice *per se*. Since one of the definitions of the humanities may be partially (and inchoately) the interrelation of the arts of communication, history, and philosophy, it is relevant that these disciplines be discussed within the context of medical practice. I agree and have attempted to do just that in the pages of this book.

The man possessed of knowledge of the humanities in ancient Rome, Hanlon reminds us, was believed to be "liberated" from the doldrums of human existence. Those who were and are able to grasp the knowledge of the humanities were then, and are today, capable of being manumitted from the inanities of human existence. And, he is also correct when he maintains that the individual, the soul liberated by the knowledge of the "Liberal Arts," possesses the key to life and is blessed with the know-how to relate to society. Physicians must indeed be, likewise, possessed of this liberating knowledge for the tasks ahead.

The humanities in Græco-Roman tradition reflected the paramount and eternal Roman interest in politics, law, and government – the disciplines which were considered worthwhile professions for the patricians and later, the Roman aristocracy, the *nobiles*, of Cicero's times. Later in the medieval universities, the Liberal Arts were divided into two major segments which were assimilated and incorporated into their curricula as the *Trivium* and the *Quadrivium*. The *Trivium* included the study of grammar, rhetoric, and logic, subjects which reflected the need for the essential attributes of communication in both writing and public discourse, attributes that were valued and treasured by the Romans. The *Quadrivium*, on the other hand, incorporated arithmetic, geometry, astronomy, and music.

Marcus Terentius Varro (116-27 B.C.), the Roman Man-of-Letters of the late Republic, was perhaps the most influential advocate of the study of the seven Liberal Arts, and perhaps his pedagogic impetus was most responsible for the preservation and later incorporation of these disciplines in medieval educational curricula of the nascent universities of the Middle Ages.(45)

This is an important point because, as we shall see in the next section, one of the great achievements of the Middle Ages was the birth and rise of the medieval universities, and associated with it, the genesis of the first medical schools. Architecture and medicine would later be formally added to the academic curricula.(44) All of these interrelated disciplines became inveterate parts of the curricula of the universities and thence, *de facto* components of the educational curriculum of the "learned professions."

In his cogent discussion of the interrelation between surgery and the humanities, Hanlon appropriately quotes E.D. Pellegrino's statement that "medicine is the most humane of the sciences, the most empiric of arts, and the most scientific of humanities."(46) This is indeed a memorable citation, for it is well substantiated by relevant medical history and certainly affirms the inclusion of medicine in the realm of the arts, the humanities, and the sciences.

But, if this is so, why is the art and science of medicine so deprecated by today's so-called health care experts? Clearly because they are statist bureaucrats and technocrats who know little of history, and their prime motivation is simply camouflaged self-interest masquerading as altruism because by militating for the government takeover of the American health care industry, they not only safeguard their own bureaucratic jobs but they augment their own positions of power whether in the private sector where they are hired to deal with government regulations or in the government hierarchy writing them.

Hanlon, in his article, calls for the revitalization of Western culture and quotes the scholar, Gerald Sirkin, who wrote: "American culture...is the belief in the self-reliance and independence of the individual; the belief in the Golden Rule, the spirit of fair play; the dedication to honesty, humanitarian decency, equality of opportunity; freedom from government meddling; the habit of working out differences by agreement and compromise."(44) The ancient Greeks not only recognized the differences between knowledge and wisdom, but they also recognized differences, nuances, and similitudes of knowledge. Here Hanlon makes a valid comparison between the accumulation of raw knowledge and the attainment of refined wisdom: "Knowledge is not the same as wisdom, the distillate of knowledge that comes with thoughtful logical analysis of information and its application to life."(44) For instance, *epistemé* refers to factual and theoretic knowledge, whereas *techné* refers to applied practical knowledge. The Greek word for wisdom was *sophia* which took into account the moral aspects of knowledge.

We must strive for quality medical education, individual ethics, and individual rights, and if that means more emphasis on the humanities in medical school, then we should all clamor for it. I have always believed that physicians should be well-versed in the humanities and conversant in the Liberal Arts, as they should be expected to be well-rounded citizens involved in learning, teaching, writing, or engaged in the civic affairs of their communities. Today, it is even more imperative that practitioners truly be Renaissance physicians in the classical sense. Yet if the emphasis on the humanities is only a pretext to de-emphasize science as a devious way to lower standards or provide affirmative action (quotas), then the policymakers would be perpetrating an intellectual travesty and a most serious affront to professional honesty.[107]

I bring this point up because along with the criticism of the medical profession and the see-sawing of the health system reform debate, I would be saddened but not surprised if in the future, the profession being less appealing, medical school admission requirements would be lowered to accommodate less qualified applicants – a move that would ultimately result in lower caliber physicians. Some recent data suggest that already many of the new enrollees' motive for entering medical school, given the present defamation and adversarial legal climate, is not answering a calling but moving towards assured financial protection from "bad economic times."(30,47-49)

Suffice it to say that physicians as members of a heretofore independent and honorable profession should look after the interest of their patients and refuse to go along with any government scheme that stresses cost containment at the expense of quality of care, or the establishment of health care rationing in order to pacify bureaucrats who have neither the interest of the profession, nor that of the sick and vulnerable at heart. I am convinced that in the present political climate, government priorities are being set under a doctrine of anomalous utilitarianism and bureaucratic pseudo-altruism that physicians in good conscience may not be able to support.[108] As we shall see, we have good reason to take these socialist, utopian ideals with great skepticism, for what we may get instead is more stifling bureaucracy, along with the deterioration of medical care, and the sapping of our own health by the actions and inactions of government providers. But what about our current crisis of conscience and the declivity of American culture precipitated by our march toward socialism (more onerous regulations, increased taxation, not to mention industrial policy in the making, etc.) led by the government elites who long for even more government control whilst giving lip service to democracy and free markets?

---

[107] Moreover, the government has in the wings plans to limit the number of specialists and because minorities are "underrepresented" in some of those high-tech, limited specialties, positions in those highly sought after disciplines will be reserved for favored minorities or allotted as to achieve proportional racial and gender equity. You will not know whether your heart specialist or neurosurgeon obtained his/her degree based on merit and achievement or was handed his/her degree to fulfill a quota. Not only is the public deceived but the intended beneficiaries stigmatized by such outrageous and unfair social engineering.

[108] Utilitarian ethics are derived from Jeremy Bentham's (1748-1832) utilitarianism that held that the greatest happiness to the greatest number is the fundamental principle of morality. John Stuart Mill (1806-1873) used utilitarianism to advocate political and social reform and thus came closer to the new fallacious brand of utilitarian ethics embodied in modern socialism. I, having lived under the reality of its full implementation in Cuba (during "its golden age") characterize it as pseudo-altruism.

The conservative writer Russell Kirk has admonished us: "we are stumbling into a new Dark Age, inhumane, merciless, a totalist political domination in which the life of spirit and the inquiring intellect will be denounced, harassed, and propagandized against: George Orwell's *1984* (1949), rather than Aldous Huxley's *Brave New World* (1932) of cloying sensuality." He believes that the affliction affecting Western culture, particularly American civilization, is a "decay of religious belief." He argues that "if a culture is to survive and flourish, it must not be severed from the religious vision out of which it arose."(50)

Likewise concerned with the disintegration of American culture, the late conservative thinker, Malcolm Muggeridge wrote:

As the astronauts soar into the vast eternities of space, on earth the garbage piles higher; as the groves of academe extend their domain, their alumni's arms reach lower; as the phallic cult spreads, so does impotence. In great wealth, great poverty; in health, sickness; in numbers, deception. Gorging, left hungry; sedated, left restless; telling all, hiding all; in flesh united, forever separate. So we press on through the valley of abundance that leads to the wasteland of satiety, passing through the gardens of fantasy; seeking happiness ever more ardently, and finding despair ever more surely.(51)

Not only are drugs, fast living, and violence contributing to self-destructive behaviors leading to poor physical health and soaring morbidity and mortality statistics, [109] but these behavior patterns also lead to the dehumanization and demoralization of American society.

Kirk maintains that the new attitudes – "scientism" and its view of the human condition, *reductionism*, a liberal ideology that denies the existence of the soul – are substantially responsible for the disarray that we experience in our personal lives, along with the decline in culture and religion in American life. He defines "scientism" incisively and precisely thus: "the popular notion that the revelations of natural science, over the past century and a half or two centuries, somehow have proved that men and women are naked apes; that the ends of existence are production and consumption; that happiness is the gratification of sensual impulses; and that concepts of the resurrection of the flesh and the life everlasting are mere exploded superstitions."(50)

As a result of these attitudes and the parlous state of human existence, we find ourselves at a perilous juncture. Kirk cites the accomplished historian, Christopher Dawson, who in 1949 wrote:

The events of the last few years portend either the end of human history or a turning point in it. They have warned us in letters of fire that our civilization has been tried in the balance and found wanting—that there is an absolute limit to the progress that can be achieved by the perfectionment of scientific techniques detached from spiritual aims and moral values....The recovery of moral control and the return to spiritual order have become the indispensable

---

[109] Perhaps these poor lifestyle and self-destructive behavior patterns are reflected in the recently released mortality statistics (U.S. 1990) which revealed that tobacco abuse resulted in 400,000 deaths; poor diet and sedentary activity patterns 300,000 deaths; alcohol 100,000 deaths; and firearms 35,000 deaths; sexual behaviors 30,000 deaths; motor vehicles 25,000 deaths; and illicit use of drugs 20,000 deaths.(52)

conditions of human survival. But they can be achieved only by a profound change in the spirit of modern civilization. This does not mean a new religion or a new culture but a movement of spiritual reintegration which would restore that vital relation between religion and culture which has existed at every age and on every level of human development.(53)

Yet Kirk does not feel that this decline is irreversible. Although American (and Western) civilization "stand in peril," restoration and renewal are possible by "true learning, humane and scientific; the reform of many public policies; the renewal of our awareness of a transcendent order, and of the presence of an Other; the brightening of the corners where we find ourselves – such approaches are open to those among the rising generation who look for a purpose in life."(50) Kirk cites the British statesman and patriot, Edmund Burke (1729-1797), who believed that the future cannot be foretold and that nations' destinies are not fixed, for even when nations "seemed plunged in unfathomable abysses of disgrace and disaster...they have suddenly emerged." Burke surmised that perhaps these changes in fortune were the work of Providence.(54) Kirk's example of a nation in crisis was Britain which, despite her precarious political and military existence in 1796 *vis-à-vis* the might and zeal of revolutionary France, emerged victorious and triumphant after the War of 1812 to become the preeminent power in the world until the advent of the 20th Century.(50)

THE PIG'S PEN

Lured and successfully enticed by the sirens' songs of government promises of financial remuneration *quid pro quo* providing medical care to the indigent and the elderly in 1965, physicians became ensnared by the web of government bureaucracy. Rather than recounting in detail this well told story, let me relate to you an analogous parable that comes to mind.

This allegoric tale concerns wild hogs, soon-to-become domesticated pigs, which I first heard from a retired colleague, Dr. L.E. Dickey of Macon, Georgia.[110] Dickey related the story as follows:

Years ago in a great horse-shoe bend down the river, there lived a drove of wild hogs. Where they came from no-one knew, but they survived floods, fires, freezes, droughts, and hunters. The greatest compliment a man could pay to a dog was to say that he had fought the hogs in Horse-Shoe Bend and returned alive. Occasionally a pig was killed either by dogs or a gun – a conversation piece for years to come.

Finally, a one-gallused man came by the country store on the river road, and asked the whereabouts of these wild hogs. He drove a one-horse wagon, had an axe, some quilts, a lantern, some corn, and a single barrel shotgun. He

[110] In the HCA Coliseum Medical Center's Bulletin, Dr. Dickey wrote, "I am reminded of a story that I have kept over the years told by the late Dr. J.G. McDaniel of Atlanta...and recorded on the pages of the Fulton County Medical Society bulletin in 1961. The story is attributed to the Honorable Stephen Pace, a highly regarded Georgia Congressman, and is said to have been told at a barbecue on the banks of the Ocmulgee [River] in response to a bill in Congress providing that farmers would be given money if they did something. Congressman Pace opposed the bill and offered the...plausible story, entitled, " *Whose Bread I Eat" – His Song I Must Sing.*"(55)

was a slender, slow moving, patient man; he chewed his tobacco deliberately and spat very seldom.

Several months later he came back to the same store and asked for help to bring out the wild hogs. He stated that he had them all in a pen over in the swamp.

Bewildered farmers, dubious hunters, and store-keepers all gathered in the heart of Horse-Shoe Bend to view the captive hogs.

'It was all very simple,' said the one-gallus man. 'First I put out some corn. For three weeks they would not eat it. Then some of the young ones grabbed an ear and ran off in the thicket. Soon they were all eating it, then I commenced building a pen around the corn, a little higher each day. When I noticed that they were all waiting for me to bring the corn and had stopped grubbing for acorns and roots, I built the trap door. Naturally, said the patient man, they raised quite a ruckus when they seen they was trapped, but I can pen any animal on the face of the earth if I can jist get him to depend on me for a free hand-out.'(55)

Understandingly, Dickey exhorts us to make our own moral conclusions regarding this highly relevant parable.

ETHICISTS, PHILOSOPHERS, AND TECHNOCRATS

A seemingly cryptic truth in medical ethics is that many of today's medical ethicists are not practicing physicians or even medical doctors. Yet they presume to know what is right or wrong, ethical or unethical, in both the practice of medicine and in the patient-doctor relationship – without having ever treated a patient or borne the responsibility of being a physician. Some are philosophers, others are professors in various other disciplines, or theologians, who have stepped in, ostensibly to fill a perceived social need in the field of bioethics.

Semi-retired or retired physicians who have served in the trenches of the health care delivery system should be encouraged to enter this burgeoning field. Active or retired members of the surgical high-risk, liability-prone specialties, unfortunately, seem to be conspicuously underrepresented in this field. Yet it is they who are frequently involved in some of the most complex medical-ethical decisions that are made in clinical practice and who are receiving the brunt of the medical-legal enfilade and the government barrage of stringent regulations and controls under the guise of questionable ethical practices. It is they who are also coming under the ever-increasing scrutiny in the process of data collection, pattern analysis, and clinical outcomes of care, under the guise of overutilization of medical services, or utilization of services that reviewers deem "inappropriate" or "not medically necessary." Make no mistake about it. In the very near future, this data collection and analysis will be used against physicians by the Orwellian government bureaucrats for their own schemes, such as economic credentialing for fiscal control of physicians.(16)

So it should be surprising to no one that these medical ethicists, filling this real or perceived vacuum in the field of ethics, and despite the best intentions of some, are nevertheless, having difficulty understanding the realities of the complex ethical dilemmas confronting present-day medical practice.

In effect, we have come to a critical area where physicians need to get involved: Medical Ethics. Active or retired physicians who have a surfeit of experience in the ethical and intricate practice of medicine and the mechanics of the patient-doctor relationship need to become involved in the evolving fields of bioethics, and the related and increasingly complex discipline of health care management. Ideally, all physicians should be well-versed in medical ethics and have some working knowledge of medical practice management. Physicians need to be more than modern-age technologically-minded *medici*, but also *enlightened physiks*, and as we shall see, they will have to become Renaissance physicians who can properly balance abstract idealism with tangible reality.

Medicine needs physician-ethicists to teach young physicians and medical students from real-life, personal experiences (in both Socratic and Hippocratic fashion), not from the vantage point of detached arm-chair philosophers who, regardless of intentions, have never had any actual experience in medical practice or the patient-doctor relationship. With this in mind, it is appropriate to recall the wise words of the eminent transplant surgeon Alexis Carrel (1873-1944) who said, "A few observations and much reasoning lead to error; many observations and a little reasoning lead to truth."

Saturated with daily, biased, sensationalist news[111] from a liberal media who espouse the leftist viewpoint on most social and economic issues (56-58), the public resents what they have come to believe is the persona of physicians, namely, that of greedy and uncaring providers who make way too much money. A view that, by in large, is neither true nor justified in the vast majority of cases. But who can blame the public, given the constant media bombardment with biased reporting, and the constant flip-flopping in "scientific and ethical pronouncements" from publicity-seeking and self-styled health care "experts" who want to score political points with the Establishment, rather than promote the dissemination of true science? A recent trend, in fact, has been the reliance placed by a growing number of the public on what the health care "experts," particularly public health workers, opine. Since these opinions are often contradictory and politically motivated, you have the basic ingredients for the public policy disarray that we so frequently experience when we turn on the news.

Meanwhile, amidst all this confusion, the health of our nation hangs in the balance. The physicians, the healers who have effected miraculous cures and brought us medical wonders in the scientific era of medicine, are plagued by incertitude and guilt. They know they are losing control of their patients to middlemen who want a piece of the action and to a growing bureaucracy with an insatiable thirst to control and regulate. Moreover, doctor-bashing has become what *Time* magazine has called, "the bloodsport of America."(24) Suddenly, physicians are the bad guys and a good topic for strangers to start conversations. Never in the history of this great nation has a whole segment of the most productive, industrious, and beneficent members of society been so much assailed, disparaged, and denigrated

---

[111] This media bias has been amply documented by such academicians as Professors Robert Lichter and Stanley Rothman; media watchdog authorities as Reed Irvine and Joseph Goulden at Accuracy in Media (AIM); and journalists as William A. Rusher, former publisher of *National Review.*

because of incipient resentment of their prosperity, justified by the proverbial "bad apples in the barrel."

So the story goes that because of the few bad apples, the whole barrel has been called spoiled and therefore, the entire profession is being blamed, accused, indicted, tried, and convicted as a whole for every ill afflicting the health care system, as an ignominious group, rather than judged as single fallible individuals. All Americans who value industriousness, entrepreneurship, private philanthropy, and self-reliance are poised for a rude awakening unless we change the present course. For in this trajectory, we are not poised for a rendezvous with a glorious destiny but for a cheap tryst with socialist injustice that we will long regret.

PHYSICIANS UNDER SIEGE

I believe there are more instances of the abridgement of the freedom of the people by gradual and silent encroachment of those in power than by violent and sudden usurpations.
James Madison (1788)

For the closing decade of the 20th Century and beyond, Americans in general and physicians in particular must contemplate the priceless dual legacy of Græco-Roman humanism and Judeo-Christian culture. Renewal of this inheritance is essential, for survival of one pillar depends upon the integrity of the other. Moreover, these two pillars must be fortified to deal with the increasingly corroding and outright hostile influences of the unabashedly liberal cultural zeitgeist of our times and the egalitarian socialist ethos of the entrenched political establishment. This does not mean that total socialization of the health care delivery system is inevitable, but it does mean that physicians will need to get the message out to their patients and to those in the media who might still listen. The message: that physicians are still the best advocates for their patients. As always, they must stress the fact that by law and by oath, and by training and experience, they are responsible for their patients' health.

As always, they must stress the fact that, day in and day out, they place their patient's interest above their own. Yet physicians should not be asked and expected to militate for total self-effacement, either in their daily personal lives or in their collective professional lives. This is neither desirable nor realistic. Physicians may be extraordinary human beings, but they are still human. It has been not by birthright, but by hard and diligent work and self-discipline that physicians have achieved a commendable status in society, a pedestal position from which now sundry, envious malefactors hope to knock them down, and undeservedly so. The integrity of the medical profession is not only fundamental to physicians, but salubrious, essential, and indispensable to society. Ethical physicians (which comprise the vast majority of physicians) must be allowed to practice the best medicine that human resources and the nation can provide for all.

Obviously, since medicine is an inexact science and physicians themselves differ as to their schools of thought, training, and abilities – conventional wisdom should lead us to believe that despite the eventual achievement of universal access, care, like everything else in life, may not be equitable. Even if practice parameters (cookbook medicine) become universally applied, the mere fact that medicine is an

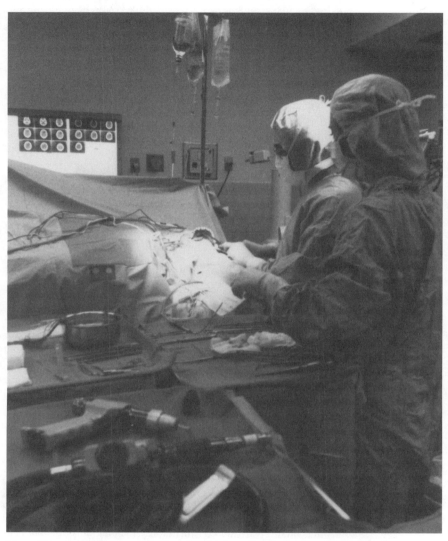

Plate 21 – Author shown performing high-tech, life-saving (high-risk) intracranial microsurgery assisted by his scrub nurse, Mrs. Lyn Sanderson, R.N. and circulating nurse, Mrs. Cathy Street, R.N. (not shown) at HCA Coliseum Medical Centers, Macon, Georgia, 1992.

art and a science, practiced by individual physicians with different backgrounds, would mean that treatment plans will be expected to differ. Moreover, as the old medical adage goes, "no two cases are completely alike." There are just too many variables to consider in each individual case to prognosticate outcome, except within the context of statistical data collection and valid scientific research.

The pursuit and use of scientific data in rigorous investigations as in research and development for the advancement of science and the betterment of mankind is one thing. The use of practice parameters to limit treatment options solely for the sake of cost reductions, indiscriminate data collection for the evaluation of the cost-effectiveness of care, and the filing of dubious clinical outcomes (e.g., patient satisfaction) is another. It goes a long way to give the state the power to call doctors "guilty" whenever it likes. In short, I fear that indiscriminate data collection of previously privileged information, like redundant rope, will be used to hang physicians merely to serve the purpose of economic credentialing [112] or to satisfy the bureaucrats in search of fulfillment of their government-assigned quotas of provider-victims.

At least for now, the Professional Review Organizations (PROs) have expressed the desire to use and review data emphasizing *pattern analysis* of physician's medical practice, rather than case by case review. But even this shift may be deleterious to physicians and patients. Dr. John D. Wilkinson, an internist in charge of utilization review at HCA Coliseum Medical Centers in Macon, Georgia, recently wrote: "All of the announcements [by the PROs] regarding 'appropriate documentation' are intended to serve as a clever distraction. Their hidden agenda has been a well-kept secret. Specifically, the focus of review is shifting from our individual *processes* of medical care to our outcomes of care. In other words, our statistics are now more important than the details of the care provided to any specific patient."(59)

Today, data collection and practice parameters are double-edge swords for physicians, although they can be used as research and educational tools, theoretically, to benefit patients; they can also be misused. Therefore, physicians, as always, will have to bear the responsibility for individualizing patient care and doing what is best for his/her own patients despite collective data and guidelines.[113]

Furthermore, bureaucratic decrees such as the well-intended Americans With Disabilities Act (ADA) have placed further constraints upon a physician's decision-making process, as it relates to their future role in cost containment and rationing of health care, as based on quality of life and disability. Medical decisions in recent years, at the behest of health care pundits and high-profile ethicists, have been based upon *cost-effective analysis* and other economic considerations, such as the *proper allocation of finite resources*. Now, under ADA rules, physicians' medical decisions will "come under ever more scrutiny, and perhaps investigation, if they involve disabled persons."(61) Specifically, physicians who treat disabled persons, regardless of clinical outcome data or practice parameters, must make sure that individualized, sound, clinical judgment enters the clinical decision making process, otherwise the mandates of

---

[112] Economic credentialing is the term used to describe hospitals' increasing use of utilization review data about physicians' medical practices not for quality of care, but for financial impact. Thus, economic factors may be primarily considered in deciding for or against physicians when they apply for new, additional, or renewal of clinical staff membership in hospitals, or membership or renewal status in health care networks such as HMOs (Health Maintenance Organizations), PPOs (Prefered Provider Organizations), etc.

[113] Available data reveal that there are at least 1,300 existing practice parameters nationwide, with an additional 200+ under development. Moreover, many of these parameters were not developed by physicians and thus may actually be inaccurate and ultimately detrimental to clinical practice and patient care.(60)

the ADA will make practitioners ever more liable for violating patients' civil rights and will consequently increase their chances of facing civil and criminal liability.(61)

One final note on this subject of data collection, practice parameters, and clinical outcomes as it relates to utilization review and quality assurance, and that is the new concept of *provider reimbursement contingent upon clinical outcome* (and patient satisfaction). If this concept becomes reality, it will be another nightmare for physicians and another health care crisis in the making, for it will open another window of opportunity for the attorney-litigators: every suboptimal result or surgical complication would be subject to litigation under the false presupposition that treatment outcomes can be guaranteed. For then, every clinical, therapeutic plan would be expected to result in a satisfactory outcome, every operation a success, every patient cured, every customer satisfied.

Obviously, the health policy experts concocting this brew of grandiose expectations have not considered human nature, nor learned any lessons from the pages of history. Namely, the fact that the practice of medicine is a marriage of art and science, and as Sir William Osler (1849-1919) once declared, "Medicine...a science of uncertainty and art of probability. Absolute diagnoses are unsafe and made at the expense of conscience." Whilst physicians must ever pursue excellence and the advancement of science for the betterment of mankind, physicians (and the health expert gurus) must not forget their own human limitations or the fleeting and evanescent nature of our existence.

As we have seen, the ancient Roman *medicus*, Scribonius Largus, placed some responsibility squarely on the patients as consumers in selecting their physicians. Moreover, he recommended that a physician's track record, as to integrity, competence, and ability, be ascertained prior to patients undergoing treatment. This suggestion is valid, as over 90% of patients seen in physicians' offices are not emergencies.(62) So patients, in most cases, do have the time to check their doctors, their reputations, and their qualifications. Medical qualifications and areas of expertise can often be ascertained from the county medical societies.

Moreover, the public can check credentials with the state medical boards [114] and find out whether physicians have been sanctioned by the disciplining process; whether physicians are board-certified can be ascertained from the specialty boards. Perhaps the best way to find out about physicians, their medical practices, and their qualifications are from present or former patients, and from family members or friends who may be familiar with a particular physician by way of previous treatment. One can also ask physician friends about other physicians or specialists.

Patients do not shop for physician services as they do other services or commodities. In my opinion, the essential ingredient that is missing is the lack of proper economic incentives that encourage patients to act as prudent consumers of medical care, not only in finding the best doctor for them but also in getting the most medical care for their own health care dollars. Today, since medical care does not follow free-market forces, patients do not act as prudent consumers when seeking medical care. You see, only 10%-20% of patients' health care bills are out-of-pocket expenses, and patients do not perceive that they are spending their own money. Consequently, in the present system, demand continues to out-strip supply, and there are no brakes to slow down health care costs. At this pace, unless true free-market principles are introduced,

---

[114] In fact, these disciplining bodies' updated lists of sanctioned physicians are frequently sent to newspapers to be published. Newspapers publish these lists at their discretion.

costs will continue to sky-rocket and rationing will ultimately have to be implemented.

I believe that Scribonius' admonition for *caveat emptor* in medical care may have been the first exhortation for freedom of choice in health care, whilst preserving professionalism and compassion in medical care. Most physicians and the public agree with this concept.(60)

The aim of medicine has always been the healing of the sick and the amelioration of suffering. This has been ascertained since Greek classical times. It is also true that "vulnerability...of the patient is always part of being sick." But I disagree that "exploitability of the patient is always part of being sick." It may be so with unethical physicians and unscrupulous "providers" but not as a truism or as a fair assumption to be made for the vast majority of men and women who chose medicine as "their calling."(39)

In fact, it may be worth repeating that in today's environment, physicians are relatively more "vulnerable" to the machinations of ambulance-chasing attorney-litigators and more "exploitable" by the entrenched bureaucracy and the increasingly prosecutorial mode of the federal government in the guise of searching for "fraud and abuse," than any patient calmly waiting in a doctor's office in the usual (90%) non-emergent private setting of quality, ethical medical care.

The problem today is that with the decline of culture and religion and the concomitant ebb in spiritual and moral guidance, Americans have been left with a great void that they are not capable of filling in their daily lives. They are restless, distrustful, and increasingly cynical. Doctors, as a relatively successful and prosperous group, have become fair game because of jealously and envy in an increasingly secular society which worships in the cult of victimhood and the intolerant political establishment which frowns on success and self-reliance. American doctors today, as the European Jews of ages past, have become the perfect scapegoats for a troubled society. It has been estimated that in the U.S. today, physicians spend between 25-40% of their time doing paperwork (13,25,60), not only to satisfy government regulations but also to document minutiae to protect themselves legally from the very same patients they are striving to heal.

Most ironic of all is the fact that patients' interests are best served by their doctors who, despite all the media hoopla and all the self-serving bureaucratic talk to the contrary, remain their genuine advocates. To quote from the Medical Association of Georgia's proposal for health care reform: "We are responsible – by personal commitment, by professional training, by law and by oath – for medical care....More than any group, physicians see people when they are sick and most vulnerable. We observe their needs not in a theoretical vacuum, but in the realistic world of pain and hurt. To us, people are not numbers, but individuals requiring compassion, respect, and healing. We are advocates for these patients and for all those who seek or need medical care."(60)

But the medical profession is opposed by a myriad of self-seeking opportunists, including consumer advocates both within and outside the government bureaucracy who can find nothing right with medicine today, because it is convenient for them to find it so. Bluntly, their jobs depend on it. Amongst these self-proclaimed guardians of the sick is Dr. Sidney Wolfe, head of the Public Citizen Health Research Group (an organization founded by consumer advocate Ralph Nader), who is one of those experts who maintains a high profile criticizing the work of physicians and making a living at it – thanks, in part, to the visibility accorded him by AMA publications. Dr. Sidney Wolfe, a medical internist, to my knowledge, has never practiced medicine following completion of his training; yet he is most vociferous in his criticisms of the current practice of medicine.(63)

From the new administration of President Bill Clinton, we can realistically expect even less than their predecessors, as far as improving the health care system. From the time of the 1992 Presidential campaign, it has become clear that physicians can expect more government intervention in medicine, whilst entertaining minimal, if any, proposals for solving the intolerable medical liability crisis. The First Lady, Hillary Rodham Clinton, brilliant and articulate, is also an attorney-advocate of a myriad of liberal causes (e.g., Children's Defense Fund). She headed the Health Care Task Force that drafted the President's proposal for health care reform, which if implemented would dictate how doctors will practice medicine in the U.S. The present Secretary of HHS, Donna Shalala, a former Chancellor of the University of Wisconsin, who was said to have been the priestess of political correctness on the university campus, has had no previous experience in health care matters. She does possess a Ph.D. in political science which might serve her well in further politicizing HHS, enforcing central planning, and shoving statist health care policies down the throat of the practicing physicians, but in my opinion, she is certainly not sagacious in health care issues, as her briefings on the Clintonian health care proposals have amply demonstrated. Yet this is perhaps the most complex issue that this administration has set itself to tackle.

THE NATIONAL PRACTITIONERS DATA BANK

You may have heard much about the blacklisting of artists in the Hollywood movie industry of the 1950s. But I doubt that you have heard much about the government's present-day version of blacklisting of physicians. It is an unconstitutional entity called the National Practitioners Data Bank (the Data Bank). The National Health Care Quality Improvement Act enacted by Congress in 1986 established the Data Bank supposedly to keep track of physicians guilty of professional misconduct, especially those going from one state to another. Purportedly, the Data Bank would not only accomplish this policing task but would also promote peer review activities and thereby improve health care. It has failed miserably on all accounts.(64-71) By virtue of being filed in this infamous blacklisting entity, physicians may carry a permanent blot on their professional records and their reputations. Statistics from the Data Bank strongly suggest that physicians in the high-risk specialties who perform the latest high-tech and most complex procedures, and necessarily extend the horizons of knowledge – not the proverbial "bad apples" – are disproportionally represented in the data bank's "malpractice" statistics.(28,64-72) It is, therefore, the doctors who minister to the sickest and treat the most seriously ill or injured patients who get sued the most and end up blacklisted in the infamous Data Bank.

This 1984-Orwellian agency is in business to track physicians and other health care providers, despite the fact that medicine is already the most scrutinized and policed profession in America. Physicians are being sued, regulated, sanctioned, intimidated, harassed, and blacklisted, and frankly, I see no end in sight to these offenses and civil rights violations. I suspect that this harassment will continue inexorably, as it is a deliberate attempt to force the capitulation of physicians and compel them to swallow the bitter pill of socialized medicine. Moreover, if this unconstitutional entity is allowed to stand, it will establish a beachhead for the landing of similar blacklisting agencies for other professions whose members' civil rights and privacy will likewise be violated.

THE AMA – A WILLING ACCOMPLICE?

Physicians have become easy prey, the scapegoats responsible for whatever ails our morally decadent society and pains our health care system.[115] All of this happened whilst physicians have been struggling to properly care for their patients in the trenches of the health care delivery system. Most of them assumed that as dues-paying members of the AMA, their interests were being represented. Yet the AMA,[116] unfortunately, has wittingly or unwittingly aided and abetted medicine's descent into government enslavement, more interested in appeasing government than in standing for firm convictions and stated principles. The AMA appears to be more interested in selling books which describe all of the new rules and government regulations, (many of which are updated annually and have to be repurchased by physicians year after year in order to comply with the ever-expanding list of draconian government decrees) than in representing the interests of its trusting members. And when the AMA leadership negotiates, you can be sure that it cooperates and appeases, thereby accommodating government and sanctioning its further intrusion into the medical field.[117]

The AMA's policy of "nonconfrontation and cooperation" of the last several years has not worked for the best interests of physicians or their patients. The AMA's intense but misdirected lobbying efforts, not to mention their public relation campaigns, have been utter failures. To underscore this point, recent events have shown that the AMA's call for a "New Partnership" with government was a dismal public relation fiasco. I am talking about the embarrassing situation whereby the AMA was denied "a place at the table" with Clinton's Health Care Task Force, even when it was obvious to health care experts that the AMA would have entered into any Faustian transaction for a vacuous seat at that table. In the words of AAPS Executive Director, Dr. Jane Orient, "The rebuff is especially

[115] The image that the mass media has projected of physicians (within this context usually referred to as "providers" so as to place them in the same mixed bag with others in the health care field from hospitals to suppliers of durable medical equipment), assisted by dubious data provided by government bureaucrats, is that of callous and greedy "providers" who are in it only for the money, commit egregious acts of malpractice against unwary patients, and engage universally in "fraud and abuse" by referring patients unnecessarily to facilities in which they have a vested financial interest.(21,24,25,28,30,73-77)
[116] By the AMA, I mean its overtly pragmatic leadership: the Board of Trustees; the Executive Committee; the AMA's perhaps most influential policy-making body, the Council on Ethical and Judicial Affairs; and the AMA's Executive Vice President.
[117] As recently as December 1993, the House of Delegates of the AMA, frightened by the upheaval and immediacy of health care reforms (in a situation analogous to the times approaching the death knells of the Roman Republic when the people gave up their right to vote and their right to representation for the security and *panem et circenses* of a dictator) voted to give the Board of Trustees more powers – "the ability to independently make policy decision" and be able to act "in between the bi-annual Interim and House of Delegates meetings of the AMA – as to be proactive and to be able to negotiate elements of health system reform with the policymakers (as reported by the AMA: 'This Week,' December 6/13, 1993)."

painful because the AMA was willing to trade practically every principle for a seat at the table."(78)

As many physicians in the trenches see it, the AMA no longer represents them and is too eager to please the enemies of the profession (79) who have already tasted blood and are going for the kill with the Health Security Act of 1993.(14-17) So it is no wonder that only approximately 40% of U.S. physicians belong to the AMA, despite the raised awareness and veritable brouhaha of health systems reform and a vigorous membership campaign (launched in 1991 with the modest goal of enlisting half of all physicians by the end of the decade). Of 718,000 American physicians, only 293,988 are members of the AMA, and little progress has been made increasing its membership. It goes without saying that with the clamor for health care reform and the uncertain times for medicine, physicians should be flocking to join the AMA. That has not happened. And frankly, despite the wish-fulfilling headlines in *American Medical News*, significant membership expansion has not taken place.(80)

The delegates to the AMA do their duty, pass resolutions, and conduct business, but much of their work is often, sadly, to no avail, for the work gets dissipated as it winds up in the laps of the AMA's pragmatic, appeasement-prone leadership. Point of fact is passage of a momentous resolution calling for abolition of the Data Bank during the Interim House of Delegates of 1991.(68) In the fight that physicians have waged on and off against the unconstitutional Data Bank, AMA delegates, representing the expressed wishes of their colleagues, have militated for the AMA position to be outright abolition of this entity. How, then, did the AMA Board of Trustees respond to the expressed wishes of the AMA membership via their delegates with the passage of the momentous resolution? Namely, by pleading for the insignificant provision that medical malpractice payments of less than $30,000 be exempted from inclusion in the Data Bank! This anemic, effete, and spineless response by the AMA leadership is one major reason that organized medicine finds itself so divided.

The AMA would have best served the interests of its members by contesting the constitutionality of entities such as the Data Bank in court (21,28,64,65,81-84) than by wasting large amounts of money ineffectively stuffing the political campaign chests of the very enemies of medicine. Yet despite spending large amounts of money, the AMA is now bogged down in the morass of the health care political debate; scoffed by politicians like Congressman Fortney "Pete" Stark (D-Ca); used as a punching bag by self-styled consumer advocates like Dr. Sidney Wolfe; and rebuffed by the Clinton Administration. And so we still have the infamous Data Bank which remains fully operational.

Enemies of the House of Medicine are now openly and eloquently calling for expansion of reporting requirements and calling for public access to Data Bank files. If in doubt, ask Congressman Ron Wyden (D-Or) who is pushing hard for the implementation of these policies.(69,85) Moreover, the Health Security Act of 1993 dictates that "repeat offenders" (the final definition thereof has not yet been fully elucidated), presumably physicians with at least two reports filed in the Data Bank, be revealed to the public. "Yet repeat offenders don't always equal repeat offenses; sometimes they [the violations] are all on the same case." Thus, this rapidly expanding list would include 6,800 American physicians presently delivering precious medical care.(85)

THE ORWELLIAN USE OF ADMINISTRATIVE LAW

Administrative law has become a veritable fourth branch of government, a gigantic unconstitutional bureaucracy created by the federal government and purportedly deriving its powers from the 1887 Act which gave birth to the first regulatory agency, the Interstate Commerce Commission (ICC).(86) Today, a myriad of government agencies have gone amok writing rules and regulations which simply become law by their publication in the *Federal Register*. Many affect health care and medical practice and encroach on the constitutional rights of physicians as U.S. citizens.(21,28,81-84) As John F. McManus, publisher of *The New American*, has pointed out, these regulations and administrative laws have mushroomed in the last two decades. For example, in President Carter's years, edicts of the federal regulatory agencies filled approximately 88,000 pages annually of the *Federal Register*; the Reagan years, 47,418 (1986); and the Bush years, 67,715 pages of edicts (1991).(86)

Physicians who have been accused (not convicted) of the ubiquitous charge of "fraud and abuse" are repeatedly threatened and sometimes sanctioned via unconstitutional administrative laws which effectively abrogate their civil rights. They are threatened not only with unlawful seizures of confidential medical records but also with the application of asset forfeiture statutes (28,73,74,83,84,86,87). These allow the federal government to seize a physician's personal property (from office records to his/her home, or family car) without a conviction, but merely the accusation of "fraud and abuse." Asset forfeiture proceedings began as a weapon to fight the drug trade, and initially these laws were used against drug dealers. Unfortunately, these laws are increasingly being used against ordinary Americans, notably physicians, who have only been accused of and not convicted of any wrongdoing. Asset forfeiture proceedings have increased dramatically each year since their inception. In fact, federal law enforcement officials have now "seized $4.1 billion in private property – more than the $3.8 billion that burglars carried away in 1992" – by invoking asset forfeiture laws as a vehicle to confiscate private property, effectively circumventing constitutional principles.(88)

The much ballyhooed government campaign against "rampant Medicare fraud and abuse" in the "provider" community was the brain-child of former Inspector General Richard Kusserow who blamed the health care industry in general and the physicians in particular for every problem, real or imagined, concerning fiscal aspects of the American health care system. He made a big issue of "fraud and abuse" by "healthcare providers" and out of his hat pulled a "10 percent rate of health care fraud," which remains the universally cited figure, although it remains unsubstantiated and unproven. Yet it has been used to intimidate physicians and to justify further intervention in the health care industry. The charge of fraud and abuse was initiated (and remains) a calculated threat of coercion and intimidation looming like a dark cloud over the integrity of American physicians, to force them to cooperate and collaborate, as protection against the smearing of reputations and the endangering of livelihoods. And so far, this intimidation campaign has been largely successful at keeping individual members of the profession at bay. (73-75,81,83,89)

The time has come for physicians to counter-attack; it is imperative that they do so. Otherwise, this venerable and noble profession will be emasculated and transformed into a veritable government trade union. If fact, this transmogrification is already taking place to the detriment of the profession, patients, and society. If it is a consolation, presumably physicians would be able to use their unions' power to strike, as has been proposed by the medical writer Harry Schwartz, Ph.D., in a recent article.(90)

As concerned colleagues, physicians should applaud the efforts of others in the medical profession who have stood for truth, warning us about what was (and still is) happening to medicine. In an article entitled, "Medical Practice Has Lost It's Glamour," Dr. George Bohmfalk, a neurosurgeon from Texas, vividly and realistically described the difficulties that conscientious physicians experience as they go about their professional lives practicing high-quality medicine in high-risk specialties, whilst at the same time, being besieged by sundry insurance companies, unscrupulous attorneys, paper shuffling bureaucrats, Medicare officials, and the like.(22) Dr. Bohmfalk not only expressed the views held by many solo-practicing neurosurgeons but also the views held by an increasing number of physicians in other specialties nationwide.

Physicians, as always, must place the patients' interests ahead of their own[118] and continue to advocate for their patients. They must comport themselves with the utmost professionalism. Yet when the occasion requires it, they must learn to fend off unjust criticisms and be proactive rather than reactive in health care policy matters. Physicians owe a duty to the public and to themselves to be well-versed on health care matters, so that they may always be able to discuss and, if necessary, debate crucial health issues with the media, health care experts, or any other influential members of society, whether they be attorneys, business leaders, or politicians.

Physicians need to speak out with sincerity, clarity of purpose, profundity of knowledge (and thought), and moral conviction. They must sharpen their rhetorical abilities and writing skills to write effective editorials and letters to newspapers and magazine editors so that they can reach the public, who thirsts for health system reform information from practicing physicians.(91) As the old adage says, "The pen is mightier than the sword."

Physicians must remember that despite the barrage of bad press and the rife practice of doctor-bashing, physicians still stand head and shoulders above most others professions in the public's regard. Despite the bad publicity, physicians remain at the top of every poll in public trust and admiration, and when it comes to either liking and trusting their own individual physicians, there is virtually no dissent – almost universally, citizens praise their own physicians. But to make the public at large truly sympathetic to the cause of medicine – which parallels their own as patients and consumers of health care – physicians will have to regain their collective public trust as a healing profession. Practitioners will have to counterbalance what they read and hear in the media and challenge any media piece disparaging the profession, especially those incited by jealousy and resentment and unsubstantiated by facts or statistics. The public must be given accurate information to be an informed and vigilant citizenry, and thus won over to the cause of medicine.

THE FUTURE OF MEDICINE

Dr. Reuben P. Bell, who retired at age 42 from the private practice of medicine because of "what he saw as a deterioration of the medical profession,"

---

[118] This primal and supreme ethic should be eternal and immutable – for if it ever changes, there would no longer be a sacrosanct patient-doctor relationship.

writes, "without question, doctors were in charge of their own destiny and that of their patients. Respect for physicians was a necessary component of medical care."(92) All of these facets of the physician's role have changed. He goes on to envision a grim future for American medicine in an increasingly "totalitarian society." He and many other physicians still in the trenches of health care delivery believe that medicine will change for the worse. "The doctors of tomorrow...unlike the aggressive, independent people who took medicine to its pinnacle...will do as they are told, through government decrees, practice guidelines, and peer review. Private practice will disappear because of the new immorality associated with the profit motive."(92) In his estimation, the profession and the work of doctors will decline because doctors will become unhappy working in an adversarial atmosphere and penalized for violating vague and incomprehensible administrative decrees. Furthermore, physician incentive to work will decline and thus, with decreased output from physicians and an increase in the aging population, medical rationing will ultimately be necessary and universal. He writes, "long hours, night and weekend work always has been the bane of doctors. But these problems have gone with the territory, along with the reasonable income and a sense of well being."(92)

Here it would be appropriate to interject that the sense of gratitude that formerly emanated from the community is either no longer present or is on the wane. It is also reasonable to deduce *a priori* that these changes are adding woes to the physician's sense of dissatisfaction, and, given the mounting pressures on physicians, in time, this situation will no longer be tenable or meaningful to doctors who, as human beings, are responsive to incentives as well as obligations.

Bell then quotes Gustave Bischoff, a former faculty member at the City University of New York, School of Engineering: "The professional person is unique among workers. He is free to choose the terms under which he will serve and assumes the attendant responsibility for his actions. This generally acknowledged autonomy flows from liberal education and long preparation in various disciplines. It also stems from the confidential relation to client and official certification of character and competency."(92) This assertion about professionalism appears to be no longer valid for physicians, although it may still be alive and well in the practice of other professions, including society's cutting edge of opportunity as evinced in the totally unregulated legal profession.

Unless physicians mobilize – first, as a moral imperative to protect their own besieged enlightened and beneficent self-interest, and second, to protect their own civil rights as private citizens – one can legitimately deduce as a *fait accompli* that the total subjugation of the medical profession to the state will be accomplished. As I've already mentioned, the profession will then become either a trade union and forced to unionize, or become another self-serving, special-interest group that will collaborate with further socialization *quid pro quo* their piece of the pie.

Unless physicians speak with one forceful voice, forsaking their inter-professional petty rivalries and individual professional jealousies, and unite against the common enemy, they will be sacrificed on the altar of political expediency and for "the public good." Such sacrifice would be extremely detrimental to physicians but even more so to the public who as patients, would be left to the mercy of arbitrary government rationing and the rapacity of government bureaucrats dedicated to perpetuating the cycle of dependency on intended beneficiaries so as to preserve and protect their positions of power and influence.

CHAPTER 24

A SAMPLING OF EGALITARIAN ETHICS AND OTHER SOCIALIST SCANDALS

I hope we shall never be so totally lost to all sense of the duties imposed upon us by the law of social union as, upon any pretext of public service, to confiscate the goods of a single unoffending citizen. Who but a tyrant...could think of seizing on the property of men unaccused, unheard, untried...

Edmund Burke (1729-1797)
Reflections on the Revolution in France (1790)

THE SOVIET CODE OF MEDICAL ETHICS

Recently, an elucidating essay by the Soviet writer A.M. Kozlov came to my attention. In this essay, Kozlov describes medical deontology as it pertained to the physicians of the former Soviet Union. He goes on, in some detail, to explain how "the Code of Soviet Medical Ethics" was passed by the Soviet legislature, adopted by the Supreme Soviet, and incorporated into the USSR Constitution in 1969. According to Kozlov, in 1961 there was a debate entitled "The Law for the Medical Profession" in which he participated and recorded the following passage:

> *all the speakers referred to the humanitarian and noble character of the physician's activity...to the fact that the medical profession is most honorable but linked at the same time to the highest responsibility. A physician must harmoniously blend high professionalism, a wealth of kindness, moral purity, and physical perfection. A great many speakers reminded the words of the great Russian writer and physician, A. P. Chekhov, who stated that 'the medical profession is an act of heroism, demanding self oblivion, purity of soul and thought, that a physician must possess a clear mind, moral purity, and a neat physique,' a fact which is not within anybody's reach.(93)*

It is only in an authoritarian, socialist state, such as the former Soviet Union c.1960-1989, that a government would have the audacity to pretend that ordinary human beings, even when they are members of the "noblest of professions," can be molded into a sort of pliable material and, by shear communist alchemy, transformed into useful fools in the service of an atheist, omnipotent state. Whether this grotesque transmogrification is accomplished by subjective intent or by objective decree, the end result is the same: the incontestable subordination of the individual physician and the subjugation of the profession to serve the all-mighty state, in the name of humanitarianism.

Kozlov informs us that on March 26th, 1971, "by a decree of the Presidium of the Supreme Soviet of the USSR, the text of the Soviet Union's

Physician's Oath was approved. The oath, "which mirrors the moral principles of socialist society," was *obligatory* for all practicing physicians of the Soviet Union:

> *Obtaining the high title of physician and treading on the path of medical activities, I swear solemnly,*
> *– to dedicate my whole knowledge and my strength to the protection and the improvement of Man's health, to the treatment and the prevention of disease, to work conscientiously where the benefit of society asks for;*
> *– to be always ready to give medical assistance, to have an attitude wholly concerned and careful with the patient, to keep the medical secret;*
> *– to continuously improve my knowledge and my medical skill, to contribute by my work to the development of science and of medical practice;*
> *– to ask from my professional colleagues' advice if this is for the benefit of the patient, not refusing advice or help if asked for;*
> *– to observe and develop the noble traditions of the country's medical status, to act in all circumstances according to the principles of communist morale, never to forget the high status of the Soviet physician, his responsibility towards the people and the Soviet state.*
> *I swear to preserve this oath my whole life long.(93)*

As an aside, it should be said that the subordination of science and the subjugation of the medical profession to the State inevitably has led to the corruption of both, as we shall see from examples of the Soviet Union (particularly psychiatry) and hard-Left socialist states, as well as in the soft Left social democracies.

Let us now analyze the tenets of the Soviet Oath. The second, third, and fourth swearing statements are innocuous enough, in that they could be part of a Western democracy's code of medical ethics (or a constitutional republic's, for that matter). The language reflects benevolent ideas inherent to the profession. Nevertheless, the first statement includes..."to work conscientiously where the benefit of society asks for." This phraseology needs some exposition and explication. It asks that the individual physician subordinate himself/herself to the will of society. This is unconditional surrender of the individual's will to the supremacy of the State – for unlimited government and state control is what totalitarian governments mean by "society." This locution is contrary to the instinctive individualism of Americans, the Western concept of limited government, and the ideals of true charity and compassion of the Judeo-Christian patrimony. The phrase, "the benefit of society," has been used by totalitarian and collectivist states to oppress and incarcerate individuals and members of oppressed ethnic minorities throughout this century.(94) In these oppressive *régimes*, "society" is a veritable synonym for the powerful state itself and is used to trounce the civil rights and liberties of individual citizens. Our legacy of natural rights that we treasure, such as life, liberty, property, and the pursuit of happiness, are nonexistent. Or, if granted at all, are qualified out of existence by the power of the state, as was the case in the constitutions of all the former communist states, and still is the case in the United Nations Covenant on Civil and Political Rights.(95)

Another related moral dilemma is summarily resolved in the clearly stated fifth statement: "To act in all circumstances according to the principles of communist morale, never to forget the high status of the Soviet physician, his responsibilities towards the people and the Soviet state."(93) This swearing statement should not be surprising for, as we have seen, in the former USSR, the collectivist and authoritarian state granted physicians their medical "privileges," as well as assigned their responsibilities to society. The physician's individual effort and ability went unrecognized, unless, of course, recognition was of benefit to the state. The physician becomes merely another useful state tool for the control and appeasement of the masses. He or she is manipulated like a chess pawn and used at the discretion of the state for social engineering, or any other unspecified purpose that the state may later decide is "for the good of society." Cultivation of individual initiatives or provisions for voluntary action, personal philanthropy, and true charity are nonexistent, because the omnipotent totalitarian state takes over all these functions.(96)

All of this should become clear to those who make the effort to read history. What is not so easily determined is the forthcoming relationship of a supranational, socialist utopia to be fashioned by the New World Order (*Novus Ordo Seclorum*) vis-à-vis the rights of the individual citizens within this microcosmic world government. The prospects are as staggering, the ramifications as overwhelming as they are frightening. Regardless of body polity and ideology, what should be clear is that total control of the medical profession by any government will be ominous, not just for physicians but even more so for the uninformed public who are the consumers of health care and have the most to lose. Patients are poised to suffer greatly from the government takeover of medicine. Unfortunately, they will only realize that the much touted sense of security is but an illusion that vanishes, when they have the misfortune of falling seriously ill. Only then will they be confronted with the tragic realities of socialized medicine: medical shortages, substandard care, medical rationing, and ultimately outright denial of care and government-sanctioned euthanasia.[119]

Moreover, history, with abundant examples, teaches that only inequities and iniquities are gained when professions such as the clergy, law, and medicine become tools of the state. Prime examples, as we shall soon discover, were the Catholic Inquisition and the equally brutal Protestant persecutions of the late Middle Ages and the Renaissance. Even during the humanism-imbued Renaissance era, religious leaders, incited by zealotry, cheered by the ignorant masses, and aided and abetted by the legal scholars and jurists of the age (as occurred in Catholic Spain, Protestant Scotland, and Calvinist Geneva), participated in collusion with secular authorities in the brutal mock trials, legal tortures, and agonizing burnings, not only of witches and heretics, but also quite conveniently, of political enemies of the state.

Another flagrant example of this perversion, namely the use of professions as tools of the state, of a much more recent vintage was Nazi Germany (National Socialism). It is no secret that during World War II, German physicians under the aegis of the Nazi government committed nefarious acts for the omnipotent state and for what the Nazi government had then decided would be for "the greatest good of society and the Fatherland." German medicine became totally subordinated to the state. Not only did biologic scientists abandon genuine medical

---

[119] Although ethicists argue that active euthanasia does not take place without patients' permission, the truth is that in the Netherlands, where active euthanasia is commonplace, "mercy killing" by physicians takes place routinely in the chronically and seriously ill, frequently without their consent. Even patients with mental disorders (whose competency should be in question) are euthanized in this nation with socialized medicine and literally "cradle-to-grave" benefits.(83)

research but also, covered by the darkness of their pseudo-research, descended into the abyss of barbarism in what came to be known as the Holocaust.(97)

I am not alone in noting the historic parallels between what is happening in America today and what occurred in Nazi Germany during the Holocaust. In an inspiring essay, Anna Scherzer, M.D., an insightful psychiatrist from Scottsdale, Arizona, notes:

> [In America today] the patient is no longer the central individual around whom and for whom the art of healing was developed. Our function is no longer primarily to care for a person. We are now managing covered lives, ostensibly for some greater national or budgetary good. Is this so different from what was demanded of physicians in Hitler's Germany? During that era, it was with the help of the physicians that the efficiency of Nazi extermination was refined. Even before the establishment of systematic, massive killing machines, the scene had been set. Resources were scarce in the post World War I era....The nation had been through terrible financial losses, and the country's morale was at a nadir. After World War I in Germany, physicians were seen as servants of the state, rather than independent practitioners. Their primary allegiance was pledged to the government. At this same time, the chronically ill were viewed as a tremendous economic burden on German society. The sickly, the impaired, the homosexual, and the undesirable were seen as being maintained at the expense of precious and limited resources of the larger community. During that time of national crisis, pressures on the national economy were simply to be eliminated. Medical care was to be rationed.(98)

How, you might ask, does the present situation in America compare to that of Nazi Germany? How could physicians be transformed into dark angels of death for the socialist Nazis? Joseph M. Scherzer, M.D., a dermatologist and President of the Arizona Chapter of the AAPS, has answered both of these questions precisely: In the highly civilized society of Germany, physicians participated in "direct medical killing and systematic genocide" because of *lebensunwertes leben* ("a life unworthy of life")—an "ethical" concept forced by the state upon German physicians and the people. "Physicians were no longer caretakers of an individual patient, but rather promoters of the general health of the German people. Physicians were servants of the state rather than independent practitioners."(99) Moreover, he explains:

> You may find what I am next about to tell you unbelievable – it may seem that I have made it up – but the next few words are all too frighteningly true. The following statement appears in the manifesto of the Arizona Affordable Health Care Coalition, the group of citizens and corporations – including Cigna, Intergroup, Blue Cross and Blue Shield – which is designing my own state's managed care plan. I doubt these people fully realize how closely one of their main policies mimics the paradigm shift in medicine which occurred in Nazi Germany. Their (confidential) "Vision Statement" maintains that: "The physician gradually will need to accept a necessary change of ethical focus from the biomedical mode (intervention without regard to cost if there be any chance of success) to a biosocial model that considers not only the health needs of individu als, but also the health needs of populations, including those members of the population who do not seek medical care...." The methods being used to

successfully turn doctors into servants of the state are designed to substantially decrease, if not destroy, the ethical incentives intrinsic to the proper practice of medicine.(99)

This dark descent into barbarism, a product of doctors cooperating with a brutal, socialist state, should not be allowed to happen. One sure way to avoid the formation of this unholy alliance is to keep medicine independent and separate from government. Now, more than ever, with the growth of socialism at home, it is imperative that medicine frees itself from the government's stranglehold to prevent its impending suffocation. And if all fails, let these words be a statement of what was, and what could have been, if physicians had united and courageously demanded health care enhancement measures that would truly have benefited the health of the American people...and the world. If the American people would again rise to the occasion by becoming an informed and vigilant citizenry in pursuit of the American dream, rather than a dependent mob galvanized by envy and resentment looking for the false illusion of government security – by sheer will and determination they could force this government to once again do what is right for America.

THE ROLE OF GOVERNMENT

Government does have a role in American medicine, and that is to provide the means to equitable and universal access to quality, affordable medical care for all Americans via the private sector. This can be done fairly and efficiently by the establishment of tax-free medical savings accounts (MSA) as promoted by John C. Goodman Ph.D. and associates at the NCPA and the Cato Institute.(25,62,100-104) But this role should not be perverted as to allow further government interference in medical practice and meddling in the patient-doctor relationship – perversions contrived so as to bring about the utter and complete socialization of American medicine. Government has provided valuable assistance in public health and epidemiology (with the tracking, combating, and eradication of infectious diseases), and the promotion of research and development (e.g., the exemplary work at the National Institutes of Health, NIH). These areas of government involvement should be welcomed, for they have in the past truly advanced the health of the nation.[120] The state, too, must recognize that it is in society's best interest to preserve the integrity of the medical profession.(105) Toward this end, government must confront the insufferable liability crisis, a veritable litigation juggernaut, that is engulfing not just businesses (product liability) and the medical profession (medical liability) but our entire society as well. This is the real culprit, the real dragon roaming the land, wreaking havoc amongst the citizens, and it must be stopped.

Major tort reform is urgently needed to genuinely "promote the general welfare" of the nation. Physicians, more than any other group in our society, have suffered the most, personally and professionally, from the devastation wrought by this litigation juggernaut. The same liability crisis that stifles competition in the marketplace, in businesses and in commerce, also hinders the development of new drugs, vaccines, and medical appliances in the medical marketplace – to the detriment of both healthy consumers and sick patients.

---

[120] The historic resources at the National Library of Medicine are also truly outstanding. This is particularly so for the History of Medicine Division of the U.S. Department of HHS, Public Health Service, NIH.

As part of providing "domestic tranquility and promoting the general welfare," not to mention the preservation of the fabric of society and the rubric of its institutions, the time is ripe to proceed with substantial and meaningful liability tort reform and put the brakes on what Walter K. Olson, Senior Fellow at The Manhattan Institute, correctly calls, "the sue-for-profit litigation industry," which is eroding the foundations of our Judeo-Christian heritage.(106) We come back to this issue repeatedly, since as Johann Wolfgang von Goethe (1749-1832) once declared, "the truth requires constant repetition because error is being preached about us all the time."(34)

EGALITARIAN ETHICS

Professor S.R. Benatar asserts that individuals and society demand the best medical treatment available, whilst at the same time they resent the status and prestige of those who provide it, the physicians.(107) This fact, combined with the manifest erosion of religious influence, which has traditionally emphasized duty, obligation, and personal responsibility, has created a conflict, a societal tension, that needs to be addressed as we grapple with the issue of health systems reform. The tendency has been for a steady pull in the liberal direction, resulting in greater power to patients, or rather their self-appointed advocates, bureaucrats, and attorneys. This trend has also eroded the status of physicians and encumbered their duties and responsibilities as the nation's healers and has been compounded by the modern trend to malign physicians and blame them for many of the ills afflicting society, most of which are not even within the purview of physicians.

Moreover, no longer do patients assume that unfortunate medical outcomes occur as a result of natural occurrences which are statistically expected to occur in a given fraction of the population or as acts of Providence. This, despite the fact that the majority of Americans claim to believe in God and affirm that they regularly attend their chosen place of worship. Yet today, a physician can safely assume that if a medical treatment does not yield the expected result and an attorney-litigator is consulted, there is a high likelihood that the erstwhile patient and his/her attorney will convince themselves of "the fact" that malpractice has been committed as a result of negligence on someone's part — either the physician, or the hospital, or both — and a lawsuit will follow.

Members of the legal profession are attempting (and competing with consumer advocates) to replace the physician, the patient's traditional advocate, as the true protectors of the allegedly disenfranchised patients. And to a significant degree they have succeeded. With the new ethics of the legal profession implemented in the 1960s, the ethos of society have encouraged more and more patients to push litigation to the hilt, providing raw material to Olson's sue-for-profit litigation industry.(106) Attorney-litigators have the dubious distinction of making millions of dollars, whilst pretending to be involved in a holy crusade fighting for the destitute, disenfranchised, and downtrodden! As Olson is quick to point out, the litigation industry has made fortunes for the litigators, but at a terrible expense: the erosion of moral values and the corruption of ethics in the legal profession.(106)

The time has come for the medical profession to recognize the fact that the survival and enhancement of traditional ethical medicine and the reinvigoration of the noble ethos of the profession depend not only on practicing medicine compassionately and competently but also on the political activism of its members (21,22,28,29,59,64,65,70,71,78,79,81-84,89,108-117). The alternative will be the complete subordination of the profession to the state. Physicians will then be compelled to practice with veterinary medical ethics,[121] using government-written guidelines, under government-mandated fees, and acting in the best interest of the state, rather than the patient's. Moreover, bureaucratic inefficiency, red-tape, medical delays, and other practices, as are commonplace in fully socialized systems, would be the rule. True compassion, the incentives to work harder and more efficiently and to strive for excellence will be conspicuously missing. Patients would lose their freedom of choice of physicians and place of treatment. Deterioration in the quality of health care and rationing would follow.

As we approach the 21st Century, it is becoming evident that the survival of the medical profession as we have known it will depend on at least three crucial factors: (1) The reinvigoration of the ethics of the profession, with emphasis placed on the need for virtue-based ethics, whilst recognizing the necessity and reality that physicians' enlightened self-interest is healthy rather than detrimental. (2) A restatement of the medical ethics principle that recognizes that in considering treatment options and medical decisions inherent to the sacrosanct patient-doctor relationship, the interest of the patient – and not the state, or "society" – will always be paramount. (3) Physicians, either as individual members of society or as members of organized medicine, must become actively involved in the political process to militate for the availability of quality health care for their patients via the private sector. Not because health care is a constitutionally-guaranteed right, for it clearly is not (unless it becomes relegated to the status of a welfare "entitlement"), but because this tenet, namely taking care of the needy, has always been an unwritten article of faith in the medical profession. It must be recognized that whilst physicians have always been generously and handsomely rewarded by the affluent and able, they have also been recompensed for their charity work with gratitude by the indigent and less fortunate.

As we near the end of the 20th Century, it is patently clear that to overcome the government-created (and exacerbated) health care "crisis," the consumer-oriented, free-market approach [122] offers the best methodology to deal with the complexities of the health care delivery system of the future.(25,62,100-104) It is the only approach that deals with the issues of universal access and cost containment *without rationing*, by empowering patients rather than government bureaucracy. These attributes are exceedingly important as a larger share of our population continues to grow older and live longer. Ironically this increased longevity has been the result of improvements in the standards of living and the wonders of scientific medicine. The proposed alternatives, including managed care

---

[121] Veterinary medical ethics is the term used by the Swiss medical philosopher Ernest Truffer who has decried the increasing interference of third parties between patient and doctor which "amounts to a rejection of the [traditional] medical ethic, which is to care for a patient according to the patient's specific medical requirement, in favor of a veterinary ethic, which consists of caring for the sick animal not in accordance with its specific medical need, but according to the requirement of its master and owner, the person responsible for meeting any costs incurred."(101)

[122] I call it the *patient-oriented, free-market approach* when coupled with a reinvigoration of medical ethics and the resurgent virtues of compassionate caring physicians imbued with human (and humane) enlightened self-interest, as well as accompanied by meaningful medical liability tort reform.(25)

and its more refined but still oxymoronic cousin, managed competition, are unstable entities that will eventually collapse under their own bureaucratic weight, ultimately giving way to socialized medicine and total government control. Then will we be jolted from the utopic reverie of free health care "that will always be there" to the harsh realities of waiting lists for diagnostic studies, treatments, and surgeries; rationing of specific services; and, as we have already mentioned, active euthanasia. If in doubt, one only has to look to the Netherlands. Today, under Dutch Euthanasia statues, between 10,000 and 12,000 persons are put to death annually, some even without their consent. The *AAPS News* reports that, "up to 81% of Dutch family physicians already participate in active euthanasia."(83) Some ethicists call this practice "self-determination." Some of it may be but much of it is not – all of it is rationing by death. Wherever medicine comes under total government control, as we shall see, the results have been as perverse as they have been disastrous.

SOVIET SCIENCE IN THE 1930S AND 1940S

Subversion of the biologic sciences by the Marxist-Leninist Soviet state began soon after the triumph of the October Revolution under Vladimir Ilyich Lenin (1870-1924) and intensified under the Red Czar, Joseph V. Stalin (1879-1953). The true Russian scientists who did not believe in the new collectivist Soviet science and Marxist genetics (and in being disposed at the service of the communist state) were purged, either expelled from their teaching or research positions, or consigned to the depths of the gulags. Some were even exterminated as enemies of the Soviet Motherland.

At the helm of Soviet science was Trofim Denisovich Lysenko (1898-1976), a Soviet agronomist who, as President of the Lenin Academy of Agricultural Science (1938-1956) and Director of the Institute of Genetics of the Soviet Academy of Sciences, became the supreme leader in Soviet science and agriculture.(118)

Professor Lysenko began another sorrowful chapter in the perversion of science, now placed at the political whims of a totalitarian state. Lysenko vehemently rejected what he called capitalist "bourgeois" genetics and repudiated the fundamental laws of genetics as proposed by the famous and celebrated Austrian monk, Gregor Johann Mendel (1822-1884), which had been accepted and used by the West in the theoretic as well as applied biologic sciences. Lysenko proscribed "bourgeois genetics" and during the immediate post World War II period, assisted by plant breeder I.V. Michurin, began a series of preposterous crossbreeding experiments based on the theory of the inheritance of acquired characteristics, a theory first promulgated in 1801 by the French biologist and naturalist, Jean Baptiste Lamarck (1744-1829). The Lamarckian theory of inheritance, although a forerunner of Darwin's theory of evolution, held that new traits in organisms developed as a need to adapt to the environment and could be inherited by the offspring. The hypothesis had been rejected in the West by the systematic, scientific observations and the sound, rigorous experimentation normally conducted by Western scientists.(118,119)

According to the historian, Fr. James Thornton, Lysenko's experiments promised to make Siberia a huge granary at the disposal of the Soviet Union, and for this purpose he created new hybrid plants through extensive crossbreeding experiments.(119) He envisaged creating new plants – with lush foliage, juicy stems, palatable leaves resembling lettuce or cabbage, and fruit-like tomatoes above ground. Comrade Lysenko also expected this new hybrid to have tuberous underground roots, with plump, nutritious, subterranean vegetable-like potatoes. In short, the entire plant was to be edible – and a monument to Soviet genetics and agriculture. Instead, he created a new hybrid, certainly a new species, that had thorny stems, withered leaves, no fruit above ground, and rudimentary and inedible roots below ground. The plant that was to resemble leafy lettuce above ground and plump potatoes below ground was the perfect opposite. Comrade Lysenko's new plants that were to feed the masses of the Soviet people were only weeds that had no nutritional value and were not fit for human consumption.

Needless to say, vast fields cultivated with these hybrid plants were lost. The promising Soviet science controlled by the state and headed by the great Lysenko proved a disastrous fiasco. He, Michurin, and his willing and collaborating colleagues were suddenly dethroned and consigned to the dustbin of bogus scientific theories, but not before exposing Marxist biology as deliberate quackery and the tool of the Soviet state.(119) Soviet science which had attempted, no less, than to manipulate the environment to create a *norus homo*, a "new man," had failed miserably.(120)

Lysenko's legacy should not be readily forgotten, for it denotes a particularly sad chapter in the history of science. It reveals science's dark descent into the chasm of ignorance, intolerance, and totalitarian control by the most powerful of former "cradle-to-grave" socialist states. Millions of Soviet citizens died during this period under Stalin as a result of bogus science, the failure of central planning and collectivization policies, and state-created famines to break the spirit of the kulaks, Georgians, or Ukrainians.(121)

We should not forget these gruesome legacies of the former Soviet state, and we must remember the hard-learned lessons that support the contention that science must remain divorced of and above politics and never become a pliable tool of government. For the nature of science is the quest for verifiable truths; the nature of government is to uphold the law (which in its essence is force). The purpose of science is and should remain the accumulation of knowledge for its own sake, or better, for the betterment of humanity, not for the promotion of government statism or to advance the social policies of the state.

More recently, we have witnessed the perversion of psychiatry by the Soviet state. In this context, it is worth remembering that whilst in constitutional republics people have civil liberties and are free to choose, e.g., to uphold and conform to the laws and be undisturbed or to break the laws and face punishment, authoritarian states allow no such choice. In the former, transgressors are punished usually by imprisonment and thus isolated to protect society. In the latter, they are "rehabilitated" or eliminated.[123] Social (-ist) democracies today want to follow the "rehabilitation" path and want no more prisons. They do not want transgressors to be punished and made responsible for their criminal conduct, but instead more

---

[123] We have already alluded to journalist Alan Stang's admonition about deliberately vague laws being proclaimed by dictators so that they can call you "guilty whenever they like."(18) In addition, there is the old communist imperative: "Show me the man, and I will find his crime," which is actually the motto of the former Soviet Committee for State Security, the KGB. Furthermore, it should also be recognized that "in a state of anguish, fear, and anxiety, a potential victim can be influenced and manipulated...impossibly complex rules are the grist of tyranny."(122)

taxation and social spending and more "rehabilitation," whilst blaming society. For today, at the crux of society's problems, lie permissiveness, egalitarian ethics, lack of individual responsibility and accountability, and the disintegration of the basic traditional family.

So from the former Soviet Union we have numerous examples, including the case of dissident Bladimir Bukobsky, who spent 10 years in Soviet prisons being "rehabilitated" on psychiatric wards. Despite the indoctrination and brain-washing sessions during his intensive "rehabilitation," he survived and lived to see the day in 1992 when he was able to return to Russia from exile in England to testify in Russia's Constitutional Court. The testimony of this Russian dissident and author is important to us because it corroborates many of the stories of civil rights abuses and crimes against humanity perpetrated by the communist state previously recounted by others *emigrés,* including the Russian patriot and writer, Alexandr Solzhenitsyn (*The Gulag Archipelago*, 1970). Moreover, Bukobsky's testimony also corroborated that psychiatry had been used as a political tool by the Soviet Union until well into the late 1980s. As had Solzhenitsyn, Bukobsky had also spent many years in the gulags in the 1960s and 1970s, whence he was able to collect the important documents that provided essential proof and solemn testimony that Soviet psychiatry was a strident instrument of repression by the Soviet communist (socialist) state.(123)

CUBA AND THE REVOLUTION

Since the revolution that swept Fidel Castro Rúz (b.1926) into power in Cuba on New Year's Eve 1958, Cuban physicians have also become instruments of the state. And although in Cuba it is true that everyone has access to a physician, the lesson to be learned here is that this does not equate with proper medical care. For what Cuban physicians can do for their sick patients is quite limited and has been so, even before the collapse of the Soviet Union in 1991 and the end of Soviet economic aid. Lack of medications, supplies, medical appliances, and proper medical care was the rule rather than the exception – even during the mythic "golden age" of Cuban socialism (in the mid-1960s through the 1970s) as proclaimed by Cuban apologists and gullible journalists. Even then there were similar shortages of the most basic commodities: food, medicines, clothing, and shelter. Much of what doctors are prescribing for their patients in Cuba today is being sent from Miami to those fortunate enough to have relatives in the U.S.

There is no doubt that the situation in Cuba has deteriorated considerably since 1991, following the collapse of the USSR and Eastern Block communism, which has acutely exacerbated an already miserable economic situation.[124] As a Cuban-American, my heart aches for my countrymen and relatives who remain in Cuba and who are suffering under these extreme scarcities and are barely surviving. To make the economic and medical situation even worse, thousands of Cubans have gone blind – later correctly diagnosed by humanitarian American physicians as

---

[124] The Cuban economy in the 1980s was propped up with an estimated $4 billion dollars of annual Soviet assistance, in addition to an inestimable amount of assistance from other Eastern Block countries.

being due to a lack of thiamine and general malnutrition.(124) "As we drive through the lush countryside," wrote two *Time* magazine journalists, "we are stunned that this island cannot feed itself. But the perversions of Soviet-style agriculture have left their legacy."(125)

The perversions these journalists decry is the central planning of socialism that transformed an island of riches into an island of poverty. The same policies that most of the world is struggling to escape from, the U.S., despite all the free-market talk, is steadily marching towards. In fact, what I witnessed as a youth in socialist Cuba in the better half of the 1960s, including mass indoctrination and socialization via violent revolution, I now see happening like a nightmarish *deja vu*, step by step, in America via evolution.

With this fact in mind, the reader can surmise my astonishment and disbelief when, for at least the last two decades, American leftists and socialist sympathizers have continued to cite Cuban progress in the areas of health care (socialized medicine) and public education. They routinely cite bogus Cuban-government sponsored statistics which have not been rigorously scrutinized or peer reviewed or subjected to any of the scientific standards to which we have become accustomed in America, especially when dealing with the dissemination of supposedly valid scientific information. And even though, we are now finding out that these statistics were "phony" and part of the charade of deception and disinformation, some die-hard apologists still try to perpetuate the myth; even the *Time* magazine article that so vividly described the Cuban socialist woes mentioned the nonexistent "golden age."(125) "The truth of course," as Gary Benoit, editor of *The New American* corrected, "is that Cuba has been a living hell ever since Castro came to power."(126) And believe me, I know. I was there for a 6-year ride. Needless to say, the Western media actually came to believe what it wrote and to view Cuban medicine "as exemplary in Latin America."

Let us take a brief look at some of the Cuban government-created and promulgated figures and statistics that were used in this country by reporters who knew better, and even by Congressional committees that should have known better.(127-132)

What were the facts? For one thing, in 1958, just prior to the revolution, Cuba had three times as many doctors as all of the Central American countries combined. Life expectancy between 1950 and 1955 was 58 years and rising at the pace of industrialized countries. Yet from 1980 to 1985, life expectancy in Cuba rose at approximately the same rate as three of the four Caribbean countries that started from about the same base.(128,130) Infant mortality in 1960 was 35.4 deaths per 1000 births – the lowest in Latin America. And soon after the revolution, between 1960 and 1964, infant mortality was lowered by 42%, to 15 deaths per 1000 births. Although this improvement appears significant at first glance, upon closer examination we discover that in fact this rate was no better than that of any other country in Central America, not even Honduras, one of the poorest countries in Latin America.(128,130) Today, as we shall see, infant mortality in Cuba has climbed to 18 deaths per 1000 births. (The U.S. infant mortality rate was 8.9 per 1000 live births in 1991 according to the National Center for Health Statistics.) What all of this means is that the Cuban health care advances of the 1960s through the early 1980s were not the great feats that American journalists made them out to be.

Let me point out some other pre-Castro statistics. According to the U.S. Department of Commerce, Cuba had one of the highest standards of living in Latin

America. In fact, the eminent Cuban attorney and author Mario Lazo, in his book *American Policy Failures in Cuba*, writes, "although Cuba lived under the blight of Spanish colonial rule seventy-six years longer than any other country in Latin America, by the 1950s, in the incredibly short span of half a century, *it had attained the highest standard of living of any semitropical or tropical country in the world, except possibly for Venezuela"* [his emphasis].(130)

Moreover, Cuba's transportation system was the most highly developed in Latin America. For example, in 1956, "Cuba had three times the U.S. railway mileage per square mile of area," according to American statistics compiled by the Department of Commerce.(131)

The same report showed that Cuban workers received 66.6% of the gross national income, compared to 57.2% for Argentina, 47% for Brazil, and 70.1% for the United States.

Despite what one may have read about the purported existence of a great many *latifundia*, the truth is that the average size of Cuban farms in 1946 was 140 acres, as compared with 195 acres in the United States in 1945. With regard to the U.S. media reporting American exploitation of the Cuban sugar industry, the reader may be surprised to learn that U.S. control of the Cuban sugar industry had declined from about 70% in 1928 to about 35% in 1958.(132)

It is an irony of history that one year before the so-called triumphant socialist revolution, Cuba, in 1957, had its most prosperous year. It was not until the end of 1958 that the economy began to decline, as a result of sustained rebel attacks. Thus, per capital income figures, "although considerably lower than in the United States, rose to the second highest level in Latin America in 1957."(132)

In Cuba, the middle class was one of the largest in Latin America. In 1957, under President Fulgencio Batista (dictator, 1933-1944 and 1952-1958) factory workers "averaged twice the wages of Mexicans, even more than the average industrial worker in Japan, and more than the workers in Australia."(133) In 1992, the same report noted that each Cuban was authorized, by monthly rationing, the following items: 6 lbs. of rice, 4 lbs. of potatoes, 12 oz. of chicken, and 10 oz. of beans. Yet by socialist sleight-of-hand efficiency, such items that used to be in great abundance in pre-revolutionary Cuba became rationed during the "golden years," and are today unavailable in Cuba's empty and dilapidated stores – unless of course, one is more equal than others, possessed of the proper Communist Party credentials or U.S. dollars from relatives in Miami, either of which enables the person to shop in special tourist stores.(125,134) Today, even cigars and sugar, the mainstays of Cuban exports, are rationed and hard to come by. Even at the height of zeal for the Cuban revolution, during the years 1965 to 1973 (during the ethereal "golden years"), meat, eggs, and most vegetables were scarce but at least available on the black market. Today, conditions have deteriorated even further; life is considerably worse and these basic necessities are hard to come by, even on the black market.

Yet despite the loss of Russian subsidies and the presence of the protracted 30-year economic boycott, Fidel Castro has not wavered in his determination to continue on the path of untainted, hard-core socialism. To solve the transportation crisis, 750,000 bicycles were imported from communist China and other socialist countries to replace automobiles which can no longer run due to the lack of oil and gasoline for civilian use. The environment is densely polluted because the government is using cheap oil in place of electricity. Defections are commonplace. Women, commonly referred to as *jineteras* ("galloping cowgirls"), sell their bodies for a meal. There is just no end in sight to the pain and suffering.(125,134)

Because of the lack of tractors and farm machinery, plows are today pulled by oxen to till the soil. And if necessary, Castro has threatened to use messenger pigeons for telecommunications. Recent refugees who have fled to the United States report that people are eating domestic and stray cats, and *jutias* (wild, agile, tree-climbing rodents that resemble large rats). Even pigeons, the same pigeons that would have been used in telecommunications, are being eaten.(134,136) The situation is nearing collapse, but the First Secretary of the Cuban Communist Party has pledged (January 1989) "socialism or death"(136) and has called these severe, bare-subsistence measures his "Zero Option."(136)

The year 1993 approximated apocalyptic proportions. This is how the situation was described in a July 1993 *Wall Street Journal* report:

> *Whatever the outcome, the clock is running on a potentially disastrous situation in Cuba. Numbers tell the story. Last year, Mr. Castro said Cuba's buying power had fallen to $2.2 billion, from $8.1 billion in 1989. One Havana study of the Cuban economy said the island's gross domestic product fell 24% in 1991 and another 15% in 1992. In May, a top official announced that the country's vital sugar crop, which in 1992 accounted for about 64% of hard currency exports, will fall 40% to 4.2 million tons, a 30-year low. Cost to Cuba, according to Mr. Castro: $500 million.(137)*

And another article, this time in an August 1993 *Atlanta Constitution*, report related:

> *Water, regularly stagnant in areas where rationing is most strict, has become a bacteria fermentation pool. Women are plagued by an outbreak of chronic yeast infections they must combat with homemade remedies like baking soda. Their children contract eye infections and skin rashes. In one middle-class Havana public health district, the infant mortality rate has risen to 18 deaths per 1,000 births, well above the national rate of 10 per 1,000.*
>
> *The ever-dwindling rice ration has been cut from 5 to 3 pounds a person per month. A soybean substitute replaced meat months ago. On the black market, a chicken now fetches 200 Cuban pesos – a good monthly wage. The value of the peso has plummeted from 15 to the dollar on the black market a year ago to 65 to the dollar today. The dollar's ascension has accelerated since Mr. Castro announced that holding American dollars was no longer a crime. Last week, the manager of a Havana bakery in the congested Buena Vista district refused to distribute a shipment of bread to a crowd that had begun to line up before dawn.(135)*

Compare this miserable condition with that of the entrepreneurial, staunchly free-market situation of Cubans in Miami, as reported in the 1990 Fall issue of *Moscow News* by Russian journalist, Alexander Makhov, "the two million Cubans [in Miami] living under market conditions, produce a GNP valued at $30 billion....The GNP of Cuba, with its population of ten million, amounts to a mere $8 billion."(138) This economic disparity between the two economic systems was noted by a Soviet writer, even before the final collapse of the USSR and the end of Soviet economic aid to Cuba.

But let us return to the egalitarian systems of education and public health during the "golden years" and compare it to the situation before the revolution. A report of dubious authenticity was circulated by a U.S. House of Representatives Committee in 1977 which stated that there were only 187,000 students in Cuba in the pre-Castro era and that the literacy rate was only 25%. Baloney! Cuba before the revolution had a well-developed educational system. In fact, Lazo remarks, "*in education and literacy Cuba ranked at or near the top among Latin American countries. It ranked first in the percentage of national income invested in education* [his emphasis]." Moreover, "In the field of public health Cuba surpassed the United States in some respects. It had almost twice as many physicians and surgeons in relation to population...and it had a lower mortality index, among both adults and infants....Cuba had a higher proportion of doctors and dentists, including some of the world's best, more than any other country in the Caribbean area."(130)

Why, then, did Cuba succumb to socialism? Several factors, were involved, namely Castro's perseverance against all odds, his mesmerizing power of oratory, and a prosperous but restless population with a large middle class that had been promised "change." But even these factors would not have been enough to cause one of the most prosperous countries (if not the most prosperous country in Latin America at the time) to throw it all away, if there had not been a U.S. liberal media which falsely romanticized the guerrillas, *los barbudos* ("the Bearded Ones"), exaggerating their actual military victories (which were few),[125] lionizing rebel leaders, and idolizing their supreme commander, Comandante Fidel Castro Rúz, then called, *El Caballo* ("the horse"), for his stamina, prowess, and steadfastness as Cuban leader.

The U.S. media, romanticizing the rebels and clamoring for change in Cuba; a complacent U.S. State Department; and a seduced population were the essential ingredients for an explosive concoction leading down the road to revolution and into the chasm of socialism. Lives disrupted; lives lost.

At least one-tenth of the Cuban population has now fled to the United States, Spain, Puerto Rico, and other Latin American countries to escape tyranny and oppression and to search for freedom and opportunity as well as a brighter future for their children – away from the opprobrium of socialism.

NICARAGUA SANDINISTA AND THE ISSUE OF ALLOCATION OF NATIONAL PRIORITIES

In Nicaragua, the popular revolution of the Sandinistas quickly degenerated into an obscene, authoritarian Marxist dictatorship. Here, suddenly, we had a small Central American country extending itself militarily beyond its means at the expense of the domestic concerns of its people. Even some of the Sandinista leaders recognized the wrong direction in which the government and the country were

---

[125] The most notable rebel victory was the Ernesto "Che" Guevara (1928-1967)-led siege (August-September 1958) and capture of the provincial capital of Santa Clara in the former Las Villas province on January 1, 1959, in which Batista's forces surrendered after hearing that the dictator had fled the country.(130) *El Che*, incidentally, the military strongman during the Cuban revolution, the architect of the friendship pact with the Soviet Union, and the forger of communist Cuba's economic and monetary policies, was Argentinean...and a physician.

headed and tried to redirect the course of the revolution. The intrepid Eden Pastora called, "Commander Zero," rebelled and went back to the hills to lead a faction of anticommunist revolutionaries, known as the *Contras,* to pick up arms once again – this time to fight against their former comrades-in-arms who had betrayed the popular revolution by turning it into a militant Marxist *régime.*

The Sandinistas consolidated their hold on Nicaragua and turned it into another totalitarian state. They closed newspapers such as *La Prensa,* nationalized businesses, confiscated private property, and flagrantly violated their citizen's civil rights. They persecuted and exterminated a large portion of the Miskito Indians, abrogating their basic human rights and stripping them of their land.(129)

But what about health care in the "former" Sandinista state – that is, before President Violeta Chamorro's popular victory in February 1990? This question may perhaps be best answered by discussing a "letter to the editor" that I submitted to one of my specialty journals as a rebuttal to a propaganda article written by an academic neurosurgeon who had praised the Sandinistas.(139) That article described the primitive health care system in Nicaragua and the ineptness of the "socialist worker's paradise." The catch, of course, was that he blamed Nicaragua's misery on the United States, President Ronald Reagan, and the Contras – joining the prevalent "blame-America-first crowd" of the time.

The following is the gist of my published response: "First, the practice of medicine (and neurosurgery) would not have been as primitive as it was in Nicaragua in 1989 with the Sandinistas, if it weren't for a misdelegation of priorities. Whilst the people of Nicaragua do not have available CT scans or MRIs, or even the Seldinger catheterization technique for angiography, the Sandinistas have a standing offensive army 300,000 strong (total population: 3.5 million).

"While they cannot afford a CT scanner to diagnose a patient with a brain tumor (not to mention treatment with radiotherapy), they possess advanced helicopters, 'flying tanks,' and MIG fighters, which are expensive weapons of destruction beyond what is needed for the defensive needs of a small nation. I have a photograph of my wife holding a surface-to-air missile (SAM-7) that was captured in November 1989 from a downed Nicaraguan plane that was transporting weapons to the leftist Salvadoran guerrillas. [Now known and exposed as the covert 'Operation Mariposa' by *The Washington Enquirer*]. One can ask: Is it moral for a country to spend their national resources on such weapons when their own people go hungry and cannot afford the medical technology that is available in other similarly or less developed countries?

"In bordering El Salvador, for example, we saw an unfortunate 12-year-old, recently-quadriplegic girl who was diagnosed with x-rays and CT scanning and then treated by her private neurosurgeon with the type of care that we would have expected in the United States. Moreover, we found that in San Salvador many working-class people are covered by private insurance for unexpected disease and injuries....Let's hope that better times are ahead for neurological surgery in that poor nation [Nicaragua]. And with the advent of a popularly elected government in 1990, in time the health of the people may be given priority over military capabilities."(140)

Although the situation in Nicaragua is by no means totally clear, the people did have an election in which the Sandinistas lost by a great margin to UNO, the acronym for a coalition of democratic parties opposed to the Sandinistas and

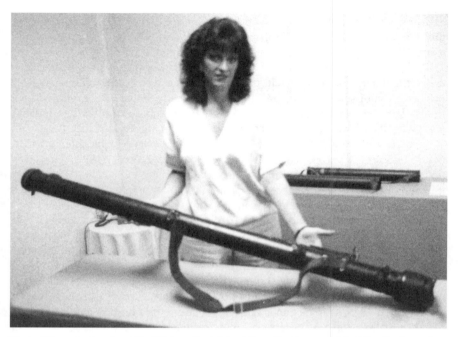

Plate 22 – Author's wife (Helen Faria) holding Surface-to-Air Missile launcher (SAM-7) supplied by the Sandinistas to FMLN guerrila forces, and captured by Salvadoran security forces. Author and wife participated in an Accuracy in Media (AIM) conference held in El Salvador, March 1990.

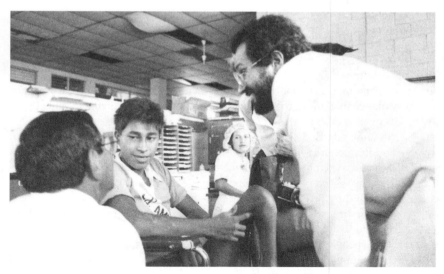

Plate 23 – Author shown interviewing wounded Salvadoran soldier at a military hospital in San Salvador, March 1990.

led by Violeta Chamorro. But despite this mandate to the opposition, the Sandinistas are still in control of the country by controlling the militant labor unions, the army, and the state's still repressive security system. Yes, the Sandinistas "continue to rule," as former dictator Daniel Ortega put it, "from below."

President Violeta Chamorro has seemingly sold out to the people who elected her. As a result, the country remains in a virtual state of paralysis, the economy is crumbling, and Commander Humberto Ortega (brother of the former dictator) remains in charge of the armed forces. The health care of the nation, like the rest of the economic sector, remains in shambles. Economic prosperity is nowhere in sight. Medical care remains primitive, one of the worst in Latin America. The leftist union infrastructure controls domestic policy and holds the country at ransom. Confiscated land and private property remained in the hand of the Sandinistas who have fortified villas and private retreats and now live in the fashion of former Eastern potentates, not Latin-American revolutionaries.(141)

Contra leaders who had returned to join the political process, such as Comandante Emilio Bermúdez, have been assassinated after responding to Chamorro's post-election "reconciliation" call. The Sandinistas used this opportunity to exterminate their political enemies and former Contra leaders who had given up arms and disbanded, as called for by the armistice negotiated by the "new" government. Although you may not have seen or heard it on television or read it in the newspapers, over 200 Contra rebel leaders have been assassinated during the disbanding and "reconciliation era."(142,143)

A SAMPLING OF LOOSE MEDICAL ETHICS IN THE SOCIAL DEMOCRACIES

We will mention briefly what I consider to be a tip-of-the-iceberg panoramic sampling of loose ethics in the "soft-Left" social democracies which are vitiated in form, nuances, or fully enmeshed in socialized medicine. The reader will be left to make his/her own conclusions as to the relationship of socialization of medicine and the occurrence and meaning of these scandals.

GREAT BRITAIN

On April 20, 1990, *American Medical News* reported the scandal of three British physicians (a kidney specialist and two surgeons) who were found guilty of "serious professional misconduct" by the General Medical Council (GMC) for their role in kidney transplantations involving four paid Turkish donors. It was reported that the British government physicians orchestrated the removal and transplantation of the kidneys from three desperate Turkish men and one woman who were paid between $4,000 to $6,000 for their organs. The GMC enunciated to the physicians, "by such conduct you have brought disgrace upon yourself and dishonor upon medical practice in the United Kingdom."(144)

But Great Britain is hardly the only Western country plagued with scandals directly attributed to state control of health care such as loose medical ethics,

blatant rationing of care, [126] a burgeoning bureaucracy, and all that this portends –
that cost controls, bureaucratic and state corruption, and economic considerations
supersede quality of care and the sanctity of human life. As Professor Eamonn
Butler, Ph.D., Director of the Adam Smith Institute in London, declared, "British
citizens are leaving the National Health Services (NHS) in droves just at the time
when U.S. policymakers seem determined to recreate it in America."(145)

FRANCE

A more recently discovered and more serious scandal embarrassed and
rocked the socialist government of France. In August of 1992, France's largest
insurance company cancelled "the policies of 25 transfusion centers because of
chilling revelations emanating from the trial of four government doctors charged
with allowing the sale of AIDS-tainted blood" in the bureaucratic, cost-conscious
French socialized health care system.(146) The blood was allegedly sold in 1985,
mind you, with the knowledge that it was tainted and posed a mortal threat to blood
transfusion recipients. Then in December of 1992, it was revealed further that the
French National Assembly had decided to proceed "to try ex-Prime Minister
Laurent Fabius and two former high-level officials in the AIDS scandal."
The scandal finally erupted after the socialist government-engineered
affair became fully known to the French public, and it became known that the state-
run Transfusion Center provided hemophiliacs with blood which was known to be
tainted with the HIV virus, but went ahead with the pragmatic and irresponsible
decision to transfuse 1200 people with it. More than 300 of those innocent victims
of socialist mishap have already died. After extensive investigations, the National
Assembly declared categorically that the bureaucratic officials in the state-run
Transfusion Center and the top government hierarchy knew that the blood was
tainted and yet proceeded with the approval of the blood transfusions based on
financial considerations.(147)

UNITED STATES VS FRANCE

Meanwhile, the National Cancer Institute has finally acknowledged that the
virus that was isolated in 1984 by Robert C. Gallo, M.D., had in fact, come from a
sample sent to him by French researcher Luc Montaigner, M.D., of the Pasteur
Institute. Even though the National Institutes of Health has investigated and found that
the contamination of Dr. Gallo's isolates with the French virus was not intentional, Dr.
Gallo officially relinquished his claim as the first investigator to discover HIV. As you
will recall from the intense media coverage of this dispute, this controversy raged for
six years as to who was first to discover the HIV virus. Up to 1987, both Drs. Gallo
and Montaigner were referred to as co-discoverers of the HIV virus.(148)
Recent evidence points to bureaucratic mayhem as responsible for this

---

[126] For instance in Great Britain during 1978, 33% of dialysis centers refused treatment for patients over the age of 55,
and today there are over 800,000 patients waiting for surgery there.(25)

dispute, and Dr. Gallo has just recently been exonerated of any wrongdoing in the incident. In the old days (late 19th and early to mid-20th Century), scientists were able to interact and cooperate freely in the exchange of information. In today's bureaucratic environment, however, it has become virtually impossible to interact freely because of the concentric layers of bureaucracy (not to mention rules and regulations) that impede and hinder rather than assist in the transfer of scientific information.

CANADA

A lot has been said about the Canadian National Health Insurance (NHI) medical care system, and like the British NHS, we will not dwell on how it, too, operates by rationing or outright denial of care. Those facts have been well documented.[127] At this point, though, we will consider one of the biggest ongoing scandals of Canada's NHI. Here I would like to refer to an article that appeared in the September 1992 issue of *Reader's Digest* by Dr. Ian R. Munro, Director of Humana Cranial-Facial Institute and Medical City Dallas Hospital. Munro reported that the "Hospital for Sick Children under Canada's national health care system has closed hundreds of beds and consequently many sick children have died waiting for treatment." Nevertheless, he was willing to admit that "the National Health Services in Canada remains popular, especially among those who have not been seriously ill."(149) Munro then related the story of Joel Bondy, a little boy who died whilst waiting for nearly two months for an operation.

And there is more to this outrage than meets the eye: whilst the seriously ill in Canada have to wait in queues, and many of them die while waiting for treatment, Munro reported, "bureaucrats, politicians and senior businessmen jump the queues by phoning hospital administrators." These dignitaries, who in typical socialist fashion consider themselves "more equal than others," call a particular hospital, and by being who they are and stating that their case is "urgent," can get immediate treatment.

Munro also explains that the National Defense Medical Center (NDMC), a 244-bed hospital in Ottawa run by the Canadian military, though theoretically for the active armed forces, is used almost exclusively by members of Parliament, diplomats, and senior bureaucrats who belong to the "more equal than others" category. Whilst Munro was there, 61% of his patients were non-military. It is the only hospital in Ottawa equipped with a helicopter pad, a nationally renowned cardiopulmonary unit, and its own CT scanner (which is a rarity in Canada). He quotes David Sumerville of the National Citizens Coalition, "I don't think we will get fundamental reform until those with the power to make changes feel the pain of the system themselves."(149) Indeed!

This brings to mind the achievements and words of the sagacious Athenian statesman, Solon, who not only decried tyranny but also laid the foundation for the building of a true constitutional republic. It was he who postulated that a well governed state was one in which "the people obey the rulers and the rulers obey the laws."

Dr. William E. Goodman, a Canadian physician who closed his medical

---

[127]As Michael Tanner of the Cato Institute has well pointed out, in Canada "the risk of waiting for heart surgery exceeds the danger of dying on the operating table."(62) And in Toronto alone, there are an estimated 1,000 people waiting longer than a year for coronary bypass surgery.(25)

practice in protest for the way the government has taken over medical care and the brazen loss of physicians' civil liberties in Canada, has described several scandalous methods by which Canada covertly rations medical services. He calls them rationing by the "back door – by piecemeal but progressive reduction of medical benefits." These methods include queues and waiting lists; "delisting" of procedures and medications that were previously considered "medically necessary" and funded; government underfunding and progressive reductions in the funding of mandated services; and the issuing of government "guidelines" or directives, aimed at reducing medical costs at the expense of quality. (150)

Why, then, does the NHI remain popular with Canadians? Answer: Because only the 4% or so who become seriously ill annually come to personally experience the harsh reality of its shortcomings. The rest of the population lives with the illusion and false security of free, unlimited health care that will always be there when they need it. A reality which could not be further from the truth.

CHAPTER 25

MODERN MEDICAL ETHICS

He who reigns within himself, and rules passions, desires, and fears is more than a king.
John Milton (1608-1674)
English epic and lyric poet

THE EVOLVING "ETHIC OF CARING"

Let us now turn our attention to the modern evolving "ethic of caring" and the behavior of many of today's physicians in the prevailing adversarial litigious climate of health care delivery. I believe it is safe to state that daunted by the fear of possible repercussions from their patients, physicians consider medical litigation as an ever-present potential consequence of the care they give to their patients.

In this light, consider the following scenario which is played out daily in the emergency rooms across the U.S., that of an automobile accident victim who is being seen for the first time by an emergency room (ER) physician. ER physicians evaluate these patients to ascertain and/or diagnose injuries they may have sustained especially those complaining of pain, say, after being rear-ended in an automobile accident. As innocuous as the "injuries" may seem to the physician, numerous x-rays are taken of every area where the patient (let us call the patient "he") hurts. It has been the practice of physicians, encouraged by legal advice and supported by ethical pronouncements, to give the patient "the benefit of the doubt" and to treat all of the "suspected" injuries. Nothing is found in the ER, and the patient (still complaining of pain) is referred for follow-up to another physician. In the course of the evaluation and treatment, the follow-up physician (let us call her, "she") comes to suspect that her patient might be malingering, but she is not absolutely sure despite studying the tests done in the ER and performing her own evaluation.

Not infrequently, such cases go on exhausting health care dollars, even after a comprehensive negative ER examination and work-up by a subsequent treating physician – until the auto insurance policy monetary limits have been spent. Only later does it become obvious that many of the diagnostic tests were not needed and subsequent treatments unnecessary.

The physician, of course, gets blamed for the whole experience (including the second guessing as to why the tests were conducted in the first place). Did she have a conflict of interest, such as financial motives, for ordering a battery of tests, or was she just insensitive to the need for controlling spiraling health care costs? Or was she just incompetent?

Meanwhile, the patient has accomplished his purpose, leaving behind a lengthy paper trail of treatments attesting to the multiple and usually "soft-tissue" injuries (a legal term devoid of significant meaning in medicine [128] ...and of course

---

[128] I remember telling a plaintiff's attorney involved in a similar case that there were "no injuries." He quickly interrupted me to tell me, "doctor, injury is a legal term, not a medical term, and we are talking about 'pain and suffering,' anyway, I know there were no broken bones. Give your patient, please, the benefit of the doubt."

subjective "pain and suffering"), and a doctor and a hospital bill that will help the patient's automobile case in court!

For the doctor, the repeated exercises in *defensive medicine* result in disenchantment, as more and more patients abuse the system, lured by the visions of windfalls conjured up by trial lawyers in their TV commercials and reinforced by news of sensational jury verdict awards. "Injured" patients expect to get what is "coming to them" (as one local commercial so aptly puts it) out of every fall or automobile accident. More and more people, sadly, are coming to believe that they deserve what is owed them by the inference of their own existence – not by what they have accomplished in their lives.

I remember an acquittance of mine who once confided in me the fact that he was receiving adjustments from a chiropractor as well as physical therapy from a medical physician for alleged musculoskeletal "injuries" which he claimed resulted from an automobile accident. He was already feeling well, he admitted, but he would assert himself with his doctors so that he could continue with his treatments. When I asked him, why? Didn't he know the price that society paid for unnecessary medical care? He retorted, "Why not? It costs me nothing, and my attorney wants me to continue treatment as long as possible. That's why I paid my auto premiums." This dialogue took place in early 1992, during the time of a perceived recession, [129] when there were allegedly millions of Americans who had difficulty in getting access to medical care, and providers were highly criticized for spiraling health care costs, not to mention, stupefied in the midst of invetrate litigation-on-demand.

To fake illness and demand unnecessary medical care, as in these particular scenarios, illustrate two important points that sooner or later will need to be addressed in the health care debate. First, that medical care is perceived as free (or deserved, because insurance premiums have been paid); and second, the phenomenon of secondary gain, which in this case was money expected to be made via litigation which encouraged one patient to seek repeated evaluations and the other to continue to seek unneeded medical care. Most of the money spent in these scenarios is not even considered in most accounts of defensive medicine, because they are considered to be "gray-zone" expenditures. [130]

And these incidents, thoughtful reader, are not isolated cases. On the contrary, these are fairly typical scenarios encountered by physicians who treat musculoskeletal injuries related to automobile accidents or workers' compensation cases. This entitlement mentality, buttressed by what physicians call "secondary gain," fuels the fire of the litigation industry which is consuming the honesty and undermining the integrity of the American people. We appear not to notice the damage it is causing, not only in terms of the monetary costs incurred in health care delivery (projected at $900 billion for FY 1993), but also in terms of damage to the moral and psychologic fiber of the nation. Many doctors, influenced by the litigious climate and our society's evolving egalitarian ethics, on the guise of following the new altruistic "ethics of caring," have all too often "given the patient the benefit of the doubt" and stretched this principle to its limit, thus actually corrupting and

---

[129] The recession, according to government economists, actually ended in April of 1991. According to the mass media, the economy did not improve until the day after the 1992 Presidential election.
[130] According to surveys by the AMA, 84% of American physicians admit to practicing defensive medicine in order to leave a paper trail behind to protect themselves from medical lawsuits.

perverting the principle of serving the best interest of the patient. Physicians' altruism and the "ethic of caring" can be stretched to the point of abuse by patients, especially when secondary (monetary) gain is involved. Workers' compensation and automobile injury cases are two of the most blatant examples where medical ethics have been abused, convoluted, and stretched – all to the detriment of society.

Close inspection of the motives and values behind the excesses of the "ethics of caring" reveals that it engenders a "going along" attitude in physicians, concomitant with a failure to stand for the true ethics of the profession that reflect ideals of trust, honesty, truth, and justice. Over-pragmatism to avoid enraging patients (which causes lawsuits) and pseudo-altruism, to justify lying to promote the patient's welfare, is amoral and counterproductive, leading ultimately to the loss of self-respect and the moral disintegration of the profession.

Selfishness and greed have always been part of the darker side of humanity and thus may be expected to appear in the most honorable of professions. But the real culprit today is of a more recent vintage: the fear of retribution via litigation, the corrupting, awesome power of Walter Olson's "sue-for-profit litigation industry."(106) As many physicians today are amply aware, the fury of the litigation juggernaut can turn into a loose cannon of intimidation and coercion against both the unsuspecting, good, ethical physicians and the much-talked-about but minuscule lot of incompetent and/or uncaring providers – if and when, they refuse to abide by the imposing and degrading rules of the litigation industry.

This unrestrained, false "ethic of caring" in today's climate of medical practice cannot go unimpeded as normal business for a venerable profession that seeks both truth and justice and to effect healing. Yet, this exaggerated "ethic of caring," I fear, will be used increasingly by physicians as a shield to justify defensive medicine and fend off the assault of the litigation onslaught, as a matter of professional survival as long as they feel haunted by the looming specter of litigation-on-demand. What will it take for society to say enough is enough as it regards a litigation system that is out-of-control? For an answer, perhaps, we should remember the words of the former Supreme Court Justice, Felix Frankfurter (1882-1965), who, despite his liberalism, believed in judicial restraint and said, "The court's authority – possessed of neither the purse nor the sword – ultimately rests on substantial public confidence in its moral sanctions." Physicians should also find ample thought and solace in Seneca's words, "injustice never rules forever."(34)

THE TRANSFORMATION OF ETHICS THROUGH TIME

Let us look for a moment back to the past and examine the ethics of the illustrious Roman physician, Celsus. This prominent *medicus* believed in treating patients who were considered difficult clinical cases, after obtaining their informed consent, even when the therapy was deemed dangerous or risky:

> *Nevertheless it can happen that an illness may require this "bleeding," but the body seems scarcely able to allow it; but if there appears to be no other remedy and he who is suffering is about to die unless there is some relief even*

though risky, in this state it is the mark of the good physician to demonstrate
that there is no hope without bleeding and to confess how much risk there is in
doing this, and then, if it is demanded, to bleed the patient. There should be no
hesitation in that sort of case; for it is better to try a dangerous therapy
than none...(151)

Celsus' final words of advice involve transcendental ethics between patients and their independent physicians. That is a far cry from today's highly regulated health care industry, where his advice would fall on the deaf ears of government bureaucrats for whom rules, paperwork, and monetary considerations are paramount. There is, for instance, the U.S. Federal Drug Administration which continues to wage a protracted war of nerves on the victims of malignant and terminal illnesses, including patients afflicted with AIDS, who want and are willing to try anything as far as drugs and therapies in a desperate attempt to extend their lives and circumvent death. Celsus' ancient ethical advice was consistent with the ennobling ethics of compassionate, caring, and benevolent physicians, no matter how paternalistic and imbued with enlightened self-interest they might have been.

It seems that the more we learn about the evolution of medical ethics and compare the stages of ethical development with the different proposed models of patient-doctor interactions, the further away we are from finding truth. Point of fact is the exposition by Dr. Edmund D. Pellegrino, "The Metamorphosis of Medical Ethics," in which he discusses his concept of the evolution of medical ethics as comprising four "somewhat overlapping periods."(152) First, he believes that there existed a "Quiescent Period" based on the 2500-year-old Oath of Hippocrates and the supporting deontologic literature of the Hippocratic ethical tradition of the School of Cos which had been influenced by the Pythagorean principles of "beneficence, nonmaleficence, and confidentiality"; the stoic tenets of duty, compassion, love, and friendship, as well as the Aristotelian, Socratic, and Platonic moral philosophies centered "on the cultivation of the virtues."

This period thus emphasized the cultivation of such virtues as courage, temperance, and justice, with the key virtue being *phronesis*, practical judgement, the ability of the physician to discern the right choice when faced with a moral dilemma. Finally, Hippocratic ethics were further modified by elements of the Judeo-Christian teachings and scriptures, "and the *noblesse oblige* expected of a gentleman." This synthesis, according to Pellegrino, "essentially unchanged by the writings of influential physicians such as Percival and Gregory in England, and Hooker in America," led to the first ethical code of the AMA in 1847. The Quiescent Period of ethical tradition remained in effect for 2500 years until the mid 1960s.(152)

Since then, according to Pellegrino, we have been immersed in the thesis of "the School of Principlism," simply put, the principles of beneficence, nonmaleficence, justice, and patient autonomy, as guiding ethical tenets in medical practice. And later, the antithesis of the latter, "the School of Antiprinciplism," which decries principlism because of a lack of uniformity in moral theory. The result is that we are now entering a "Period of Crisis" complicated "by the parlous state of contemporary philosophy and ethics, and the strong current of nihilism and skepticism...."(152) We are left with the competing philosophies of "virtue-based" ethics and the "ethics of caring" for consideration in this "Period of Crisis." Therefore, Pellegrino opines, "I am reasonably certain that virtue and character will be part of any future version of biomedical ethics"(152); yet physicians must be careful that the prevailing "ethics of caring" intermingled with casuistry (a fallacious alternative theory of ethics) is not used by unethical clinicians to justify their way of handling litigation as we have described.

In the meantime, in arguing the questions of ethics, philosophers are demolishing the idea of the existence or relevance of any theory of basic truth or absolute reality. Moral relativism, situational ethics, and deconstructionism rule in this milieu of skepticism and nihilism. [131] Nietzsche's philosophy of ultimate truth as an illusion prevails – as do the ideas of multiple competing truths and negation of moral accountability. Nevertheless, out of this chaotic insanity, Pellegrino writes, "there are no atheists in foxholes, and there are no patients (even when they are ethicists themselves) who are truly nihilists or total skeptics when their own health or welfare is at stake." He advises physicians to be aware of "shifts in contemporary moral philosophy, if they are to maintain a hand in restructuring the ethics of their profession."(152)

THE PARADIGMS OF THE PATIENT-DOCTOR RELATIONSHIP

In a timeless article, the medical ethicists Drs. Ezekiel J. Emanuel and Linda L. Emanuel proposed four models of the patient-doctor relationship which may serve as paradigms for the future. They believe that this relationship has been affected for approximately two decades by different forces whose net effect has militated toward curtailing the primacy of the physician and augmenting patient control – thus changing the essence and dynamics of this interaction. Let us briefly discuss these models of the patient-doctor relationship as envisioned by these authors and their significance in medical practice:

> In the Paternalistic Model the physician acts as the patient's guardian, articulating and implementing what is best for the patient. As such, the physician has obligations, including that of placing the patient's interest above his or her own and soliciting the views of others when lacking adequate knowledge. The conception of patient autonomy is patient assent, either at the time or later, to the physician's determination of what is best."(153)

The *Informative Model* is considered the ethical interaction now in vogue; it is a consumer-based model which, in my view, is nurtured by the medical liability crisis. In this model, physicians give full, informed consent as "purveyors of technical expertise," but it is up to the patient to choose and select the treatment that he or she wants. Patient autonomy rules. The *Interpretive Model* aims to elucidate the patient's needs and values, and the physicians assist the patients in selecting the treatment mode that coincides with their patients' values.

And finally, the authors relate the *Deliberative Model*, in which

---

[131] Moral relativism is the theory that holds that morality depends on the circumstances of the given case, and situational ethics, similarly, maintains that the right or wrong of a particular act of commission or omission depends on the specific situation. By inference, moral relativism and situational ethics explicitly or implicitly hold that there is no absolute right or wrong or ultimate truth. Deconstructionism is the hypothesis that formulates that words, phrases, and written passages have no fixed meaning and can be interpreted contextually from the individual reader's frame of mind.

physicians help the patient determine the "best health-related values that can be realized in the clinical situation."(153) The patient's needs and values are not only taken into account but also the "worthiness" and "implications" of treatment options, as they relate to universal health-related values. The authors argue that the deliberative model is the ideal physician-patient relationship. The caveat which only becomes obvious as one reads and assimilates the mechanics of this interaction, is that when all is said and done, it becomes quite obvious that we have nearly circumambulated 360 degrees, and are now back to a model which approaches the fundamental principles and ideals of the prototypical paternalistic model of time immemorial.

The authors perceive this philosophic quandary and, deflecting possible criticism of this dilemma in advance, explain:

> *The deliberative model is not a disguised form of paternalism....And no doubt, in practice, the deliberative physician may occasionally lapse into paternalism. However, like the ideal teacher, the deliberative physician attempts to persuade the patient of the worthiness of certain values, not to impose those values paternalistically; the physician's aim is not to subject the patient to his or her will, but to persuade the patient of a course of action as desirable.(153)*

> *Yet they look to higher authority to cement their cause, and they find it in Plato who, in his book,* Laws, *distinguishes between "persuasion" on the part of the physician, as in the author's deliberative model, and "imposition" as in the paternalistic model of the patient-doctor relationship. According to this reasoning, the authors thus quote Plato:*

> *'A physician to slaves never gives his patient any account of his illness...the physician offers some orders gleaned from experience with an air of infallible knowledge, in the brusque fashion of a dictator....The free physician, who usually cares for free men, treats their diseases first by thoroughly discussing with the patient and his friends his ailment. This way he learns something from the sufferer and simultaneously instructs him. Then the physician does not give his medications until he has persuaded the patient; the physician aims at complete restoration of health by persuading the patient to comply with his therapy.'(154)*

I remain skeptical and unconvinced. It may be that when the health care and litigation crises are properly addressed and solved, the prevalent interaction will be a synthesis that would embody "virtue and character" on the part of the physician as presaged by Pellegrino (152) and encompass significant portions of the paternalistic-deliberative models.(153)

The sheer advances in technology and the forthcoming strides in science and medicine, coupled with the ancient tradition of medical ethics, will dictate that the benevolent, virtue-based ethics of caring physicians – who, like it or not, are in part motivated by enlightened self-interest within the context of the paternalistic-deliberative model of the physician-patient interaction – will likely prevail in the future. Within the paternalistic framework, there has been evolution toward awareness and recognition of the importance of individual needs and values, as well as health-related societal values (e.g., public health measures), and it is logical that, if the profession is able to slip away from the present health care morass in which it is mired, in most interactions, physicians will inevitably lapse into the beneficent, paternalistic interaction, albeit inextricably entwined with features of the deliberative model so as to be in some instances virtually inseparable.

On the other hand, if the litigation crisis is not remedied, it is my belief that the patient-doctor relationship will degenerate to the impersonal, value-free, relativistic, informative model – an approach adopted as a survivalist instinct for physicians doomed to practice defensive medicine in an adversarial climate of medical litigation. By this time of course, medicine will no longer be a calling, but a job.

I believe that it is not only advisable but desirable for the physician to be surrounded by an aura of benevolent authority that radiates trust, confidence, and competence (not arrogance or condescension) – although he/she should not give the impression of promising false hopes or guaranteeing success of therapy. Moderation, as Aristotle asserted, was (and still is) the means between extremes, and a rule that applies here. Trust, confidence, and understanding are necessary when recommending treatment, especially when confronted with serious illnesses and difficult medical problems associated with high-risk treatments and/or accompanied by significant morbidity and mortality.

This is particularly true of specialists who see patients on a referral basis for a specific treatment, which is different from the situation of primary care practitioners. Primary care physicians, in most instances, have an ongoing and sometimes life-long relationship with their patients. This is less likely to be the case with specialists, where oftentimes, due to the urgency of the situation, may only be able to see the patient once or twice before initiating invasive treatment. During that relatively short period of time, the specialist must not only build and develop a working relationship but also establish confidence and trust. Given the fact that medicine is an inexact science, and some treatments are fraught with hazards, some treatments do not always yield the expected result. And although the treatment may have been required to prevent death or disability, untoward complications or death may result. No model of patient-doctor relationship will avoid an untoward result, but the paternalistic-deliberative model (forging the best concepts of the old and new approaches) may be the most suitable and workable solution for the patient-doctor relationship in the foreseeable future. Moreover, a paternalistic-deliberative model does not exclude patient autonomy; on the contrary, it should go a long way toward enhancing autonomy, trust, and mutual understanding – but to be genuine it must be accompanied by litigation relief.

Ethicist Ian E. Thompson's assertion that: "Aristotle's definition of prudence as 'the wise discrimination of means, in the light of principles, in the contingency of the actual situation, with a view to obtaining the best possible end' could well be taken as the motto of medical ethics"(155) is certainly valid, but it poses a conflict with physicians' professional ethos. As society becomes more knowledgeable and more demanding in their health care needs, it becomes understandable that physicians will need to have their roles as healers redefined. The ambiguous and contradictory state of affairs cannot and must not go on.

Point of fact is the gradual implementation of rationing of medical care that is already in place: The gate-keeper concept of the HMO-managed competition model. In this role, physicians are induced to restrict their patients' choice of, and access to, specialists and specialized, high-tech, and expensive treatments that are potentially life-saving – under the pretext of controlling health care cost. Thus cost considerations have superseded the basic ideals of quality of care. And for the first time in the history of American medicine, physicians are allowing themselves to be placed in the uncomfortable dilemna of putting the interest of a health care entity (HMO, PPO, etc.), or "society"-at-large, above that of their own patients and the previously sacrosanct patient-doctor relationship.

As American society confronts a veritable crisis of conscience, physicians themselves will be faced with their own professional identity crisis (will they lead or will they follow?) – both crises fomented to a significant extent from outside the medical profession by political activists cheering for more government control and pushing us ever closer toward the abyss of socialized medicine. Perhaps this was best exemplified by Senator Jay Rockefeller (D-WV) who, unabashedly for socialized medicine, has assured us that, "We are on the verge of making our dream a reality once and for all....We will roll over anyone who tries to stop us."(156)

Moreover, the professional crisis of physicians faced with the prospect of losing control of their medical practices and anticipating the demise of their profession as they have known it, and the layman's personal identity crisis of seeing the void within them, concomitant with the cultural disintegration of our society, heralds that the time of reckoning is fast approaching when we must tackle the intricately interrelated problems of health care delivery and the gargantuan medical liability crisis.(25,157,158)

We have been forewarned about the dangers intrinsic in a pendulum swinging too far in one extreme as it relates to the "ethic of caring." Let us now touch again upon the opposite extreme: the relinquishment of physicians' responsibilities to their individual patients ostensibly for the good of society, a society incarnated in the ever-increasing power of the federal government. Physicians should not allow either one of these extremes to become the norm, for like Aristotle, they must pursue the mean between extremes. And citizens should be aware that the new pluralistic ruling elite's consensus that is emerging out of this post-Modern age seems to be leading us inexorably toward conformity (despite diversity and multiculturalism); toward the concentration of political power in the politically connected and favored special interest groups; toward central planning in the guise of free-market capitalism; toward democratic socialism (excessive rules, onerous regulations, and heavy taxation) masquerading as compassion and philanthropy; toward the concentration of economic power in the hands of the corporate internationalists in cahoots with a thoroughly interrelated socialist world government; and toward the loss of the erstwhile concepts of rugged American individualism and self-reliance in which this nation was founded. Small businesses and entrepreneurs will be swallowed up by the new corporate magnates and internationalist industries protected by a nearly omnipotent government.

Society owes a debt of gratitude to the medical profession for the self-evident miracles of medical progress. In fact, as we prepare for confrontations in the battle over health systems reform, Americans must be reminded of the truly needed changes in health care, namely universal access via the private sector with tax-free (MSA) medical savings accounts; high-deductible catastrophic insurance purchased from the MSA; portability of coverage; vouchers for those who cannot truly afford health care coverage; and substantial and meaningful medical liability tort reform. Unfortunately, these are not the reforms enumerated in President Bill Clinton's

Health Security Act of 1993.

Instead, the Clinton proposal promises to be the greatest government takeover of a U.S. industry in American history. Both *Time* and *The Economist* have expressed astonishment at the magnitude and manifest ramifications of this bold proposal.(14,15) As events today rapidly unravel, it is becoming clear that there are ulterior motives. Like Lewis Carroll's fanciful story, *Through the Looking Glass*, things are not always what they seem. One thing is for certain. As events unfold, it is becoming evident that the battle over health systems reform is not about access or coverage, quality of care, U.S. perinatal mortality, or even soaring health care costs. It is about the *de facto* government takeover of a lucrative U.S. industry. If passed by Congress, the government would effectively control 14% of the GNP which translates to a whopping one-seventh of the U.S. economy.

I suspect the real reasons for health system reform, particularly the Health Security Act of 1993, are two-fold: (1) the implementation of a socialist health care system [132] where health care decisions will no longer be made by physicians and their patients, but by government bureaucrats more concerned with budgets and control than the sanctity of human life; and (2) a disingenuous allurement for the seduction of the middle class that would make prosperous Americans (87% of whom already have adequate insurance) resemble the welfare poor, a government-dependent class. For socialist planners know that once the yoke of socialism is harnessed on the beasts of burden, it is virtually impossible to shake off as the experiences of England, Norway, and Sweden amply testify.(17)

---

[132] Since its unveiling in 1993, the Health Security Act has grown from a 239-page proposal to a massive 1,342-page document.

PART SIX: MIDDLE AGES

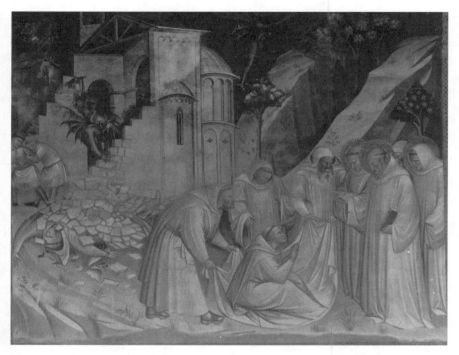

Plate 24 – St. Benedict of Nursia, founder of the Benedictine Order (c.529), in a fresco dating c.1387 by Spinello Aretino. Canali Photobank, Italy.

CHAPTER 26

THE DARK AGES: MONASTIC MEDICINE AND THE ORIGIN OF THE BARBER-SURGEONS

Punishment in this world, may be redemption in the next.
St. Benedict of Nursia (c.A.D.480-c.543)

THE DARK AGES

Rome, the "Eternal City," had fallen, and the once mighty Roman Empire had been veritably overrun by fierce barbarian hordes. The feelings of anger, uncertainty, and the general despair of the Dark Ages which had settled over humanity was well encapsulated by St. Gregory I, (Pope Gregory I, "the Great," A.D.590-604). St. Gregory writing even whilst another swarm of barbarians, this time the Lombards, descended upon Rome in the year A.D.593-594, elucidated the gloomy atmosphere of the times.[133] He writes in his eleventh homily on the prophet Ezekiel:

> *Everywhere we see sorrows, everywhere we hear laments. Cities lie destroyed, fortresses overthrown, harvests ravaged; the land is brought to desolation. No peasant in the fields, scarcely a dweller in the cities is now left; yet even these little remnants of the human race are still smitten today unceasingly. The scourges of Heaven's justice have no end; for not even through these scourges are guilty actions turned to right. Some of our people we see led away prisoners, some mutilated, some slain. What, then is there to please us in this world, my brethren? If even thus we still love it, we love now not its joys, but its wounds. Rome herself, once mistress of the world, how do we see her now? Worn out with mighty griefs, bereft of her citizens, trodden down by enemies, full of ruins....Where now is her Senate? Where her people? Their bones lie rotting, their flesh consumed, all the pride of her worldly glories is dead and gone.(1)*

St. Gregory I, who began his career as a Roman magistrate and later joined the priesthood, became one of the founders of monasticism and climbed the ecclesiastical hierarchy to become pope. As pope, he brought the power of the papacy to unprecedented heights with his enforcement of the doctrines of the temporal powers of the pope and papal supremacy. He strengthened the power of the Church in temporal affairs, reformed the administration of the clergy, and boldly proclaimed the Papacy as the head of all Christians. He anticipated the coming conflict between the Church and the State, and availed himself of power to fortify the Church's position in the struggle. He reserved the Church's right to try and

---

[133] For simplicity I have divided the Middle Ages (A.D.476-c.1400) between the Dark Ages occupying the period A.D.476-c.1000 and the Medieval period, c.1000 to c.1400.

punish clerical transgressors and sent Benedictine monks to evangelize the surrounding Italian territories, England, and North Africa. It is said that his successors' claim to absolute power was derived from this last of the Church fathers' austere authority.(2)

MONASTICISM AND MEDICINE

The failure of Greek medicine as practiced in the Byzantine Empire to contain and control the devastating plague of Justinian in the 6th Century, just as Byzantine armor failed to institute law and order in the chaotic West, veritably wrought the death knell of the Roman West – there would be no resurrection of the Western Roman Empire. Yet like a phoenix, Græco-Roman medicine, albeit in rudimentary form, would rise from the ashes of the Western Roman Empire in the form of monastic medicine. Monastic medicine emerged to alleviate the suffering of the ill and to cure the sick during the time that the horrible pestilences afflicted mankind. Monks of the 5th through the 7th Centuries treated the sick out of the sense of Christian charity.

Monastic medicine, therefore, became the charitable but primitive form of medical care rendered to the sick by the early founders of monasticism and was later crystallized by the Benedictine monks in the monasteries of the West.[134] In these monasteries, for treating the sick and ministering to those in their last hours, the monks relied heavily on the strengthening of faith and the repentance of sins, along with the service and comfort provided to those in need of food and shelter. Prayer, penance, contact and veneration of sacred relics (such as the bones of revered saints), ingestion of herbal remedies, supplication to venerated saints, and the anointing of unctions as in shriving or other healing rites were all part of the healing arsenal used by the Benedictine monks. Although the monks possessed only meager knowledge of physiology and anatomy, they nevertheless performed such procedures as the cleansing and dressing of wounds; tooth extractions; the setting of broken bones; simple surgery, such as incision and drainage of abscesses; and the suturing of lacerations.

In the Dark Ages, lay physicians were essentially forgotten. The monks residing in the monasteries became the new healers, following in the steps of the pious St. Benedict (Benedict of Nursia, c.480-c.543) who founded one of the earliest communities of monks. It is written that St. Benedict went to a cave 50 miles from Rome and lived there as an ascetic hermit for three years. When he emerged, he devoted his life to preaching, healing by intercession and divine intervention, and set himself the task of establishing monasteries where monks could live austerely, could pray for spiritual strength, and divorce themselves from temptations of the flesh and other earthly distractions – as well as be close to God.

According to the scholar Eleanor S. Duckett, in her book, *The Gateway to the Middle Ages*, St. Benedict founded the monastery in the mountainous terrain of

---

[134] In its essence, monasticism embodies the retreat from worldly life for the total devotion to religious life. The monks subscribed to vows of poverty, chastity, obedience, and in some cases, asceticism. Western monasticism was founded by St. Benedict, and its hallmark was devotion to learning and to preserving manuscripts containing the essence of Græco-Roman civilization. This latter fact, more than any other, separates Western from Eastern monasticism, or monasticism as is found in other religions. In Eastern monasticism, Basil the Great (c. 330-379), one of the four Greek Doctors of the Church, formulated the rules of conduct, manual labor, and liturgy in accordance with the tenets of the Greek Orthodox Church.

Monte Cassino after having wondered aimlessly in southern Italy, and having survived one attempt on his physical life. A group of monks, indignant over St. Benedict's austere ways, tried to poison the devoted monk, eager to get rid of him. Another attempt, this time on his spiritual life, was made when an envious priest who resented St. Benedict's piety and wisdom tried unsuccessfully to tempt the pious monk by arranging to have lascivious, half-naked wenches parade outside his cell window.(1) Despite these trials and tribulations, the good monk's spiritual strength did not waver, and he went on to found the great monastery of Monte Cassino. This is how Duckett relates the events leading to the founding of the famous monastery:

> *The Abbot [St. Benedict] had started out and would not now turn back. He continued his journey in search of a new home until he reached the foot of the great mountain of Casinum, half way between Rome and Naples; from the point where he stood the rough trail led up two thousand feet of rocky cliff to an ancient fortress, still dedicated even at that time to pagan worship. We can imagine the brethren toiling up. Once at the summit, they hurled down the images of the heathen and the altar of their rites; then more slowly they changed the pagan sanctuary into a Chapel of Saint Martin of Tours, that the thought of Martin's monastery at Marmoutier might inspire the dwellers in this Christian retreat. At the very top of the mountain, where the altar of idolatry had stood, Benedict built a place of prayer dedicated under the name of Saint John the Baptist, in the desire that simple austerity might also be the hallmark of his own solitude. Here, then at Monte Cassino, was rooted and grounded the great Benedictine Order. Here, little by little with immense toil and difficulty the brethren built their first cloister, adding, as the years went by, the different portions needed for their life and work.(1)*

The Monastery of Monte Cassino was constructed under St. Benedict's direction, and his Benedictine Order was formally established in A.D.529.[135] Western monasticism and monastic medicine were born in this solemn and austere setting. [136]

The Benedictine monks subscribed to the idea of illness stemming from sin and divine retribution. Thus, as cures, they espoused asceticism, repentance with penance, and prayer in an attempt to obtain forgiveness from God, expecting and forever hopeful that, through God's boundless wisdom, infinite grace, and incomprehensible mercy, they would be granted the power to heal by divine intercession, effecting cures, and granting miracles. It should be noted that the Benedictine Rule, by the late 5th Century, included a rudimentary plan for medical education and treatment based on the available treatises of Hippocrates and Galen, which were to be used in conjunction with spiritual discipline and prayer. Thus, it was during this incipient period of the Middle Ages that elements of both a spiritual and scriptural Judeo-Christian tradition and a classical Græco-Roman legacy were forged to

---

[135] Other famous monks of the Benedictine Order included St. Gregory I (pope, A.D.590-604; Rome), St. Augustine (Archbishop of Canterbury, d.A.D.605; England), and St. Boniface (c.A.D.675-754; Germany) – all of whom disseminated the teachings of the Order across Europe and fostered Western monasticism in its various forms.(2) Moreover, in England, most of what we know about the Dark Ages is derived from the Venerable Bede (St. Bede, c.A.D.673-735), a Benedictine monk who was a devoted historian. He wrote in Latin the informative, *Ecclesiastical History of the English Nation*, a primary source of English history from A.D. 597-731.(2)

[136] Nevertheless, generally the Benedictine Order stressed moderation more than austerity.

establish the basis for monastic medicine as practiced at Monte Cassino.

At the onset of the barbaric invasions of the Dark Ages, Monte Cassino remained a bastion of Roman Catholicism and a repository of knowledge, whilst surrounded by a sea of heretical Arianism, chaotic ignorance, invasions, and wars. This is how Duckett describes Monte Cassino during this period:

> *If we turn back once again from this point to the onset of the Dark Ages, we find that Monte Cassino held high a torch of learning and scholarship which was to lighten the shadows of the world when culture entered eclipse. The wise and practical ritual with which Benedict wrought the marriage of faith and intellect, of things contemplative and things practical in one sacrament of daily life within the cloister, bore its fruit steadily, through all the years of barbarian terror, through all the succeeding vicissitudes of invasion and recovery. It still bears its fruit wherever the sap of the branch of science rises day by day within the Tree of Life. (1)*

Yet even before the time of St. Benedict, during the barbaric onslaughts surrounding the events leading to the fall of Rome, other priests tended to their flocks and tried to ameliorate suffering as best they could. Here again, Duckett recounts the life and time of one such pious and courageous monk, Severinus (d.A.D.453), who lived on the south bank of the Danube in the Roman province of Noricum along with a band of priests and his flock of lay followers. It was during these perilous and uncertain times in the closing days of the Roman Empire, during the repeated attacks and invasions by the Germanic barbarians, that the indomitable monk led his weary and demoralized band of Roman followers to safety.

Duckett recounts that just as weakened Rome, "relaxed her grasp, her provinces were left unprotected, to defend themselves as best they might against the invaders who were steadily encroaching here and there, step by step...." Severinus found himself the spiritual as well as earthly protector of his people. Yet for the monk, leading his flock during this time "was a hard calling for, like all the saints, he longed for solitude."(1) Nevertheless, in spite of all the confusion and chaos of the 5th Century, Severinus trained his followers to survive and persevere in the face of unremitting famine, pestilence, and death: "Prayer, repentance, alms-giving and fasting were the means by which he tried to lead both himself and his people to God, and these, too, were the means by which he taught them to meet their enemies."(1)

As previously intimated, in the monasteries of the Middle Ages, diseases were mainly attributed to witchcraft, demonic possession, transgressions of the flesh, and other earthly sins which were thought to be punished by divine retribution. Even though the monks relied on faith and divine intervention as the mainstay of healing, it should be noted that they also applied natural remedies. As late as the 12th Century, the abbess St. Hildegard of Bingen treated illness and disease by strengthening the physical body so that "one might withstand the attacks of the Devil."(3,4)

And another founder of Western (or Roman) monasticism in continental Europe (at Vivarium in southern Italy), the learned monk Cassiodorus (d.c.A.D.575), provided baths for the sick, and "admonished those who cared for them to be sympathetic, thinking more of their brother's trouble than of their own," and to "understand the properties of herbs and study authorities on medicine, such as Hippocrates and Galen in a Latin translation. But let him remember, withal, to trust in the Lord above all simple [sic] and potions of human device."(1)

Besides the development of monastic medicine, it must be noted that the monks performed another extremely important function and that was the copying and preservation of priceless manuscripts. In this light, the great monk Cassiodorus, who considered the travails of perpetuating the works of holy scholars a glorious task, should be given due credit for this painstaking and momentous endeavor. In fact, for the important task of copying and preserving old and archaic manuscripts, he not only encouraged the monks but also provided study aids for them such as oil lamps "ingeniously constructed to replenish their own fuel from a little reservoir, sundials for daytime and water-clocks for cloudy days and the hours of night. Thus no one would miss by concentrated study the more direct work of God."(1)

And Cassiodorus understood that this tedious and demanding work was not for everyone in the monastery. Monks who could not intellectually fulfill Cassiodorus' eminent task of copying or translating works of antiquity (i.e., from Hebrew or Greek to Latin) were given other tasks:

> *[They] were sent to till the fields and to tend the gardens and orchards. Such manual labour, Cassiodorus admits, is not unfitting for monks nor without its blessing: 'To give fresh fruit to the weary and to nourish the hungry with sound meat is, indeed, a work of heaven, though it may seem to savour of earth.' Even these sons of toil, however, are to seek for enlightenment in the written page; from Columella, or from other authors, if he be found too difficult. More glorious, nevertheless, is the task of perpetuating works of holy scholars. 'Happy is the aim, praiseworthy the eagerness, to reveal tongues with the fingers, silently to give salvation to men, to fight with pen and ink against the attacks of the devil. Satan receives a wound in every word written by him who makes fresh texts of the ancient law of the Lord....'(1)*

Cassiodorus, a devout and saintly monk, taught his novitiates at Vivarium "to link the things of God with the things of men, mindful that all things are of God...only let Reason ever be obedient to Faith."(1)

Amongst the giants of monasticism, we also find the Bishop Caesarius (c.A.D.469-542) of the diocese of Arles in southern France, who prescribed fasting and abstinence from wine and meat, with consideration and "tolerance of human frailty...for no one is obliged to do more than his health will allow...." Moreover, the good bishop placed great importance on charity and alms-giving, and earnestly "inculcated with great vehemence. Not only the tenth[the tithe] is expected, as a matter of course, but from the remaining nine-tenths each is bidden give what he can for the aid of the poor." Caesorius also strongly believed in the rewards of penitence, "as a basis of all progress in Christianity," and the existence of "mortal sin, which causes the death of the soul and leads, if not repented of, directly to eternal fire, [and] was found in murder, fornication, robbery and theft, false witness, pride, envy, greed, consulting of sooth-sayers, attending indecent or sanguinary entertainments, and anger or drunkenness, if persistently indulged."(1)

Nevertheless, the sagacious bishop (and abbot) was well aware of those who lived in sin, postponed their penitence, and only on their deathbeds confessed their sins. In this vein, Duckett notes:

Many people, however, though their consciences were by some grave matter,
deliberately postponed penitence till they lay dying in their beds, when the
Church naturally counselled private confession before the priest rather than a
bad death. Such sinners, when hale and vigorous, had preferred to run the risk
of dying unshriven rather than ask guidance of the Church, lest, as was proba-
ble, the public ordeal be recommended. On such deathbed penitence Caesarius
preaches a specially sane sermon. If genuine, it is better than nothing: 'But, O
man of intelligence, do you really think it decent that you should be a slave to
vices and failings all your earthly life, and then at last try to pull yourself
together to gain eternal life when you are only half-alive to do it? You wouldn't
stand such conduct from your servants!'(1)

For those who have committed repeatedly any of the seven cardinal or venial sins, the dutiful bishop declared, "Never despair; rise quickly from your sins. But never presume upon God's mercy, and never imagine for a moment that penitence without good works is worth anything. The last day of our lives must find us further on the road to Heaven than the day of our Baptism did, innocent though we were then." And in his sermons, Caesarius preached the value of prayer and solitude found in monastic life. He counselled, "If a man does not try to free the wings of his soul from the hindrances of this world and the sticky mire of sins he will never come to true rest. Let us try to cut down something from our worldly occupations that we may gain a few hours for prayer and sacred reading."(1) On humility and bad thoughts he cautioned his monks: "Don't grumble at rebukes in sermons; a priest is a physician, and must administer medicine nasty as well as pleasant. Of course you can't always be actually thinking about God; I know you have all those daily duties to think about. But you can leave some little time free. And don't deliberately embrace a low thought. You wouldn't want to embrace a public prostitute in the streets if all your friends were there watching."(1)

THE FIRST HOSPITALS

In the West, the first hospitals were built by the Romans at the time of the Republic. These were military field hospitals which tended to the sick and ministered to the wounded soldiers of the mighty Roman legions. And later during the Empire, the best hospitals, not surprisingly, remained the military hospitals which took care of the sick and wounded Roman legionaries. In fact, some of the greatest Græco-Roman physicians, including Dioscorides and Galen, served with the Roman army – the most ubiquitous of Roman institutions.

For the indigent, the first hospital for which we can definitely account was founded on an island in the Tiber river in 293 B.C. at the site of a temple consecrated to Æsculapius.(5) The great Roman historian Suetonius (c.A.D.69-c.122) says, "On this island of Æsculapius certain men exposed their ill and worn-out slaves because of the trouble of treating them." Exposure as used in the above statement had a certain connotation which was no part of physicians' practices. It usually meant the practice of leaving unwanted or malformed infants to die of starvation. Suetonius continues, "The Emperor Claudius however decreed that such

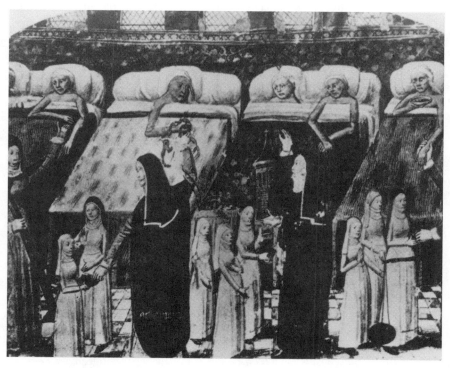

Plate 25 – Medieval monastic hospital where charity care was provided by monks and nuns. World Health Organization, Geneva.

slaves were free, and if they recovered, they should not return to the control of their master."(6) Care, although rudimentary, was given to the sick, the infirmed, and the poor who went there, and thus in that sense it deserved the denomination of a "hospital." Moreover, it was during the reign of Claudius (Roman emperor, A.D.41-54) that the first general public hospitals were founded. The early hospitals were more like alm houses than real hospitals in the modern sense, and even though there were no professionals, or even trained practical nurses, the sick were provided with clean, comfortable surroundings, food, water, and shelter.(4) All their shortcomings, notwithstanding, these primitive hospitals must be considered the first systematic attempt at treating diseases in hospital-like surroundings.[137]

Charity care to patients began in the Roman Empire only after the rise of Christianity and the founding, by Ladies Fabiola and Marcella (fl.A.D.4th Century), of the first true misericordia hospitals in the Western world. These two famous Christian ladies of Rome, imbibed with the Christian spirit of compassion and true charity, refurbished their pristine palaces, and converted them into misericordia hospitals to house the old, ill, sick, and infirmed and to provide them with the much needed service of nursing care. This Christian tradition of running charity hospitals would come of age later during the Crusades, as we shall see, when hospitals sprouted up along the routes the Crusaders took to provide the Christian holy warriors with potable water, food, shelter, as well as medical care during their journey to the Holy Land.

The first truly modern hospitals in the West were founded in France as two Hôtel-Dieu sister hospitals. The first was founded in Lyon in A.D.542, and the other in Paris in A.D.660. These hospitals arose out of the need to isolate lepers from the communities and therefore were named *Lazarettes* – after the leper's protective patron, St. Lazarus. In England, St. Cross Hospital in Winchester and St. Bartholomew's Hospital in London, were both founded in 1123.[138] These ancient hospitals, later during the Renaissance, became teaching hospitals *par excellence*.

Unfortunately as I write these words, the very existence of these venerable institutions is threatened as a result of mismanagement in Britain's socialized health care system (NHS). Unless a financial or administrative miracle takes place, their doors will soon be closed to the public by the British government.

THE CRUSADES AND OTHER MEDIEVAL TALES

Another important phenomenon of the Middle Ages was the organization and conduction of the Christian Holy Wars, referred to as the Crusades, when all of Christendom united, not under any political emblem, but under the banner and aegis of the Christian church, to seize and rescue the Holy Sepulcher from the Moslem infidels. As H.W. Haggard writes, "Chivalry in its flower was to strike at the heart of the Saracens."(5)

---

[137] In addition to the innovation of hospitals, as you would remember, the Romans excelled in other public building projects that were associated with public health, sanitation, and medical care. The Romans were superbly adept at building majestic aqueducts and ingenious sewer systems. The construction of modern aqueducts furnished ample water supply to the cities, and the sewer systems provided proper disposal of human wastes – fostering clean water, sanitation, and consequently, better health.

[138] St. Bartholomew's Hospital, in fact, is one of only two extant originally Norman churches in London, the other one being Tower Chapel.(7)

The rivalry between the (Christian) infidels and the (Moslem) Saracens (as the holy warriors styled each other) began after the Turks seized the Holy Land from the more tolerant Arabs and refused Christian pilgrims passage to visit Jerusalem. To add insult to injury, the Holy Sepulcher itself was desecrated. The Holy Land was thought to have been further profaned by the torture of Christian pilgrims who had attempted to visit Jerusalem in spite of Turkish proscription.

Despite the best military efforts, devotional exertions, religious zealotry, or any other reasons that might have motivated Europeans to join the religious-military campaigns in the faraway Holy Land, only the First Crusade (1095-1099) was completely successful. It began shortly after the Council of Clermont, when Pope Urban II (pope, 1088-1099) began exhorting the Christian world to rise up in arms against the Saracens to reclaim the Holy Land.(2) This victorious campaign resulted in the capture of Jerusalem in 1099 and in the formation of the Latin kingdom of Jerusalem. It also encouraged the organization of the Order of the Knights Hospitalers and the Knights Templars.

We have already mentioned the fact that as a result of the Crusades, many hospitals were built along the route to the Holy Land. In addition, there were also monasteries founded nearby those routes, and within their walls monastic medicine was being practiced. Pilgrims and crusaders alike sought the refuge of monasteries for clean water, food, shelter, rest, and medical treatment. And like those monastic hospitals, the quasi-military hospitals which sprouted up along the routes of the Crusades were organized by religious orders, such as the Knights Hospitalers, a military-religious order also known as the Knights of St. John (also the Knights of Jerusalem, of Rhodes, of Malta); and as.the latter names imply, the Knights of St. John established themselves and their hospitals in Palestine (Jerusalem in the 11th Century), and later in the Mediterranean islands of Rhodes and Malta.(2,8) All of these hospitals, incidentally, were attacked by the expansionist Ottoman Turks in later centuries and bravely defended by the Knights – of particular renown was their heroic and successful defense of Malta.[139]

The Third (1189-1192) and Sixth (1217-1221) Crusades were only partially successful; they led to truces which permitted Christian pilgrims temporary access to the Holy Land. The Sixth Crusade, for instance, led by the gifted and indefatigable Frederick II (1194-1250), King of Sicily, Germany, and later Holy Roman Emperor, would have been considered successful, but for its short-lived gains – for it was as a result of this campaign that Frederick II gained a most symbolic title as King of Jerusalem in 1227.

Let us now relate other tales that took place at about the time of the Crusades. As we have seen, between the 6th and 9th Centuries – that chaotic period in the midst of the Dark Ages – Western Europe reached its nadir in intellectual activity and human progress. Very few people could read and write. This situation had not changed much for the common people in the Medieval period. Literacy was not only a cherished commodity but a social and legal privilege. In fact, under medieval jurisprudence, a very special privilege called *benefit of clergy* was extended to the very fortunate few who were literate. This extraordinary privilege

---

[139] The Knights were expelled from Rhodes in 1522 by the Ottoman Sultan, Sulayman the Magnificent (reigned, 1520-1566). However decades later, in 1565, the aged Sultan failed to take fortified Malta from the courageous Knights, despite a terrible siege and massive attack.(8)

afforded a defendant the right to be tried before an ecclesiastical court rather than a civil court – except in the case of treason, which was as much a capital sin in civil court as heresy was in ecclesiastical court. Both treason and heresy carried a death sentence (and since the church "abhorred the shedding of blood," heretics were burned at the stake, and witches were frequently drowned). Nevertheless, heresy aside, since the church considered most transgressions sins of the flesh caused by the frailty and weakness of human nature (and therefore forgivable), atonement could be achieved with penance through God's boundless compassion and mercy.

Cases of heresy were a different matter, because heresy was a sin of thought that threatened the foundation of the Christian church. Heresy was tried by the Inquisition which used torture as a means to obtain legal confessions. Nevertheless, barring cases of witchcraft and heresy that were generally tried by the Inquisition, the penalties imposed by the church were relatively mild. The civil courts, on the other hand, ordered the death penalty freely for crimes such as thievery, pick-pocketing, robbery, and murder. *Benefit of clergy* was therefore a cherished privilege and one that would save many unruly students attending the medieval universities.(5)

It was in the medieval universities that the title of *doctor scholasticus* was used for those students who graduated in the study of Law and Theology. And surprisingly, it was not until the 14th Century that the term *doctor* was used as an appellation for physicians. In the United States, medical doctors were referred to as "Mister (Mr.)" as late as the 18th Century, and even today in England surgeons are still referred to as "Mister."(5,9) It was also during the Medieval period that a clear distinction was made between a *physicus,* a physician who was inclined to approach medicine from a philosophic perspective, and a *medicus*, a practitioner who actually treated his patients with either medicine or surgery.(11)

During the Medieval period Galen's and Avicenna's erudite writings reached maximum appeal for both physicians and surgeons because of their dialectic reasoning, power of persuasion, and intrinsic "dogmatism" – over the earlier Greek, or for that matter, the pure empirical observation method of Hippocrates. Thus, it was Aristotelian humanism and Galenic "dogmatism" – both tempered by Christian theology which was built upon a Judeo-Christian tradition – that held sway throughout this period, until the upheaval of the Renaissance.

Leprosy, which came to Europe from the East, was also associated with the earliest Crusades (c. late 11th Century). The dreaded disease was finally contained and nearly eradicated by the isolation of lepers. As inhuman as it may seem today, this practice wiped out the disease in the Middle Ages in Europe, except for a few remaining isolated clusters.

It was towards the end of the Black Death epidemic of the 14th Century that *quarantining* was first used to contain the spread of infectious diseases. In fact, we can categorically state that it was as a result of the Black Death that the first major advance in public health was made. In 1374, the Venetian Republic appointed three officials to inspect and exclude all infected vessels from the ports as a public health measure to control infectious diseases, and three years later, by 1377, it had become customary that travellers coming from infected places be detained for 30 days, and when this period was found to be ineffective, for *quaranti giorni* ("40 days"), referring to the period of isolation from which our modern word *quarantine* derives.(10) The practice of quarantining passengers *per se* is believed to have originated at the Mediterranean port at Marseilles in southern France.(5)

THE FEUDAL SYSTEM

Under the feudal system that gradually emerged from the smoldering ruins of the Western Roman Empire, feudal lords became not only the rulers and nominal protectors of the local people but also the owners, or rather, holders, of feudal domains or fiefdoms. The feudal lord was also the head of the economic unit of the landed state, which in England was referred to as the manor. Feudalism, then, comprised both a political and an economic order, whereby vassals rendered service to their feudal overlords from whom they received not only protection but also land granted in return. Later, as kings began to unify nations and sought to rule by *divine right*, they strove for the consent and support of the church to attain and maintain royal power, and to curb, and whenever possible, curtail the power of their ambitious and sometimes unruly feudal vassals – the landed nobility.

Therefore, it was this feudal scheme that finally imposed needed law and order on the chaos that had reigned during the Dark Ages. Impoverished peasants seeking protection from the landed lords under this feudal (political) and manorial (economic) system became indentured servants or serfs, bound to the land and owing allegiance (fealty) to their feudal suzerain. For, as history teaches us, order is always preferable to chaos.

From the 12th to the 14th Centuries, feudalism gave way to the rise and development of central authority in Europe, an event propelled by the growth of cities, the founding of the medieval universities, and the gradual loss of the temporal power of the church. In reality, though, the kings supplanted the old suzerains, becoming the supreme feudal overlords, at the very top of the feudal hierarchy. In the name of the people and empowered by divine right, they broke the power of the nobility and began ruling the emerging nation-states of Europe.

Christianity flourished during this period of the Middle Ages, and continued to play a major role by preaching faith, good works, charity, and self-sacrifice, and linking these religious and philosophic ideals to the old Græco-Roman concepts of philanthropy and humanitarianism. Whilst some pious Christians interpreted these benevolent ideals in the extreme, such as the goodness and purity inherent to leading the lives of hermits – undergoing rites of penance and self-mortification, suppressing mundane pleasures, and denials of the flesh, etc. – others interpreted the notions of charity and self-sacrifice as meaning a devotion to caring for the poor, providing comfort to the sufferers of bodily or spiritual pain, and providing care to the sick and the ill. And it was, I believe, this later interpretation that inspired the Christian ladies, Marcella and Fabiola, to found the first Christian charity hospital in Rome shortly after the Roman Empire's mass conversion to Christianity.(5)

During the Medieval period, the prevailing view remained that the etiology of disease was halfway between the natural and the supernatural. External injuries were treated with natural remedies, whereas internal diseases were still considered to be the result of sin and retribution from God. Therefore, cure was to be effected by prayer and penance; preventive medicine was to be effected by the omission of sin. When witchcraft was believed to be responsible for disease, exorcism was performed under the aegis of the church. Life on earth was only but a brief preparation for the afterlife – a heaven of peace and security, or a fiery hell of everlasting torment. Thus, capital punishment was feared less than excommunication, for excommunication from the Christian church carried the certainty and celerity of eternal suffering and everlasting damnation.

THE INVESTITURE CONTROVERSY

Two kings raised themselves from the Dark Ages and above feudal society and aligned their rule with those of the ecclesiatical power. They were the strong and determined Frankish monarchs, Pepin the Short (A.D.714-768) and Charlemagne (A.D.742-814). As such, they endowed exemplary donations upon the church which deserve mentioning, not only because of their direct beneficial effect on Christendom but also because of the way they affected the emerging geopolitical power, such as church protection by the state [140] and the claims of temporal authority by the Church. We have already discussed the apocryphal Donation of Constantine. Let us now consider the case of these two monarchs.

In A.D.753, Pepin the Short was officially given the title of King of the Franks *quid pro quo* his generous "Donation of Pepin" that ceded to the Pope territories around Ravenna that erstwhile had belonged to the Byzantine Empire, as well as lands bordering Rome. These territorialities were thus added to the titular head of "the states of the church," and became the Papal States, ruled directly by the Pope as its sovereign. [141] Pepin's son was none other than the energetic Charlemagne, Charles "the Great" (King of the Franks, A.D.768-814), the powerful Carolingian monarch who brought the alliance of church and state to its apogee. The story goes that on Christmas day A.D.800, Charlemagne was crowned Emperor of the Holy Roman Empire by Pope Leo III (St. Leo; pope, A.D.795-816), thenceforth establishing not only a dangerous precedent that would have profound ramifications in the relations between pope and emperor during the Middle Ages but also establishing what would later become a much sought-after service – that of being crowned Emperor by the Pope as a Christian ruler. Conversely, the power to crown emperors gave the Pope the authority of papal investiture – namely, the power of making (or breaking) emperors.

It would also be the Western (Holy Roman) Emperor Charlemagne who first reunited many of the countries of Western and Central Europe and rebuilt and consolidated the biggest empire in the West since that of Rome. During his time, Charlemagne also made the first concerted effort to establish and extend Latin learning and liberal education to all of the subjects in his realm. He not only built cathedrals but also decreed that monastic schools, the forerunners of the medical universities, be established in the monasteries. He militated for the study of reading, writing, and the pursuit of the Roman concept of the liberal arts in these schools, thereby challenging the old notion that liberal education was inconsistent with church teaching. As a result, the rise of the universities in the Medieval period resulted in a resurgence of learning following the long and deep intellectual slumber of the Dark Ages. [142] This learning was particularly fervent in the newly

---

[140] The policy of imperial protection of the Holy see of St. Peter was championed by Pepin the Short and Charlemagne throughout their reigns.

[141] Today, the Pope's temporal title is Sovereign of the State of the Vatican.(2)

[142] Whilst the establishment of universities was truly the crowning scholastic achievement of the Medieval period, the humanitarian *tour de force* remained the founding of charity hospitals spurred by the Crusades.

resurgent liberal arts in both the trivium and quadrivium,[143] as well as in general medical education in the form of Græco-Roman medicine.

Following the example of Pepin and Charlemagne, papal investiture was avidly and eagerly sought by rulers and royal claimants to the various thrones of Europe.[144] The power and prestige vested upon monarchs by the act of being crowned by the pope, especially later in both French and German dominions, would give rise to major disputes amongst European rulers, from the Middle Ages up to the Renaissance. What began as a cozy church-state relationship would later degenerate into a protracted rivalry and recalcitrant feud between popes and emperors. Let us briefly foray into one related and notable episode that took place in the midst of the Middle Ages.

The need for rulers to obtain not only acceptance but also approval from the pope was indeed exemplified in the lay-investiture controversy which reached its dramatic climax in A.D.1077, when Holy Roman Emperor Henry IV (reigned, 1056-1105) defied and engaged in a dangerous and escalating struggle with the pope, the powerful and insightful Gregory VII (St. Gregory VII; pope,1073-1080). Upon the emperor's insistence on the power to preside over the investiture of bishops, and the pope's equally intense and obdurate opposition to this policy, a great dispute arose between them. The emperor proceeded with his intransigent imperial policy, and in return, Pope Gregory declared Henry's election as emperor "null and void" – even worse, the emperor was excommunicated. The tables had suddenly turned for Henry who now, facing the dual prospect of civil strife amongst his restless populace and the potential revolt of his vassals, found himself in an untenable situation.

Indeed, his feudal vassals not only feared the possibility of their own excommunication if they sided with Henry (the equivalent of certain perdition) but also saw Henry's troubles as an opportunity to defy imperial rule and resurrect feudal dominion. Henry, then recognizing the fact that his vassals would acknowledge the authority of the pope over his own authority and realizing the danger of his predicament, set out to salvage the potentially disastrous situation in which he found himself mired. The Emperor appeared on a cold, dark night outside the castle at Canossa where the Pope was temporarily residing. "Henry declared himself a penitent, and Gregory kept him waiting outside the castle for three days, barefoot and in sack cloth. When he was finally admitted, he did penance and Gregory absolved him."(12)

THE ORIGIN OF THE BARBER-SURGEONS

As fate would have it, a seemingly inconsequential edict of the Church began a cascade of events that changed the course of medical history. This obscure and early edict required that monks and priests be clean-shaven (though in those days most men wore beards) – prompting many itinerant barbers to take up

---

[143] As previously denoted, the great inspiration for the establishment of the seven liberal arts (grammar, dialectic, rhetoric, geometry, arithmetic, music, and astronomy was Marcus Terentius Varro (116 B.C.-27 B.C.), the illustrious man-of-letters of the Roman Republic, who advocated classical studies to "liberate" the mind of man from the toils of existence and the doldrums of everyday living.

[144] As students of history know, the issue of papal investiture culminated with the crowning of the majestic and immensely powerful monarch, Charles V (Hapsburg King of Spain, 1516-1556; Holy Roman Emperor, 1519-1556).

permanent residence in the monasteries in order to be of service to the monks. In the monasteries, the barbers were exposed to the rudiments of medicine and surgery. The monks, ministering to the sick, not only spiritually but also medically and surgically, in the presence of the barbers, served as teachers, and thence as conduits by which the earliest of barber-surgeons came into existence. In due time, barber-surgeons and monks would come to exchange medical and surgical knowledge, for there were only a very few lay, scholarly physicians in those days.

This was, in fact, the prevailing situation when the ecclesiastical Council of Clermont in 1130 forbade the practice of medicine by monks. And in 1163, the Council of Tours further curtailed the practice of medicine by priests and monks with a proclamation specifically proscribing the clergy from practicing surgery. As a result and out of necessity, the practice of medicine and the task of performing surgical procedures logically fell to the barber-surgeons who had learned medicine and surgery from the monks. In fact, the barber-surgeons had become quite adept at bleeding patients, lancing and draining abscesses, setting broken bones, amputating limbs, and even performing dentistry.(5,7,9)

In 1215, the influential and powerful Pope Innocent III (pope, 1198-1216) issued his famous bull, *Ecclesia Abhorret A Sanguine*, "the Church abhors the shedding of blood," which in effect, confirmed and clarified the Church's previous edicts and summarily forbade the practice of surgery by the clergy. Since many physicians at this time were also members of the clergy, the proclamation barred the practice of surgery by those physicians who were also clerics. Most of them complied, with the only general exception being the physician-surgeons of northern Italy and southern France who, living in relatively isolated communities, continued to practice medicine and surgery unimpeded by the rulings.(3,4)

These well-intentioned papal bulls and church edicts had been proclaimed to prevent the accidental death of a patient during surgery in the hands of the clergy. The church maintained that the possibility of death as a surgical complication was too great a responsibility for clergymen to assume.(3,7,13) That responsibility would have to fall on the shoulders of the few scholarly, lay physician-surgeons and the intrepid barber-surgeons.

Given the content of these ecclesiastic proclamations and the fact that many learned men, including the venerated and influential Persian physician, Avicenna (A.D.980-1037), and most of the other influential Islamic physicians (except Abulcasis), considered surgery inferior to medicine, it was not surprising that the bulls and edicts were interpreted erroneously as forbidding the general practice of surgery. Consequently, these rulings of the Church accidentally created a professional rift, a virtual separation between the practice of medicine and surgery and contributed to the delineation of what actually comprised these separate specialties.

Nevertheless, it must be recognized that the generally accepted demarcation between the two disciplines has been ascribed primarily to the writings of Avicenna, chief physician for the Baghdad Caliphate, who avidly supported the separation of the two specialties and firmly believed that theoretic and diagnostic medicine was superior to practical, and what was then, painful and bloody surgery.(3,7,13) Except for a few physician-surgeons, notably, Guy de Chauliac (1300-1368), the separation of medicine and surgery remained fairly well demarcated until the Renaissance, when enlightened Renaissance physicians, recognizing the important interrelation between the two disciplines, argued the advantages of having knowledge in both fields. These physicians practiced medicine and performed surgery in their private medical practices.

REGULATION OF MEDICAL PRACTICE IN THE MEDIEVAL PERIOD

In 1140, the Norman king, Roger II (King of Sicily, 1130-1145), promulgated a decree that legitimized the medical profession by conferring a professional degree on medical practitioners. Furthermore, he encouraged medical education and specifically stipulated that physicians could not be trained unless they had completed three years of studies in the liberal arts – a wise proclamation, indeed!

The crusading King Frederick II (Holy Roman Emperor, 1220-1250), grandson of Roger II, went one step further and effected needed reforms in the practice of medicine during the Medieval period. Frederick was the right man to do this, for he was not only a brilliant lawmaker and administrator but also a noted patron of the arts and sciences. He consolidated the School of Salerno in his domain as the leading medical university of the period, and in 1224, founded a university in Naples. He personally supervised translations of Greek and Islamic works into Latin.(14) As a patron of the School of Salerno, the Holy Roman Emperor issued a proclamation proclaiming that only physicians from that school "had exclusive rights to the practice of medicine in his empire." The proclamation also elevated the status of all physicians so licensed to the status of "doctors."(7) Frederick II established medical examinations which placed medicine and surgery on equal footing (at first temporarily in his kingdom, and later in his empire).

Additionally, this revolutionary proclamation called for two classes of surgeons: the "surgeons of the first class" who were to be examined by three university professors in Latin, and if successful, they were then given a diploma to practice both medicine and surgery; and the "surgeons of the second class" who were to be examined by two teachers in the Italian vernacular who then endorsed the applicants' diploma if they passed and became "qualified." The later candidates, the proclamation required, "must take an oath never to treat internal diseases and they could not receive the title of doctor."(9)

As Holy Roman Emperor, Frederick was another early and active participant in what we previously noted had become the seemingly endless and protracted struggle between pope and emperor which raged throughout the Middle Ages.(2,12) In 1245, Frederick was even excommunicated by Pope Innocent IV (pope,1243-1253). He fought ardently for the centralization of the power of the emperor, as opposed to regional autonomy, which was sought by the nascent Italian and German towns that strove towards political as well as economic independence.[145]

In France, after the Council of Tours forbade surgery by the clergy, the learned university-trained surgeons began to organize into what gradually became known as the Confraternity of St. Côme whose members were designated Master

---

[145] In the later Middle Ages, this papal-emperor rivalry coalesced in the fierce struggle between the opposing political parties in Germany and Italy. Those who supported the pope were designated *Guelphs*; and those who followed the Holy Roman emperors, the *Ghibellines*. It also denoted the two rival German families whence the appellations derive, the Welfs (Guelphs), and the Hohenstaufen (of which Frederick II was a member). In Italy, the recalcitrant feud spilled over into open warfare between the rival factions of the independent Italian city-states amidst the Renaissance.(2,12)

Surgeons. In time, the Confraternity would evolve to become the Royal College of Surgeons. Though still considered one or two notches below the physicians, the Master Surgeons nevertheless occupied a lofty status, especially when compared to that of the humble barber-surgeons. The Master Surgeons were university trained and literate in Latin; the barber-surgeons were not. The Master Surgeons taught at the universities, and directed their apprentices and the barber-surgeons in the actual performance of surgery. They pointed at structures and followed surgical texts, as the barber-surgeons performed the actual operation.(9,11,15) The Master Surgeons were called the Surgeons of the Long Robes, as opposed to their apprentices and the barber-surgeons who wore short robes. Interestingly, this tradition, whereby professors of medicine and surgery and medical faculty members wear long robes whilst students, interns, and residents don short robes, survives even today at certain institutions in the United States.[146]

GUY DE CHAULIAC: MEDIEVAL SURGEON

Guy de Chauliac (1300-1368), the famous French surgeon, who studied at such great medical centers of learning as Toulose, Montpellier, and Paris, was one of those physicians of southern France who was not only a cleric but also a physician-surgeon, although for him, surgery was his primary vocation. Just before the time of the Great Schism of the Western Church (1378-1417),[147] he rose in Avignon to be chaplain and personal physician to popes Clement VI (pope, 1342-1352), Innocent VI (pope, 1352-1362), and Urban V (pope, 1362-1370).(3)

As a physician who practiced both medicine and surgery, Guy de Chauliac helped to elevate surgery to greater heights, enhanced the esteem and prestige in which both physicians and surgeons were held by the public, and through his medical contributions and surgical achievements, advanced the progress of medical science during the Medieval period. He promoted advances in general surgery as well as in other disciplines in the surgical arts: dentistry (teeth replacement and artificial dentures), the use of traction with pulleys and weights for reduction and immobilization of fractures, amputations and description of surgical techniques, and compilation of principles of wound healing.(16-18)

In 1363, Guy de Chauliac published his *Grand Surgery*, the most comprehensive medieval compilation of surgical principles and techniques – a veritable encyclopedic textbook – which was extensively referenced, citing more than 100 previous medical authors. At the top of the list was Galen, with 890 citations, followed by Avicenna, with 661.(3,19) This clearly written and well-organized text has

[146] In fact, this tradition was still in practice at the time that the author obtained his neurosurgical residency training (1978-1983) at Emory University School of Medicine.
[147] Following the Babylonian Captivity and Pope Gregory XI's (pope, 1370-1378) return to Rome in 1377, a struggle ensued after his death with the contested election to fill the seat of the see of St. Peter. The Great Schism (or Schism of the West) was a splintering of the Roman Catholic church. Urban VI (pope, 1378-1389) was elected pope, but soon he estranged many in the church with his violent and unbecoming behavior. His election was declared null and void by the cardinals, and another pope was elected. Thus, there were two popes: Pope Urban VI who reigned in Rome and the antipope Clement VII who had his court assembled in Avignon, France. They and their successors forged two lines of popes and antipopes. The schism was finally solved by the Council of Constance (1414-1418) which accepted the resignation of the pope at Rome, deposed two reigning antipopes, and finally elected Martin V (reigned, 1417-1431) as pope; Pope Martin V restored the prestige and unity of the papacy.(2)

been praised for its scholarly contribution to the art of surgery and belatedly earned him the title of Founder of Didactic Surgery.(3,5)

In surgery, de Chauliac used the surgical knife for extirpating tumors and the cautery for controlling hemorrhage as advocated by Islamic physicians. Although de Chauliac had a conciliatory tone when it came to different schools of thought in surgical practice, he was uncompromising when the need arose, as for example, in the treatment of wounds with a new method. He strongly argued for the "dry method" for treating simple, clean wounds by allowing healing by primary intention; thus he specifically approximated the edges of the wound or surgical incisions with sutures (stitches) for better healing. Yet he was experienced enough to advocate Galen's "wet treatment" with the use of packing and draining of wounds, and promote healing by allowing suppuration for wounds that were deep, draining, and contaminated – "wounds altered by air which must be purified [for healing]."(16) In these cases, he believed that the old "wet method" was necessary, espousing the conventional view.

Moreover, de Chauliac discussed the use of the soporific sponge, an invention attributed to an earlier physician named Theodoric (1205-1295). It is most likely that this early attempt at surgical anesthesia was comprised of opium impregnated onto surgical gauze and in this manner used as a topical anesthetic. The idea went unnoticed, perhaps because it was too revolutionary for its time. There is no doubt, however, that this practice made surgery slightly more palatable for the unfortunate patients who underwent surgical procedures during this era.

Most importantly, Guy de Chauliac set an example in the history of medical ethics when, as a physician-surgeon, he voluntarily stayed behind to treat those afflicted with the bubonic plague of 1347-1348, the Black Death – that great killer of humanity which assailed Europe, parts of Asia and Africa, and the littoral Mediterranean. This was the time when many in the clergy, as well as some physicians, deserted the sick and the afflicted, for fear of contracting the dreaded disease for which there was no cure. At the height of the Black Death of 1348, even the see of St. Peter, Pope Clement VI, refused to admit and see visitors or to mingle and minister to his flock. Instead, he locked himself in his papal study in Avignon and kept a flame burning to purify the air in an attempt to avoid getting infected with the plague. Yet, Guy de Chauliac, the pope's own physician, was making house calls, treating the sick, and tending the afflicted.(3,5)

CHAPTER 27

THE SCHOOL OF SALERNO AND MEDIEVAL MEDICINE

We are like dwarfs seated on the shoulders of giants. If we have seen more and farther than
they, it is not due to our own clear eyes or tall bodies, but because we are raised on high and
upborne by their gigantic biggness.

Bernard of Chartres
English Chancellor, 1119

The city of Salerno is located south of Naples on the tranquil Bay of Paestum, on the sole of the boot of the Italian peninsula. During imperial Roman times, the city was famous for its healthy climate conducive "to rest and cure."(7) Even the Roman emperors and their retinues were believed to have enjoyed Salerno's Mediterranean climate. It was also said that the salubrious city had become a melting pot of different cultures, races, and religions – where its diverse inhabitants lived in total harmony.

The primal school at Salerno was the first nonecclesiastic institution of learning to rise in the West after the fall of Rome. Legend has it, in fact, that the medical school that developed there was founded by four physicians, each of different backgrounds and cultures: A Greek, a Roman, a Jew, and a Moslem.(7) Unlike other nascent church-sponsored universities that sprouted later, Salerno was a secular university which attracted students from far away, as early as the 9th Century (the century in which the university was thought to have been founded). Salerno reached its pinnacle of glory between the 11th and 13th Centuries, at the height of the Medieval period.(7,20)

During the transition between the Dark Ages and the Medieval period, we discover, in one of those antiquated passages wherein obscure historic events tend to merge imperceptibly with legends, the exploits of the learned and enigmatic figure of Constantine Africanus (1010-1087). It is said that under his tutelage, the School of Salerno flourished. We do know that the man Constantine, who was later christened "Africanus," was born in Carthage and that during his formative years he traveled extensively in the Middle East. It is surmised that during those long journeys, he learned about different cultures and customs, as well as studied languages (including Greek and Arabic) and medicine. Not surprisingly, he was an avid collector of old medical books.

It was because of his extensive knowledge (he was also literate in Latin) that he was accused of practicing magic and of being a sorcerer. Facing a charge of sorcery, a forbidden practice, he hastily left Carthage, which he accomplished by dressing as a beggar, ultimately settling quietly in Salerno. One must remember that is those days, eccentric men possessed of learning were suspected of being magicians or sorcerers, and this almost universal peculiarity of equating knowledge with magic contributed further to the stagnation of learning that impeded scientific investigations during this time.

In Salerno, Constantine practiced and taught the art of medicine at the university. Yet his true passion (and in which he avidly immersed himself) was the study of languages and the translation of old medical books he had acquired during his long treks through Islamic countries.

In 1076, after many journeys, he took up residence at St. Benedict of Nursia's remote and mountainous monastery at Monte Cassino.(7) It was there that the enigmatic Constantine immersed himself entirely in the translation of old medical works. In fact, Constantine Africanus is reputed to have translated no less than 30 medical treatises, including Islamic works, as well as writings of Hippocrates and Galen. These translations, as we shall see later, were immensely important during the rediscovery of the Greek and Roman classics at the outset of the Renaissance.[148]

During his years at Monte Cassino, Constantine Africanus lead the life of a simple monk, where he eventually died in 1087.[149] Suffice it to say, that during the turbulence of the Dark Ages (and the early Medieval period), many of the great Greek and Roman classical works survived because they had been preserved, not only in the continuing tenebrous monasteries and the dusty libraries of Constantinople but also in the hands of scholars in the Islamic East, scholars who kept the invaluable manuscripts safe from the deprivations of the barbarians in the chaotic West, where many would have been certainly lost. Because of the Moslem and Hebrew scholars, the precious information contained in those manuscripts returned to the West at a more propitious time. These Arabian medical works proved to be veritable fountains of knowledge, although to a significant extent they were based on preceding Greek and Roman works which had been forgotten in the West after the fall of the Western Roman Empire.

And during the incipient Medieval period, it was Salerno that held the spark of knowledge which would later light Europe. The founding of the universities at Salerno and then Bologna in Italy, and at Montpellier in France, rekindled the fire of learning that spread incessantly during the Medieval period.[150] The medical university at Salerno excelled not only in the studies of the Greek and Roman classics but also in medical ethics and medicine. The *Regimen Sanitatis Salernitatum,* which was published anonymously in the mid-13th Century, was a popular collection of home remedies and health rules composed in poetic verse to maximize memorization by the common people, who for the most part remained illiterate. The *Regimen Sanitatis Salernitatum* was used by all, the common people, the nobility, and even royalty. Legend proclaims that the manual was actually written for the benefit of Robert II (Duke of Normandy, 1087-1106), the eldest son of William the Conqueror, who, according to a popular yarn, had a brief romantic sojourn in Salerno on his return trip from the First Crusade. The book contained 350 rules which in later editions was richly and amply illustrated to further assist the populace

---

[148] Perhaps inspired by the example of Constantine, translations of the great Islamic physicians Rhazes, Avicenna, and Albucasis (of whom we will have a great deal more to say later) began in earnest in Toledo under the guidance of the scholar Gerhard of Cremona (1114-1187), supplementing the work of Constantine Africanus, and keeping alive the knowledge and preserving the wisdom of the great Persian and Arabic physicians.

[149] A.D.1087 was the same fateful year that the great conqueror, William of Normandy (1027-1087), sustained his mortal injury whilst riding his horse and died an agonizing death in Rouen, the capital of his native Normandy.

[150] In due time, Montpellier, perhaps because of its proximity to the Western Arab Caliphate, emerged to compete successfully first with the university at Bologna and then with Padua, for the honor of carrying the torch of knowledge during the transition period between the closing of the Middle Ages and the dawn of the Renaissance.

in understanding the health advice and remedies therein contained. It is also known that as faraway as England, and as late as Elizabethan times (1533-1603), this practical health guide was still being used to educate the royal children of the English court in cleanliness and hygiene.

Another important medical document, the Bamberg Manuscript, of which only fragments survived, is perhaps the oldest surgical text produced at the School of Salerno. It was likely the work of several authors and included surgical sections based on the works of the Byzantine surgeon Paul of Aegina (A.D.625-690), as well as the Islamic surgeon Albucasis (A.D.936-1013). And it is this text that contains a description of the soporific sponge, the early precursor of the anesthetic mask, that we mentioned previously.(7)

One of the foremost surgeons of the School of Salerno was Roger of Salerno (fl. late 12th Century) who, assisted by his disciples, composed one of the first surgical texts, *Chirurgia Magistri Rogeri*, which laid the groundwork for surgical education in Europe. His *Practica Chirurgica* was another important book of the School of Salerno. In addition, two other contributions discussed the care of head wounds, the surgical management of skull fractures, and expounded on the theories of wound healing. Despite his scholarly contributions, Roger of Salerno was a child of the times who incorrectly believed that wound healing by secondary intention required the formation of pus, *per intentio secundam*. Moreover, suppuration was considered "good and laudable pus," *pus bonum et laudabile*.

A successor to Roger of Salerno was the Dominican friar and surgeon, Theodoric (1205-1296), who has been praised as one of the most original surgeons of all times. Theodoric denied the notion of laudable pus, "...And as all present surgeons maintain that pus be formed in wounds. No mistake can be greater! Such a procedure is quite against nature, prolongs illness, and hinders healing and the consolidation of the wound."(7) He therefore subscribed to the newer doctrine of primary wound healing, *per intentio primam*, and claimed, "in truth nothing is more important than cleaning a wound!"(7)

As we have already stated, one of the greatest accomplishments of the Medieval period was the establishment of the universities and their faculties which were ecclesiastical institutions of higher learning intimately associated with churches, cathedrals, and monasteries. We have discussed the School of Salerno, the oldest medical school which was likely founded between A.D. 850 and 950, and we have intimated at one of the reasons the center of medical knowledge subsequently shifted in the late Medieval period from Salerno to Bologna and ultimately to Montpellier.

Montpellier remained a hub of learning throughout this period. Its medical faculty was patronized and sanctioned by Pope Nicholas IV (pope, 1288-1294), and its university status officially granted by a specific statute in 1289.(7) Montpellier's ascendancy as a favorite medical school along with Padua was not only because of its superb faculty but also because of its location near both the resurgent Italy (which gave birth to the Renaissance) and Islamic Spain (which, given its Arabic influence, was already a beacon of learning and culture).

EARLY CHRISTIANITY AND ITS INFLUENCE ON MEDIEVAL MEDICINE

From our foregoing discussion on the early Middle Ages, especially the immediate period following the collapse of the Western Roman Empire, which we have referred to as the Dark Ages, we noted a strong tendency to attribute illness to religious or supernatural causes and to the frailty of human nature which made man vulnerable to temptations of the flesh and other worldly sins. These transgressions, in turn, prompted swift and severe retribution. Cures were sought by prayer and penance. Some sought healing and salvation by withdrawing from worldly temptations and absorbing themselves in asceticism, and, in some instances, in deprivations of bodily needs or mortification of the flesh, such as engaging in self-flagellation or some other ungodly punishment. Such punishments were believed to lead to expiation of one's sins, spiritual healing, and salvation of the soul.

Thus, asceticism, from the rejection of simple comforts to the utter neglect of bodily needs such as grooming and cleanliness, was carried to stringent extremes to avoid the corrupting influence of worldly temptations. Personal cleanliness including bathing was rejected, because it was believed to stem out of personal vanity and pride. Bodily hygiene reached a nadir during this time. Uncleanliness was equated with saintly humility and closeness to the simplicity of early Christianity.

It was unfortunate that Christians regarded cleanliness as a mundane luxury and during the Middle Ages rejected it as a vain endeavor. Diseases, therefore, were rampant in such dirty and filthy environs that were the typical European homes of the Middle Ages – where vermin infestations, poor hygiene and sanitation were universal. Not surprisingly, life expectancy was a pitiful 8 years during most of the Middle Ages – the result of these conditions as well as the extremely high maternal and infant mortalities. Unfortunately, this tragic reality would remain virtually unchanged for centuries. It was not until physicians and medical scientists proved the true nature of the contagion through scientific advances that Europeans finally accepted the notion of hygiene and cleanliness, but this, alas, had to wait until the 19th Century! [151]

Despite these obstacles, medieval medicine made some advances which took place in three forms: First, monastic medicine as practiced by monks which, as we have seen, ultimately gave rise to the itinerant barber-surgeons. Second, Islamic medicine as practiced by the great Arabian, Persian, and Hebrew physicians which thrived in the Islamic East (proving to be another great repository of medical knowledge). Third, scholastic medicine as taught and practiced in the nascent medical universities such as those at Salerno, Bologna, Padua, and later, Paris and Montpellier – which set standards, gave rise to the scholarly doctors of medicine and put the profession again on respected footing.

It should be noted that in the period of early Christianity, the teachings of the Christian martyrs of the New Testament, the canonization of Christian men and women who had performed medical miracles and devoted their lives to the betterment of mankind, and the influence of Christianity and its teachings on medical ethics proved immense and incalculable. As the examples of St. Benedict and others indicate, the division between religion and medicine remained to a significant degree blurred and indistinct. Nowhere was this as evident as in the resurgent field of medical ethics.

---

[151] By the end of the 19th Century, medical knowledge was poised to add nearly half a century to the average length of life as a result of scientific breakthroughs, medical advances, improved standards of living, and sanitation. At the time that Dr. Haggard wrote his fascinating book, *The Doctor in History*, in the 1930s, the average life span was approaching 60 years of age. Today, it approaches 80 years of age in many countries including Japan and the United States.

The concept of Christian charity in medical care was truly engendered in the care of the sick by the clergy, the physician-clerics, and subsequently, the lay physicians. Complete self-effacement and charity as exhibited by the Christian saints became the desirable goals associated with the practice of medicine and the healing arts. As the medical historian and ethicist, Professor Gary B. Ferngren, writes, "It was not curing but caring that constituted the chief ministry of the early Christian community to the sick."(21) According to Professor Henry Sigerist, the most revolutionary change in medical care during this time was the preferential social position assigned to the sick and suffering by the Christian healers which was fundamentally different from what it was in pagan times, and which was to remain unchanged henceforth.(22) It must also be noted that even though Christianity sought to heal afflictions of the body, redemption and salvation of the soul always took precedent over bodily diseases and remained paramount.(21)

Yet during the first four centuries A.D., many of the early Church Fathers, such as Origen (c.A.D.184-c.253) and Clement (c.A.D.150-c.220), asserted that pain and suffering from illness and disease were "trials of the soul," often sent as "admonition, for correction of the past, and to make one mindful of the future."(23) Yet these assertions did not preclude medical treatment, for all the wisdom and knowledge of the art of medicine had been placed in the hands of physicians by the grace of God. Medicine, after all, existed for the benefit of man.(23)

Christian saints not only were thought to intervene and effect cures by spiritual intercession, but pious and Christian holy men were believed to be dutiful replacements for lay physicians in medical treatment – in both physical and spiritual healing. The veneration of Christian saints was commonplace, as was the adoration of their relics. St. Anthony, for example, was the patron saint of those afflicted with ergotism, the dreaded malady which was then referred to as St. Anthony's Fire because of the dark, gangrenous changes preceding the dreaded falling-off of limbs of the unfortunate victims. St. Sebastian was the patron saint of those afflicted with the plague, and because arrows were emblematic of the plague, the saint was usually depicted in agonizing torment whilst being pierced by arrows. Likewise, Santa Catalina was appealed and prayed to for relief of headaches.(18)

The story of the twins, St. Cosmas and St. Damian, has been immortalized in numerous works of art and medical illustrations and vividly recounted in many texts on medical history. The brothers, born in Asia Minor, acquired medical knowledge and were proselytized to Christianity. They were said to have been practicing physicians in Anatolia, where, because of their conversion to Christianity, they were persecuted and ultimately beheaded in A.D.287. As Christian martyrs, they were subsequently canonized. According to the story, their remains became treasured relics and were taken to Rome c.A.D.526 and A.D.530, where the sacred remains were deposited in a church built in the Roman Forum.[152]

The Christian priests, unlike the lay physician-surgeons, were free of repercussions from their charitable medical work. And medicine, insofar as clinical results and medical complications of treatment, was a risky business – not only for patients but also for practitioners – in the doom and gloom period of the Dark Ages, as well as in the doldrums of the Medieval period. For instance, in A.D.580,

---

[152] As late as 1969, we were informed by the medical historian Dr. B.J. Anson that the venerated relics were housed in the same religious shrine where they could still be visited.(18)

Gutram, King of Burgundy, killed two surgeons because they could not cure his beloved queen who was afflicted with the dreaded plague, and in 1337, King John of Bohemia had a surgeon drowned by having him thrown into the river Oder because he failed to cure him of blindness.(5,24)

So it was to be, that towards the end of the period of monastic medicine in the 13th Century there was a gradual but unequivocal separation of the two professions – medicine and the priesthood – which had previously been intricately entwined. It has been said that "often Church doctrine conflicted with medical practice,"(25) and indeed this is substantiated by the conflicting edicts that we have already discussed which adamantly commanded the separation of the two. In addition, the church was concerned with the possible spiritual distractions of their priests when treating the bodily ill. There was also the insistence of church authorities in requiring priests to hear confessions before providing medical care to the sick (25), in contradistinction to the physicians' Hippocratic Oath. Moreover, the rise of the secular (and even the religious) universities during the Medieval period and their expansion during the Renaissance, cannot be discounted, for these institutions of learning added philosophic and secular dimensions militating for separation. There was also the profitability factor in the practice of medicine, which conflicted with the church's view that medicine should remain a charitable service which ministered to the sick in harmony with the church's teachings.(25,26)

It was at this juncture that physicians took necessarily different professional paths. The divergence of the two professions was not due solely to trendy market forces, as some recent authors have suggested, but adaptation and specialization between the two professions as to tending to the needs of the body with natural remedies, and the needs of the soul with spiritual comfort. There were also various other forces, not just economic, but political, historic, and social, that shaped and affected this divergence. In the end, true medical knowledge was believed to have a divine origin, stemming directly from the divine reflection of God – just as Aristotle "had clearly asserted that the intellective faculty of man's soul was divine."(27)

Perhaps just as important, if not more so, were the numerous edicts of the church and papal bulls that ultimately forced the separation. Moreover, there were ideologic, structural, and motivational differences between the tenets and workings of a Christian church that relied primarily on faith, charity, and good works, and an incipient evolving profession that provided a service as a vocation and relied on the natural sciences, as elementary as they might have been at the time. Inspired by the inquiring nature of the medieval universities, medical scholars sought facts and basic truths that could be verified by observations of natural and physical events, and later, by experimentation – and explained by logical reasoning and rational explanations.

Carrying the argument to its logical conclusion, it must be admitted that the church remained more preoccupied with God, with preparation for the afterlife, and the redemption and the salvation of the soul, whilst the medical profession directed its energy to the relief of bodily pain and suffering, the struggle against disease here on earth, and the postponement of death. In fact, this difference in priorities – that is, the physicians' tendency to treat physical ailments and diseases, and medieval Catholicism's preoccupation with the well-being of the individual's soul – remained a source of tension from the period of early Christianity to the late Middle

Ages, latent as this tension might have been.(28) Yet it was not really an "all or none" separation. Most physicians continued to believe and abide by the teachings of the church and practiced with the compassion inherent in their profession – a profession permeated by the philanthropy of the Greeks, the humanism and humanitarianism of the Romans, the teachings of the Mosaic Laws, [153] as well as the sense of compassion of the Good Samaritan, and the charity of the Christian church.

I would like to reiterate an important point at this time, and here I paraphrase Professor Darrell W. Amundsen of Western Washington University who has stated that "the flight of physicians away from plagues and pestilences during the Middle Ages was not as extensive as some modern scholars have suggested."(29) In his extensive review of pest tractates dealing with pestilential diseases during this time, he arrived at the conclusion that the number of physicians who fled epidemics was relatively small, and the majority, although taking extraordinary precautions, e.g., wearing elaborate masks and gloves, etc., continued to treat those afflicted with the plague. This despite the fact that physicians like Guy de Chauliac understood their dilemma during the Black Death: "[a physician was] faced both with extreme peril to himself and the knowledge of his own inability to be of any real help...."(29) In the words of Guy de Chauliac: "It was useless and shameful for the doctor the more so as they dared to visit the sick for fear of being infected. And when they did visit them, they did hardly anything for them, and were paid nothing."(30)

Moreover, the motives of the physicians who compiled the tractates, according to Amundsen, appear, "to have been a sincere effort to do all in their power to help in such crises." Many authors stated their reasons, and for the most part they were motivated *pro bono publico* [as were the cases of Jacme d'Agramont (1348), Johannes Jacobi (c.1364 or 1373), Francischino de Collignano (1382), etc.].(29) Towards the end of his excellent essay, Amundsen writes: "not only did the authors of the pest tractates write them generally without thought of profit, but also they attempted to make their advice employable by the poor as well as by the well to do."(29)

In due time, especially during (and after) the Renaissance, both the newly energized secular legal and medical professions became well paid and recognized prestigious endeavors, which of necessity, had to be concerned with the "here and now" rather than the "afterlife."(31) In fact as early as the Medieval period, in the 12th and 13th Centuries, scholars at the University of Paris were complaining that clerical students were pursuing more marketable scholarly subjects such as law and medicine, "which offered the prospect of well paid and prestigious jobs – [which] was leading them away from their principal area of study, theology."(27) The Judeo-Christian tradition and later, the teachings of the Catholic church, continued to expound on the concepts of the Good Samaritan, good works, and charity, particularly in providing care to the poor and the downtrodden. And to this day, a network of Catholic charity hospitals throughout the world continue to provide charity care with diligence and compassion.(26)

Thus, in our great age of science and technology in the closing years of the 20th Century, with the secularization of society and the advent of the legal age, the physicians, even with their imposing modern day high-tech medicine, remain

[153] From Judaism, particularly, stems the fundamental ethic of the dignity of man and the sanctity of life – now parts of our Judeo-Christian legacy.

suffused with the ancient ethics of compassion and charity. In today's adversarial, litigious, and egalitarian climate, this has resulted in a curious and incongruous mixture of guilt, disunity, and for a vast majority who remain silent, utter submission. So, despite their material success and prosperity, physicians have proved to be no match against their numerous battle-hardened adversaries on the field of combat.

But such are the iniquities and inequities of our times. Because of the manifest greed of a few much-talked-about "bad apples," American physicians today are both maligned if they are prosperous and suspect if they are not. A no-win, catch-22 situation if ever there was one. They are also taken to task if their behavior does not coincide with those of saints who have attained martyrdom. Their lives must be immersed with the political correctness of coercive compassion and their times saturated with the pseudo-altruistic liberal expectations of what a physician's life ought to be – namely, hagiographies nurtured in the cult of victimhood widely venerated in our uncertain age. Perception of monastic sainthood and collective self-denial – not genuine compassion, dedication, and independence, or personal integrity, or professional competence – are today the qualities that are expected of American physicians, to coax and prepare them for the planned government takeover of the profession.

Government health experts and many in the public apparently seem to forget that despite their deserving qualities, physicians separated from the clergy long ago to tend to the suffering and diseases of people...here on earth. In this so-called post-Modern age, physicians should regroup and reassert their basic traditional rights as individuals who long to practice medicine independent of government. They should be cognizant of the fact that as individuals they should not be expected to shoulder more burden than they can possibly carry in obeisance to the state. Government health experts in collusion with self-styled ethicists are stretching the concepts of charity and compassion to unending limits, so as to bring about the necessity for government intervention using make-shift (and outright false) ethics as to seemingly occupy the moral high-ground to justify change and ultimately, socialized medicine. For they conveniently ignore or choose to forget other old and proven ethical principles upon which both the profession and this nation were founded.

"Modern society refuses to accept ageing, illness, suffering and death," writes the French medical author Claude Quétel referring to the changes in attitude commonplace in the West, "as an anguish that afflicts our de-Christianized society."(32) And for the real or imagined mortal sins of the American health care system and the incipient envy of many who resent the relative prosperity of physicians, the nation is again poised to enter a new Dark Age, bringing with it the ravaging of modern Orwellian Vandals already in our midst.

MEDIEVAL MEDICAL ETHICS

Let us now return to history and discuss briefly medical ethics in the Medieval period, for ethical principles also evolved during this time. Judeo-Christian beliefs, for example, promised that to assist the sick and the needy was a sign of inner strength, charity, and moral character, not a sign of personal weakness.

During the early Middle Ages, the cauldron of medical ethics which contained both the ancient legacies of the Græco-Roman world and the Mosaic law of the Old Testament, also became infused with New Testament Christian ideals of charity and submission. Almost imperceptibly, new versions of the concepts of social duties and obligations were added during the Dark Ages and monastic medicine. In the later Medieval period, as monastic medicine gave way to scholarly medicine as taught in the medieval universities, we find lay physicians, *medici,* who practiced both medicine and surgery as closely-related learned professions. Here we see a separation of the ecclesiastical from the medical profession. And amazingly, even during those days of meager and scarce medical knowledge, great medieval physicians such as Arnald de Villanova (1235-1311) concerned themselves with medical ethics and attempted to provide practical rules of moral conduct for the lay medical "professionals" of his day who had separated themselves from the clergy and perhaps needed guidance:

> Note that the physician must be learned in diagnosing, careful and accurate in prescribing, circumspect and cautious in answering questions, ambiguous in making a prognosis, just in making promises; and he should not promise health because in doing so he will assume a divine function and insult God. He should rather promise loyalty and attentiveness, should be discreet in making calls, and he must be careful in speech, modest in behavior and kind to the patient.(33)

And with regard to Villanova's *De Cautelis Medicorum* (an outstanding treatise on medical ethics which was translated by the scholar, Henry E. Sigerist; 1891-1957), Dr. Ilza Vieth writes:

> The third part advises the physician on his deportment when making house calls. On entering the house of the patient, the physician is to inquire from the relatives about the duration and nature of the illness and about its symptoms. This is necessary because even after inspecting the faeces and urine and the condition of the pulse, the doctor might still be unable to arrive at a diagnosis. If then, however, he can enumerate the symptoms, 'the patient will have confidence in the doctor as the author of health.' Moreover, the physician is to insist that the patient confess, 'because many illnesses originate on account of sin and are cured by the Supreme Physician.' On entering the sick-room the doctor must not appear haughty or overly eager; he must also realize that the patient's pulse rate may be increased by his joy at the doctor's arrival and by 'thoughts about the fee.' After all necessary examinations of the patient's complexion, pulse, and urine are completed, the doctor is instructed to announce to the members of the household that the patient 'is very sick, for if he recovers you will be praised for your art; should he die his friends will testify that you had given him up.' The doctor is further advised not to 'look at a maid, or a daughter or a wife with an improper or covetous eye' for such entanglements interfere with the women's attentions to the patient and detract from the respect accorded to the doctor.(34)

These words on medical ethics were written by a medieval physician even before the devout Italian epic poet Dante Alighieri (1265-1321) criticized the papacy and high dignitaries of the Church for mundane and profane excesses, interference in earthly matters, corruption, bribery, and simony. [154] Indeed it is in Dante's *Inferno,* consigned to eternal damnation, that we find several prelates including the powerful Pope Boniface VIII (pope, 1294-1303) who was Dante's bitter political and ecclesiastic enemy. We should also keep in mind that these words were also written before both lay jurists and ecclesiastical prosecutors had begun in earnest the gruesome witch hunts and the ghastly witch trials which were conveniently sanctioned by ecclesiastic as well as secular legal authorities within an inimical system that called for confessions obtained by legal torture.

Moreover, with the advent of the Renaissance, medicine would return firmly to the hands of the lay medical profession, with many doctors now training at prestigious medical universities such as Padua, Paris, and Montpellier – institutions which were teaching the new learning and disseminating the newly-found knowledge contained in the venerated Greek and Roman classics. Physicians would again be preoccupied with furthering the art and science of medicine through the natural observation of the disease process, experimentation, and verification of what were considered previously assumed truths. The doctors would now follow the dictates of their own conscience and the precepts of their own (or their professional organization's) moral code of ethics. Humanism was becoming a predominant philosophy, asserting that man was the center of the universe! Nature was there so that man could conquer it, but not plunder it, for it was believed that everything in nature was within man's reach. This Renaissance philosophy served the physicians relatively well. For, as we shall see, empowered with newly-acquired medical knowledge, Renaissance physicians returned to the benevolent virtue-based ethics of enlightened self-interest and comported themselves in many ways as the model Renaissance physicians that they had ultimately become.

PHYSICIAN ACQUIESCENCE – A LEGACY OF MONASTIC OR MEDIEVAL ETHICS?

Live a life worthy of the calling you have received. Be completely humble and gentle; be patient, bearing with one another in love. Make every effort to keep the unity of the Spirit through the bond of peace.
                                        St. Paul
                                        (Ephesians 4:1-3)

From the onset of the Dark Ages, Christianity had taught submission by preaching: "Love your enemies, do good to those who hate you, bless those who curse you, pray for those who mistreat you" (Luke 6:27-28). Although these ideals rarely materialized (except perhaps in ascetic Christians), they appear to have become incorporated, consciously or subconsciously, in the unwritten, collective ethics (i.e., acquiescence, complaisance, equanimity, etc.) of the noble profession of medicine. Yet I wonder if the Judeo-Christian ideals of compassion, the Good

---

[154] A word derived from Simon Magus, a 1st Century sorcerer of Samaria discussed in the Book of Acts 8:9-24.

Samaritan, and charity – and even traces of the less generally accepted Christian concept of submission – were coupled with the ancient Græco-Roman tenets of philanthropy and humanitarianism, and have remained etched indelibly in the conscience of physicians.

This fact might just explain why, despite physicians' above-average intelligence and manifest tenacity (for those are essential qualities for successfully completing medical school and engaging in the practice of medicine), they are reluctant to participate in the present-age, rough and tumble political combat that is needed to defend their profession, and keep the fruits of their labors. It is during these uncertain and trying times, when medicine, like ancient Rome, is seemingly at the brink of being dismantled, besieged by modern barbarians amassing at her gates. Misled by an overly pragmatic leadership without vision, medicine's defense and counterattack (with a few exceptions) have frankly been too feeble for effective counteraction. Thus, as a result, the present-day barbarians are breaching her defenses, pressing on the gates of the profession, and piece by piece, effectively dismantling the centuries-old edifice of the sacred House of Medicine. Unless physicians act, the gate which is about to fall, will fall – to the detriment of the honorable fraternity and the patients entrusted to their care.

The analogy of medicine, and its belief in freely-expressed compassion and genuine charity, with the all but forgotten Christian ideals of humility and submission to authority, has influenced immensely the attitudes and ethics of the medical profession throughout the ages. The posthumous attainment of sainthood by devoted priests and pious monks, for their preeminent holiness, good works (miracles), and martyrdom during this spiritual epoch, along with the founding of religious orders and charity hospitals for the care of the indigent sick and infirm who were treated with unreciprocated charity and compassion, no doubt left an indelible mark in the collective memory of later-day physicians. This is perhaps reflected in the ethical writings of such illustrious physicians as Sir Thomas Browne (1605-1682; *Religio Medici*, 1635) and Thomas Percival (1740-1804; *Medical Ethics*, 1803). These self-imposed rules of professional conduct and medical ethics finally came to fruition with the compilation of the AMA's first Code of Ethics in 1848.

This medical ethical tradition, perhaps, explains why even today, when the profession is under siege and active participation in organized medicine is imperative (for the very survival of the profession as we know it is at stake), physicians still hesitate to participate in the political debate regarding not only the options for health systems reform but also the step-by-step process of government usurpation of their individual rights as independent practitioners. I believe it is this erroneous, misunderstood, and lingering belief by the rank and file physicians – that members of an honorable profession should not engage in the *mêlée* of political activism – that may be at work here. Notable exceptions to this rule are American physicians with more liberal views who are frequently given a forum by the mass media to express their sundry politically-correct views on the environment, nuclear war, socialized medicine, etc., as well as to deprecate their own profession.

For the most part, conservative physicians have been reluctant, immersed in acquiescence, paralyzed by guilt, and overwhelmed by self-intimated excuses about their relative prosperity. The vast majority of physicians deserve their incomes, for they have earned it by working long hours and effacing their self-interest for the health and welfare of their patients. And let me repeat: it is no longer enough to pay dues to county, state, and national medical organizations – personal commitment is necessary in this life and death struggle for the survival of medicine and the preservation of the best features of the American health care delivery system as we now know it. As *American Medical News* contributor, Robert M. Tenery Jr., M.D., puts it: "The time has come for physicians to stop making excuses for their incomes. In the vast majority of cases, they have earned it – and, what is even more important, they continue to earn it. Every time they care for a patient – in the office or the hospital, during the middle of the day or the middle of the night, on a weekday, weekend or holiday – they earn it."(35) As Tenery and medical writer, Harry Schwartz, Ph.D., have pointed out, physicians do earn more money than average, but what they earn is commensurate with the value that society places on their services. The fact has been and remains, that when it comes to their own health care, Americans want the best at any cost.(35-38)

Moreover, Tenery argues that physicians must stop making excuses: "Most physicians, or their replacements, are there either by telephone or in person for their patients any time they are needed. They are there whether the patient can pay or not. Additionally, there is the time that physicians must spend staying abreast of medical science, so they can offer their patients the very best. There is the significant amount of time spent doing paperwork, dealing with multiple problems by telephone and attending meetings to comply with accreditation requirements of their hospitals and their practices. There are also the countless days, nights, and weekends where plans are changed or abandoned completely to be available in case a problem arises, all for which there is no compensation."(35)

As regards the earning differential of various specialties amongst physicians, Tenery further opines: "Certain specialties and individual physicians will make more than others. We should not begrudge them if they earn it. Some physicians are also more in demand by their patients, because of their reputation or rapport. This is a part of life and they should not be penalized."(35) Furthermore, if physicians do not follow this latter advice, they will only make it easier for their adversaries to impose the Machiavellian maxim of divide and conquer, with deleterious effects for both the profession and patients.

Although it is true that some physicians engage in unethical practices and unbecoming professional conduct either because of incompetence, personal misconduct, or character flaw (naked greed), the fact remains that it is the government that has tied the hands of physicians when it comes to disciplining those unscrupulous or errant amongst their ranks. In the sagacious words of Tenery: "Due to several factors, but predominately the threat of anti-trust lawsuits, physicians are unwilling or unable to restrict the inappropriate actions of their errant peers. Only when the restrictions are changed into safeguards will physicians be able to adequately deal with those in the profession who are putting their own self-interest ahead of the patient's."(35)

Instead, the government relies on general fear, intimidation, and unconstitutional practices such as the implementation of an infamous and ineffective National Practitioners Data Bank which has contributed to the deleterious adversarial atmosphere in the health care system. Finally, Tenery's insight that "it is easy to be critical of those who seem to profit from other's misfortunes...remember what these individuals went through to get where they are, and what they are sacrificing to stay there...that when they are gone, there must be others to take their place, who hopefully will be just as competent and compassionate" – is illuminating and farsighted.(35)

Tenery certainly has a point. Unless the climate changes for the better, and America reverses its present course of doctor-bashing, and instead recognizes and appreciates physicians for their labors – Americans may just get what a small but vociferous and politically-motivated group has been asking for. America may in the very near future find itself with a new breed of physician, one that will be politically correct and will gladly wear a facade of government-induced (coercive) compassion, but is not as dedicated or competent as the erstwhile physician of years past.(39,40)

It was the novelist Robin Cook, a physician himself and author of the bestselling book, *Coma,* who said, "A physician experiences more stress in one day than most people experience in their life times."(41) I believe that the public recognizes the essence of this truth. Yet, physicians should realize that individuals tend to formulate opinions about their doctors based not only on the quality of care rendered but also on the attention that they receive from their physicians. They tremendously value the aura of compassion radiating from their physicians and their "bed side manners." Patients also like and want to feel that their physicians genuinely care about them as persons, not as exotic diseases or interesting cases.

Most patients like their doctors; it is the media depictions and the politically-motivated government projections of physician images that the general public has come to dislike.(36-38,42) But that egregious image is that of "someone else's" doctor. The public is generally satisfied with the care they obtain from their own physicians. In fact, they are willing to accept the status and prosperity of their *own* physicians. Many patients seem to understand (and accurately so) that this is the result of long hours of work and heavy responsibilities.

Yet because of media and government propaganda, the image of the profession has been tarnished, based largely on the undeserved projected imagery of "greedy" physicians. Doctors are in general disparaged as "greedy and uncaring providers" who are interested only in making money, accused of the much hackneyed proverbial sin of greed.(36-38,40,42)

It is time that physicians go on the offensive. How, you ask? By letting the public know the work physicians do day in and day out and combatting media bias and inaccuracies. Physicians must become part of the informed and vigilant citizenry, and even more, they must become activists for their patients, for themselves and the profession. A few years ago a wise attorney wrote an illuminating article attesting to this reality. He suggested that physicians use the media to project their authentic image. He also admonished physicians to "fight back before it is too late."(42) Mr. R. V. Wills was correct then, and his statement remains correct and applicable to this day.

Another creeping socialist ideation and philosophy that is affecting not just physicians but all prosperous and successful members of society is the fallacy that inherited wealth or even material prosperity created from one's labor is immoral, for the simple and disingenuous reason that others, who are not as fortunate, remain dispossessed. [155] If the American people have come to subscribe to this belief, then we are

---

[155] If in doubt, check the amount (already increased by President Clinton) that is today taxed and due the government in inheritance taxes (55%). The word is that this administration intends to push it even higher. In this light, we should remember that the third plank of Marx's *Communist Manifesto* (1848) which sought: "Abolition of all right to inheritance." The second plank, "a heavy and progressive or graduated income tax" has, of course, already come to pass.

surely doomed, for it will mean that Americans have been seduced by the lure of socialist ideology, despite the lessons of history.

Another facet of health care delivery that deserves mentioning within the context of the present discussion is that – along with the practice of defensive medicine (the amount of which is truly incalculable) – the proliferation of techno-logic advances that are prolonging the extent and the quality of our lives have been significant culprits in precipitating the spiraling health care costs.

The free market has been blamed for soaring health care costs, but as we have witnessed, the truth of the matter lies elsewhere. Health care costs have soared as a result of government intervention which began in earnest with Lyndon B. Johnson's spending spree in the ferment of the Great Society he inaugurated, and which brought about Medicare and Medicaid.

Both health care spending and litigation costs began to grow in the 1960s for different reasons. In the case of health care, it was the government's interven-tion in medicine with the inception of the Medicare and Medicaid Acts of 1965, which lured doctors to feed from the government trough in the manner of the aforementioned "Pig's Pen" (Part V), which reimbursed physicians for the services they formerly provided *pro bono publico* to their charity patients. In fact, the grad-ual escalation of health care costs began with and paralleled the growth of the pub-lic sector in medicine. Indigent patients who had been taken care of by physicians as a matter of professional ethics (charity) were taken over by the government, placed on welfare and Medicaid, and thereafter placed on the liberal plantation of government dependency from which they have not been able to escape.

In the case of the legal profession, the litigation problem also had its inception in the mid-1960s. It had been preceded by three decades of legal writings militating and paving the way for judicial activism and the liberalization of the U.S. courts.(43) The ethics of the legal profession began to change rapidly and have now sunk to record lows. Whereas in years past, attorneys resorted to suing as a matter of last resort, counselling their clients to settle conflicts amicably, in the 1960s, attitudes toward litigation began to change. It became more and more fash-ionable to sue in order to settle the slightest societal disputes.

Suing, which erstwhile was considered to be disruptive to society, sud-denly became good for society and a desirable goal. Lawsuits began to be filed at the drop of a hat. Advertising for legal services and solicitation became acceptable and the norm. Terms such as "ambulance chasing," "fishing expeditions," "lottery litigation," and others became commonplace, attempting to describe the nature and *modus operandi* of the various stages of civil litigation.[156] The increase in the usage of these terms also reflects the low standards of ethics to which some trial lawyers had "stooped to conquer," whilst dishonoring the ethics of another ancient and noble profession.(43-50)

To confront the health care dilemmas of our age, we must first admit that as Americans many of us have been unwittingly lured by the songs of sirens lead-ing us precariously adrift in socialist waters, navigating between the Scylla of false security and the Charybdis of "free" health care. Like sailors in uncharted

---

[156] And to the legal profession: Beware! Unless you heal thyself, you will follow suit. As a sibling profession, you, too, are viewed as elitists, and your public image is way below that of physicians. The time will soon arrive when, despite all your political power, you will succumb to the heavy hand of government authority.

waters, we have been enticed by health care experts and ambitious politicians to believe that government (a giant amoral bureaucracy gone amok) can make anything possible, including false "cradle-to-grave" security and "free" care. What we are really going to get is health care rationing, outright denial of care, and government-sanctioned euthanasia. [157]

[157] The word *euthanasia* comes from the Greek, *eu* meaning "good" and *thanatos* meaning "death," and it stands for "mercy killing." Modern ethicists claim that in active euthanasia, a person asks for death because of a painful and agonizing death, or because he/she suffers from a terminal disease for which there is no cure. In practice, this may not always be so, as the example of Holland amply demonstrates. In Holland today, over 80% of doctors engage in active euthanasia and in many cases without the patient's consent.(51) Yet it is promoted to the public as an act of "self-determination."(52) So, between 10,000 and 15,000 patients are put to death in that "progressive" country under socialized medicine. The government, of course, is all behind it, for death is the ultimate form of rationing and the most efficient method for proper allocation (preservation) of resources by the socialist central planners.

CHAPTER 28

THE ISLAMIC LEGACY

Ah Love! could thou and I with Fate conspire
To grasp this sorry Scheme of Things entire,
Would not we shatter it to bits – and then
Re-mould it nearer to the Heart's Desire!

> Omar Khayyám, Rubáiyát
> Persian poet (fl.11th Century)

Dante Alighieri composed the Christian epic poem, *The Divine Comedy*, in the closing century of the Medieval period. This monumental work, which is a voluminous and erudite encyclopedia of medieval theology, philosophy, and literature, formed the basis for the modern Italian language. Because of its early Renaissance qualities, Dante's work is sometimes used as marking the beginning of the transitional period to the "Rebirth." Yet before we immerse ourselves in the momentous period of the Renaissance, we must discuss another important legacy that enriched our Western intellectual tradition and is paramount to our story. I am referring to the Islamic legacy, which contributed immeasurably to the preservation and rediscovery of the Greek and Roman classics. In medical history, for instance, Islamic and Hebrew physicians contributed significantly to the forging of the historic Renaissance physicians – the ultimate objective of our historic quest in search for historic parallels.

Whilst in the Christian East, embodied in the Byzantine Empire, classical works of Greek and Roman authors of antiquity gathered dust on the shelves of the libraries and churches of Constantinople, monastic scribes were busy copying manuscripts in the remote and isolated monasteries of Christendom. In the lands conquered by the prophet Mohammed (c.A.D.570-632) and ruled by his Islamic heirs, the powerful Caliphs, a steady stream of medical knowledge surfaced in the writings of Arabic, Persian, and Jewish physicians, especially from the 8th to the 12th Centuries. The lights of Athens, Alexandria, and Rome had dimmed and passed with the pages of history as the hubs of ancient learning. In their stead, Salerno and Bologna were rising slowly in the West. It was left to the great cities in the Moslem world – such as majestic Baghdad, Damascus, and Cairo in the Eastern Caliphates, and Moorish Granada and Córdoba in the Western Caliphate (the latter, until it fell to the Spanish King Ferdinand c.1289) – to hold fast and carry proudly another flaming torch of learning and progress during this period.

THE ARABIC INFLUENCE

It is a tribute to the Arab Moslems that they were relatively magnanimous and tolerant towards the vanquished peoples they had overrun during their zealous conquests in the Middle East, North Africa, and Spain. Yet it must also be noted that following those impressive and astonishing Islamic conquests of the 7th and 8th Centuries, the victorious Arabs also demanded unconditional acceptance of the words of the great prophet, Mohammed, as written in the *Koran*. It was perhaps this early fanatical zeal to promote and enforce (if necessary by the scimitar) the teachings of the *Koran* as the book of basic truths, the *de facto* bible of Arabia, that may have prompted in A.D.641, the final burning and destruction of the remains of the great library of Alexandria. [158]

Arab zealots were then completing their conquest of Egypt under the leadership of the second, and one of the greatest, of all the Caliphs, Umar Ibn Al-Khattab (c.A.D.586-644). It was during his reign that the Arabs inflicted a major defeat upon the Byzantine imperial forces at the Battle of Yarmuk in A.D.636 and upon the Persian imperial armies at the Battle of Nehavend in A.D.642. Jerusalem fell in A.D.638 and Egypt in A.D.642. The greatest Arabic conquests took place at the time of Mohammed and during Umar's Caliphate. Despite the burning of Alexandria and its library and the wars, Islamic culture would repay Western civilization by serving as a preserver of knowledge and by sustaining the torch of learning at a critical and agonizing period of European history when the West reposed – palled by the shroud of the Dark Ages and the relative slumber of the Medieval period.

The Arabs forbade translation of the *Koran,* so that converts to the new faith of Allah had to learn Arabic. As a result, to this day the Arabic language is universal in Arab nations, though not in non-Arab Moslem countries such as Iran, Turkey, and faraway Indonesia. Religion and language have kept the Arabs essentially united as one remarkable culture for 14 centuries.

In Persia, under Arab patronage, the flickering flame of Byzantine medicine was rekindled and resulted in advancement of medical knowledge. This passion for the pursuit of knowledge lead to the resurgence of learning that overtook Islamic countries in the midst of the Middle Ages. It should also be noted that it was the Nestorians, the Christian followers of the Byzantine priest, Nestorius (d.c.A.D.451), who first introduced the Arabs to the concepts and tenets of Græco-Roman medicine.[159] I0t was during this time that the sciences of chemistry, geology, and algebra were founded, and the disciplines of pharmacology, botany, medicine, and surgery were advanced under the auspices of the Caliphs – the theologic and political leaders considered to be the direct successors of Mohammed. In arithmetic, the numeric system that we use today took its form from the Arabic numerals, and many modern words in our vocabulary trace their origin to the Arabic language. For example, alcohol, alfalfa, admiral, arsenal, azure, cipher, algebra, zero, zenith, syrup, julep, alcove, etc., are all derived from the Arabic that took root in Western languages during this period.(5,13)

In addition, the Arabs, as erudite and experienced herbalists, added many plants and spices to the medical pharmacopoeia, adding countless useful medicinal

---

[158] At the time of its final destruction, Alexandria and its library were already in their final decline. Today, only a small underground cellar remains of the splendor that was once Alexandria's library.

[159] Nestorianism was the 5th Century heresy preached by a patriarch of Constantinople, Nestorius, who predicated that Jesus was two distinct persons, one human, the other divine. Therefore, Mary bore only Jesus, the man, and therefore, the Virgin could not be titled "the Mother of God." The Council of Ephesus (A.D.431) and Chalcedon (A.D.451) reaffirmed the orthodox view of the Catholic church, that Jesus has "two natures, inseparably joined in one person who partakes of one divine substance."(2)

plants to those collected and described by Dioscorides many centuries earlier. Herbs which had been used originally as spices for flavoring and preserving foods were later found to have medicinal value and used as remedies. This included camphor, nutmeg, cloves, and musk. As we shall see in the final section (Part VII) of this book, Columbus' momentous voyage in search for a shorter route to India during the Renaissance was not inspired by a spice trade, but by a profitable medicinal drug trade.

THE RISE OF ISLAM

To understand the early Arabian zeal for the Mohammedan religion, a new faith partly derived from Judeo-Christian teachings, one must revisit the story of Islam.

We have already noted how the fall of the Western Roman Empire ended a chapter in Western civilization and heralded a dark age in the Western world. With the onset of the Dark Ages, spiritual healing was provided by the Christian church, and holistic healing by monastic medicine. In the same light as spiritual nourishment was provided by religion, physical security was provided by feudalism during those trying times of uncertainty and chaos. Christianity was boosted in the West by the infusion of newly-Christianized Germanic barbarians. It was consolidated in the East by the spiritual power of the Eastern Orthodox faith and the temporal might and prestige of the Emperor of the Byzantine Empire. The desolation of the countryside caused by the terrible plague of Justinian also fortified the already considerable power of Christianity, as people looked to the hereafter whilst seeking comfort in the arms of the Christian church.

During this time, the cradle of Judeo-Christian civilization also gave birth to an aggressive and fervent religion, Islam. It was on the vast, arid, Arabian peninsula that Mohammed (c.A.D.570-632), a successful merchant, founded a spiritual religion centered in the Middle East that reached its zenith in Europe, Asia, and North Africa in A.D.717.

Mohammed began his conquests in his native Arabia with a small but highly spirited band of Bedouin tribesmen who, after their initial victories, were joined by proselytized followers from throughout the Arabian desert. He reached Mecca with his followers but was repulsed and forced to flee the city. His famous flight from Mecca to Medina, the *Hegira,* took place in A.D.622. This later became the Year One of the Moslem calendar and a rallying point for Moslems everywhere.

It was in Medina, the second holiest city for Moslems, that Mohammed's religious, political, and military fortunes turned definitely in his favor. For when he returned to Mecca, he returned triumphant. Thenceforth, an impressive series of conquests awaited the Arabs and Islam. Enemies were defeated one after the other, even when Moslem forces were opposed by increasingly larger and more impressive enemies. These military accomplishments became an inspiration to Mohammed's followers and testified to the Prophet's spiritual and moral courage, as well as his personal charisma and physical stamina – for he led his armies in the field with the *Koran* and the scimitar in hand.

From Mecca, Mohammed invaded and conquered much of Arabia. By A.D.637 just five years after his death at Medina, the Arabs had defeated the Persians and broken the rule of their former overlords, the Sassanid Persian dynasty, thereby gaining control not only of Mesopotamia but much of the former Persian empire. Islam had come of age. After Egypt was conquered in A.D.642, the rest of North Africa quickly followed, and the Arab conquerors reached the Atlantic Ocean in A.D.711. Meanwhile, the lands of Syria, Persia, and Palestine had fallen in the East: The invading Arabs were now at the door of the Eastern Roman Empire. The conquering Arab armies in the late 7th and early 8th Centuries were at their peak, and their holy warriors seemingly unstoppable.

The Saracen scimitar of Islam was poised to strike at Christendom on two fronts. In the West, the Visigothic kingdom of Spain was conquered and overrun between A.D. 711 and A.D.732, whilst in the East in A.D.717, the Byzantine citadel of Constantinople had come under siege. Christendom was in great peril. Islam had now extended its borders from the Iberian peninsula in the West to the frontier of India in the East – military accomplishments, unprecedented since the time of the Roman legions of the Republic and the conquests of Alexander the Great.

In the fateful year of A.D. 732, Moslem expansion would finally be halted in the West. At the decisive Battle of Tours, Charles Martel, "the Hammer" (King of the Franks, c.A.D.688-741), at last halted and finally defeated the Islamic conquests in western Europe. Nevertheless, to the south, the Moorish, Islamic kingdom of Spain, now solidly in place, would remain for another seven centuries. During that time, it would continue to be considered by Spanish Christians an alien kingdom in their own country and perceived by the rest of Europe as a potential threat to Christendom.

In the East, the Arab threat was checked with the ascension of the Byzantine Emperor Leo III (reigned, A.D.717-741). By then, the Arabs had more or less settled down to enjoy their conquests, and Islamic culture flourished. Perhaps nowhere was this splendor of culture more noticeable than in ancient Iraq where the wise and celebrated Abbasid Caliph of Baghdad, Harun ar-Rashid (c.A.D.764-809) of the fabled *1001 Arabian Nights*, ruled. [160] The *1001 Arabian Nights* is a fabulous collection of stories imbued with Arabic culture and traditional teachings. The best known stories contain such heroes as Ali Baba, Sinbad, and Aladdin. The book was translated from the Arabic to English by the British scholar and indefatigable adventurer of the 19th Century, Sir Richard Francis Burton (1821-1890). [161]

MONGOLS AND OTTOMAN TURKS

The greatest happiness in all the world is to crush your enemies, to see them fall at your feet, and to take their horses and goods.

> Genghis Khan (1167-1227)
> Mongol Chieftan

Between A.D.750 and 1258, the Abbasid Caliphate made majestic Baghdad the beacon of the Islamic Golden Age, both in the cultivation of the arts

[160] The enlightened Caliph of Baghdad was a friend of Charlemagne, and during their reigns they presented each other with gifts. In fact, they were on such friendly terms that Harun ar-Rashid presented the Holy Roman Emperor with the keys to the Holy Sepulcher in Jerusalem.

[161] Burton not only translated the magical Arabian book, but also made a peregrination to Mecca and Medina (forbidden to non-believers) disguised as a Moslem pilgrim. He discovered Lake Tanganyika with fellow explorer, John H. Speke (1827-1864) whilst trying unsuccessfully to find the source of the Nile. He also wrote an authoritative book about swords and translated from the Sanskrit the *Kamasutra*, a book of Hindu eroticism much in vogue during the "Age of Aquarius" and the sexual revolution of the 1960s.

and in the sciences. The Abbasids were the dynastic Arab leaders who were considered descendants of Mohammed's grandson Husain, who had been murdered at Karbala. In fact, because of their distant kinship to the prophet Mohammed, the Abbasid Caliphs were acceptable to the Shiite Moslem sect.(53,54) In 1258, the conquering Mongol hordes invading from central Asia finally overran and destroyed bustling and dazzling Baghdad, but in the process of conquest the new invaders ultimately became assimilated in the Islamic culture. Even during this period of turmoil in the East, Islamic scholars remained the custodians of invaluable manuscripts of the Græco-Roman heritage, whilst most of Europe was barely beginning to come out of the abeyance in which it had been languishing throughout much of the Middle Ages.

Amidst the doldrums of the Middle Ages, there were intermittent periods of chaos, particularly along the fringes of the known world, as if to brake the spell of listlessness affecting the heart of Europe and culturally-related parts of Asia. During the Medieval period, for example, Central Asia was excoriated by Genghis Khan (1167-1227) and his Mongol hordes who overran 5000 miles of Asian steppes and Near Eastern terrain. There was also the celebrated ruler of Marco Polo's travel, Kublai Khan, "the Great Khan" (c.1215-1294), who was Genghis Khan's grandson. Kublai Khan, unlike his predecessors, became accustomed to the niceties of China. By 1268, from his capital at Peking, he ruled an empire encompassing much of Mongolia, Korea, and China. In fact, after conquering southern China, Kublai Khan turned his attention to Japan, a nation that refused to submit to Mongol rule. Two vast and heavily armed armadas were sent in 1274 and again in 1281 to conquer Japan; both failed. The Mongol invaders were repelled by the fierce Japanese Samurai defenders aided by the divine winds – *Kamikaze* – that demolished much of the invaders' fleets during their repeated assaults.[162]

A century later, almost bridging the gap of time between the Middle Ages and the Renaissance, there was a less well-known figure who again ravaged the plains of central Asia with even more barbarity and ferocity than his predecessor. His name was Tamerlane (c.1336-1405), and he was the last of the great Mongol warriors. The deeds of Tamerlane, an indirect ancestor of Genghis Khan, are indeed astonishing. After setting up his capital at Turkish Samarkand (the former Republic of Turkestan in the former USSR), Tamerlane swept across central Asia, wreaking havoc amongst its nomadic inhabitants and conquering what was perhaps the largest empire in history. Between 1380-1399, he held vast stretches of lands in central Asia, Persia, Mesopotamia, and immense territories in southern Russia. Like Alexander the Great, he crossed the Khyber Pass, and then took Delhi and conquered northern India. He was notorious for his cruelty: in the city of Delhi, he is said to have summarily slaughtered 80,000 prisoners.(2)

Tamerlane did not stop there. His nomadic warriors clashed with and decisively defeated the seasoned Ottoman troops in Turkey in the years 1401 and 1402, capturing their Sultan Beyazid I (1347-1403) and conquering most of Asia Minor. At Isfahan, Persia, he built his infamous pyramid of 70,000 skulls. He came

---

[162] And so, *National Geographic* states: "A fortress with the sea its moat, Japan has never been successfully invaded....U.S. invasion plans during World War II were abandoned when Japan surrendered. Japanese suicide pilots in that war adopted the legendary title of *Kamikaze* – divine wind – hoping to imitate the storms that defeated the Mongols in 1274 and 1281."(55)

close to challenging the citadel of Christian Constantinople. But as fate would have it, in the midst of his conquests, Tamerlane contracted a fever and died on his way to invade and conquer China. After his demise, his empire disintegrated almost as rapidly as it had been created. His death ended, once and for all, the sinew of Mongol power and the recrudescence of warring nomadic hordes from the plains of central Asia.(2,12,14)

Finally, out of the turmoil in the East, emerged Sulayman, "the Magnificent" (Sultan of the Ottoman Empire, 1520-1566),[163] who entered Baghdad in triumph in 1534 with his highly disciplined *Janissaries* and Turkish troops. Sulayman conquered Belgrade in 1521, and as previously noted, expelled the Knights Hospitalers from the Greek island of Rhodes in 1522. He annexed most of Hungary and much of the Balkan peninsula, Persia and Arabia, but despite his alliance with Francis I of France, he was unsuccessful in his warfare against Charles V and the Holy Roman Empire. He failed to take Vienna in 1529, lost Tunis to Charles V, and was unable to defeat and subdue the Knights of Malta in 1565.(2,8) After Sulayman's death in 1566, decline set into the Turkish empire, culminating in the defeat of the Turkish fleet by Don John of Austria at Lepanto in 1571.[164]

THE PHYSICIANS AND THE ISLAMIC MIDDLE-EASTERN TRADITION

Fortunately, despite the disarray of the Dark Ages, the relative slumber of the European Medieval period, and the upheaval of the Mongol invasions in the East – all knowledge was not lost. Yet relatively few Western scholars of this period had access to medical knowledge. In fact, such was the scarcity of applied medical knowledge in the Roman Empire of the East that Byzantine emperors were obliged to seek medical advice and treatment from Islamic physicians.

From the 9th to the 14th Centuries, Greek medicine other than Galenic medicine ceased to exist in clinical practice. Even in Islamic countries (as in most of Europe), autopsies and human dissections were prohibited during the Middle Ages. Medical scholars – East and West – up to the time of the Renaissance relied on Galen's ancient writings for their anatomic references. Islamic countries contributed to Western medicine by preserving and codifying Greek medical manuscripts (thought to have been lost) and translating them – into Latin by Jewish physicians and into Arabic by Islamic physicians. But who were these outstanding medical scholars and Islamic physicians who thus contributed and influenced the course of Western medicine?

Perhaps the greatest of the Islamic physicians was the Persian scholar Avicenna (A.D.980-1037). He was chief physician at the teaching hospital in Baghdad and court physician to the caliphs. His magnum opus, *The Canon*, contains dissertations in all fields of medicine and discusses such topics as meningoencephalitis, apoplexy, hemiplegia, and paralysis. It also contains a remarkable treatise on facial palsy, distinguishing clinically and anatomically between central and peripheral

---

[163] Sulayman was the son and successor of Selim I and grandson of Muhammed II, "the Conqueror" (Sultan, 1451-1481), who conquered Constantinople in 1453, and thus ended the Roman Empire of the East.

[164] Over the centuries, the Ottoman empire continued to weaken and disintegrate so that in the 19th Century, Turkey became known as the Sick Man of Europe. After World War I, under the influence of the reformist Young Turks and the overthrow of the last sultan by the Turkish leader, Kemal Atatürk, the Turkish empire disintegrated. The modern history of Turkey is said to have begun with the establishment of the Republic in 1922.(2,12)

facial paralysis. Avicenna discussed and distinguished pyloric stenosis (a constriction at the gastric outlet) from gastric ulcers. He even linked the etiology of hepatic (liver) disease to the harmful effects of alcohol. He also discussed jaundice (yellow discoloration of the skin and body tissues in disease states) and classified the clinical types of jaundice, i.e., hemolytic (from the breakdown of red blood cell corpuscles) as in systemic infections, as opposed to obstructive jaundice caused by a blockage in the hepatic-biliary system.

Avicenna, like Galen, recommended blood letting for apoplexy in plethoric subjects with the proper clinical history and who were recognized as having "a full red congested face and eyes."(20) Given today's medical impetus for volume expansion (increasing the volume of the blood) and hemodilution therapy (thinning the blood), as to improve the cerebral circulation in patients with cerebral ischemia (lack of adequate cerebral blood flow), the claim is actually not too far off the mark! Interestingly, one recent physician-scholar has indicated that the poetry attributed to the celebrated Persian mathematician, poet, astronomer, and hedonistic philosopher, Omar Khayyám (fl.11th Century), may actually have been written by the physician Avicenna.(56)

Other acclaimed Islamic physicians who were keen observers of natural processes, as well as practicing clinicians, and who left behind detailed clinical histories documenting their clinical cases include Avenzoar (1094-1160), Rhazes (d.A.D.923), and Abulcasis (A.D.912-1013). Avenzoar described pericarditis. Rhazes described the revolutionary idea that fever was merely a symptom of the body fighting illness rather than a disease process itself. Abulcasis, the famous Islamic surgeon, was born near Córdoba in the Western Caliphate which was at the time a great seat of medical knowledge. Abulcasis, credited with restoring Arabic surgery to its former glory, was not only a practicing and skillful surgeon but also a talented medical writer.(20) His book on surgery, *Altrasrif* ("Collection"), was an illustrated compilation of surgical techniques. He considered cautery, as did most Islamic physicians, an excellent method of treatment and gave specific indications for its use. He described tracheotomy (opening the windpipe to restore or maintain breathing) performed transversely between the 3rd and 4th tracheal rings.

Averroës (1126-1198), the Spanish-Moslem physician, was also a philosopher from Seville. He published *The Colliget*, an encyclopedic compilation of all the knowledge of his time. Frequently referred to as "the Commentator" by medieval thinkers, Averroës translated and reintroduced to the West the writings of Aristotle. He admired Aristotle, and as such, arduously attempted to merge Islamic theology with Aristotelian rationalism, an endeavor which resulted in the creation of a mystic and philosophic sect imbued with pantheism – *Averroism* – which made Averroës a controversial figure. Averroism was deplored by many religious leaders, and for centuries its followers were persecuted as heretics.(20,56)

Moses Maimonides (1135-1204) was a Jewish physician who also lived in the enlightened city of Córdoba. To escape religious persecution, he fled to Fez where he received protection from the Sultan Saladin.[165] Maimonides was an excellent physician who realized the importance of preventive medicine and recognized the interrelationship between emotions and bodily functions.(57) He even

---

[165] The Sultan of Egypt and Saracen warrior, Saladin (c.1137-1193), was the nemesis of the Crusaders and opponent of King Richard I, "the Lion-Heart" (1157-1199). Saladin's seizure of Jerusalem in 1187 triggered the Third Crusade.

described their physiologic interrelationship in scholarly fashion. As the most influential Jewish physician-philosopher of his age, Maimonides was able to achieve a philosophic synthesis between Aristotelian rationalism and Jewish theology in Judaism, in a similar fashion as St. Thomas Aquinas and St. Augustine accomplished in Christian theology – monumental tasks which successfully reconciled natural philosophy with religious dogma.

Like Hippocrates, Maimonides composed a code of medical ethics that is still in use today, and like the Hippocratic Oath, his oath respects individual autonomy and does not subordinate the individual physician to the power of the state, only to the service that a physician renders to his/her patients. Here is the Oath of Maimonides:

> *Exalted God, before I begin the holy work of healing the creations of your hand, I place my entreaty before the throne of your glory, that you grant strength of spirit and fortitude to faithfully execute my work. Let not desire for wealth or benefit blind me from seeing truth. Deem me worthy of seeing in the sufferer who seeks my advice a person neither rich nor poor. Friend or foe, good man or bad, of a man in distress, show me only the man.*

> *If doctors wiser than me seek to help me understand, grant me the desire to learn from them, for the knowledge of healing is boundless. But when fools deride me, give me fortitude! Let my love for my profession strengthen my resolve to withstand the decision even of men of high station. Illuminate the way for me, for any lapse in my knowledge can bring illness and death upon your creations. I beseech you, merciful and gracious God, strengthen me in body and soul, and instill within me a perfect spirit.*

Another discipline, Islamic pharmacology and therapeutics, was completely empirical. There were experiments with drugs in animals. Rhazes, for example, studied and discussed the effects of mercury in monkeys. Islamic physicians also studied botany and traveled abroad specifically to study new plants for medicinal purposes and to enlarge the Islamic pharmacopoeia.

Islamic physicians are also credited with being the first to develop clinical teaching hospitals which were founded and administered in association with great medical schools, such as those in Baghdad, Cairo, and Córdoba. At the time, those institutions of learning were unsurpassed in the Western world.[166] It was also in these Islamic teaching hospitals that the idealism embodied in the concepts of compassion and charity were reconciled with the realities of indigent care in public hospitals. Islamic physicians were the first to link the procurement and application of medical knowledge to charity medical care for the mutual benefit of medical students and indigent patients.

It has been said, and we have reiterated, that Islamic translations and the preservation of knowledge were, perhaps, the greatest contributions of Islamic and Jewish medical scholars to Western culture during this period. Unfortunately, the statement does not do these scholars full justice. They not only supplied Western scholars with material to translate and study (i.e., works of Galen, Dioscorides,

---

[166] In this context, we should not neglect to mention the library of Khalif el-Hakim II of Córdoba which was said to have contained 600,000 volumes, providing a fountain of knowledge to the physicians, medical students, and scholars associated with the teaching hospital and medical school of that splendid city.(20)

Hippocrates, Plato, and Aristotle), but they were also excellent physicians *per se*, who in their own right, contributed to the medical and philosophic heritage of Western civilization. From the foregoing, it is fair to say that to a significant extent, Islamic and Jewish scholars kept the torch of medical knowledge burning at a time when the curtains of the Dark Ages had fallen on the stage of Europe. Perhaps it is also fair to state that these Islamic contributions should be considered not apart from the Judeo-Christian Western tradition, but like the Roman culture before Constantine the Great and Christianization, an integral part of our Western legacy.

THE TRANSITION TO THE RENAISSANCE

Both the perceived frailty and vulnerability of man and the infirmity of the church *vis-à-vis* the Black Death was seen by some as evidence of the intrinsic weakness of the Christian church, which had failed to protect and heal mankind from the horrible pestilence. This fact may have encouraged man to look for more secular answers about the here and now – rather than to heaven and hell and the hereafter. The early humanists were beginning their search for fertile ground in which to plant the seeds of inquiring nature in their quests for both secular and basic truths, and for answers to more mundane and immediate matters. Ultimately, they planted the seeds of the Renaissance, sown by such Italian humanists and literary men as Petrarch (1304-1374), the poet laureate of Rome (1341), and the scholar and poet Giovanni Boccaccio (1313-1375), who in the *Decameron* recorded the death and destruction wrought by the Black Death.

There was also Geoffrey Chaucer (c.1340-1400), the Father of English literature, author of *The Canterbury Tales*, a collection of medieval stories ranging from satiric tales to religious fables told from the perspective of individual pilgrims as they traveled to the greatest of English shrines, that of the martyred Archbishop of Canterbury, Thomas á Becket (1118-1170). This pilgrimage took place during a time of pestilence and death – the same pestilence to which Chaucer himself succumbed at the age of 60.

Lastly, we should not forget Dante Alighieri (1265-1321), statesman, poet, and unbeknownst to many of us, a registered physician, whose transcendental work, the epic masterpiece, *The Divine Comedy*, has been cited as the literary landmark demarcating the earliest beginnings of that ferment that began in Italy, swept through Europe, and came to be called the Renaissance.

When the Renaissance arrived, the scholasticism of St. Thomas Aquinas was challenged and partially demoted, whereas the study of natural, observable events assumed an importance that was heretofore unknown. The rediscovery of the Greek and Roman classics and other works of antiquity did not negate the need for rational thought and experimentation. Although the ancient authorities, i.e., Aristotle, Dioscorides, Galen, and Avicenna, were still revered by Renaissance scholars, their works and writings were, for the first time, subject to scrutiny and criticism, verification and confirmation.

During the Renaissance, nature assumed a new importance. There was great interest in the study of the Græco-Roman classics, but even these works were subject to study and verification by Renaissance scholars. The Renaissance also challenged the scholastic doctrine of Final Cause which required that known observations be consistent with known or assumed truths. Observations and experimentation, rather than philosophic studies and preconceptions, led the way for progress.(31,58,59)

For instance, the manuscript tradition of the Middle Ages, for the most part, did not rely on natural observations but on earlier illustrations and descriptions that were accepted as truths. As we have seen, these manuscripts were copied and recopied over the centuries, and inevitably, errors occurred in the translations that ultimately hindered knowledge and progress. Specifically, in the study of botany, the medical pharmacopoeia was based on previous descriptions and preconceived assumptions, rather than on the actual study of plants in nature. Botanical illustrations, therefore, came to represent scenes from mythology and assumed a more decorative function than an informative one. Point of fact is Dioscorides' *De Materia Medica* that we have already discussed.(31,60)

During the Renaissance, artists began to make their own observations rather than rely on previous descriptions and illustrations from old manuscripts to formulate their own ideas regarding nature's works. This new blossoming period in history witnessed the ascendancy of Neoplatonism, Hippocratic teaching, observation of natural phenomena, and the decline of Aristotelian philosophy, Galenism, and scholasticism. Nevertheless, these philosophies, particularly Aristotelian philosophy, continued to play a role in Western thought – Aristotle was never disavowed.

Human dissection was reintroduced in the Western world during the Renaissance.(7) Although autopsies had occasionally been permitted in the Middle Ages – as in cases where the cause of death was questioned – human dissections were now openly sanctioned by the Church and were widely used to teach anatomy in the major universities. Anatomic discoveries brought on an unquenchable thirst for more anatomic dissections and experimentation which were essential to the acquisition of medical knowledge in the newly-created, burgeoning disciplines of anatomy, pathology, and physiology.

FRANCIS BACON: SPOKESMAN FOR INDUCTIVE REASONING AND SCIENTIFIC EXPERIMENTATION

The philosophy of Francis Bacon (1561-1626), lawyer, humanist, philosopher, and Lord Chancellor of England (1618-1621), provides us with an excellent point at which to begin our discussion of the transition in the way of thinking and reasoning – from the scholasticism of the Medieval period to the humanism of the Renaissance. Although Bacon was a late Renaissance figure, he exemplifies better than anyone else the philosophic basis for the transition. Moreover, he was an ardent and eloquent spokesman for the inductive method of reasoning and scientific experimentation. He promoted the concept of observation and the collection of facts, without the formation of a preconceived hypothesis, prior to the formulation of a general theory of knowledge. His philosophy insisted on the inductive approach, *a posteriori* reasoning, the search for truths derived from observed facts as is, theoretically at least, the case in modern science, rather than relying on the old deductive, *a priori*, method of medieval scholasticism which was characterized by a quest for truths derived by reasoning from self-evident propositions, whereby observations are consistent with known or assumed truths.

Bacon called for scientific experimentation in his book, *Novum Organum,* and openly opposed the theology and philosophic concepts of St. Thomas Aquinas.(61) In effect, he revived the philosophy of his namesake, Roger Bacon (1214-1294), the Oxford Franciscan, who had unsuccessfully called for scientific experimentation almost 300 years earlier.(62) Francis Bacon advised scholars to pursue the natural sciences to arrive at truth. His approach was laboring experimentation, inductive *a posteriori* reasoning, natural observations, and generalizations (from the particular to the universal), though he himself was said to have been a poor scientist.(12)

In 1621, in the last few years of his life, whilst still Lord Chancellor, Bacon was accused and pleaded guilty to charges of bribery and was proscribed from holding public office. He wrote and completed many of his works, such as his *Essays,* during his retirement. His major contribution to the world, nevertheless, remained his impetus for the use of the inductive method of reasoning used in modern science.(2)

It was this relatively sudden upheaval in learning and creative thinking that lit the fire of the Renaissance and paved the way for the great scholars, especially our Renaissance physicians, who would blaze new paths of learning toward the advancement of medical knowledge: Paracelsus, Vesalius, Paré, and others. We will meet them *tête-à-tête* in our continuing saga, as we march toward the epicenter of that great, turbulent epoch of the medical Renaissance.

PART SEVEN: THE RENAISSANCE

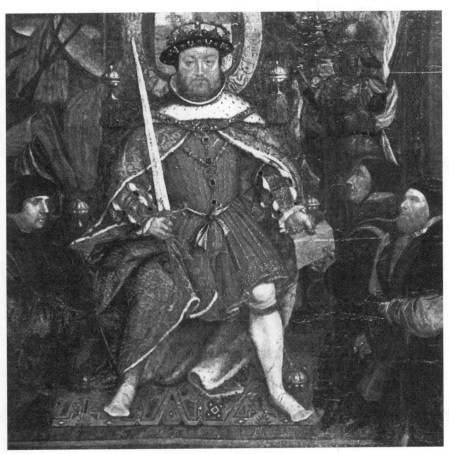

Plate 26 - King Henry VIII (1491-1547) handing to Thomas Vicary the Act of Union Charter which established the professional guild of Barber-Surgeons in 1540, an event immortalized in a painting by Hans Holbein the Younger. By permission of the President and Council of the Royal College of Surgeons of England.

CHAPTER 29

THE ZEITGEIST OF THE RENAISSANCE

Nothing great in this world has ever been accomplished without passion.
Georg Friedrich Hegel (1770-1831), from Philosophy of History
German Philosopher

THE PERIOD OF THE REBIRTH

It would be an understatement to say only that the Renaissance was a remarkable epoch in Western civilization. For the Renaissance was truly an intense period of rebirth in the acquisition of learning, leading directly from the *a priori* logic of medieval scholasticism to the *a posteriori* reasoning, and the intellectual and scientific achievements of the Age of Enlightenment. This period of rebirth was accompanied by an intellectual explosion that affected all areas of learning and human endeavor: sculpture, painting, poetry, writing, philosophy, astronomy, and medicine.(1,2)

As we have previously commented, the earliest beginning of the Renaissance dates from the time of Dante Alighieri (1265-1321), the great Italian epic poet, and extends through the time of John Milton (1608-1674) – a period spanning roughly 300 years.(3) Curiously, it could be stated that this period began almost wispily with the publication of a great Christian (Catholic) epic, Dante's *Divine Comedy* in the early 1300s, and likewise ended, fleetingly and almost imperceptibly, with another Christian epic poem (albeit a Protestant one this time) of equally heroic proportions, Milton's *Paradise Lost* (1667).

But this rebirth in the arts and sciences was more than a revival or rediscovery of the ancient Greek and Roman classics. This period also spawned new ideas that precipitated new ways of thinking and fervent discoveries that provided practical innovations for the betterment of mankind. Guttenberg's printing press (c.1452) was amongst the latter and would prove essential in the dissemination of the new ideas and erudition characteristic of the Renaissance.

The Renaissance even heralded a significant improvement over the Julian calendar when, in 1582 at the behest of Pope Gregory XIII (pope, 1572-1585), England adopted the Gregorian calendar (the United States adopted it in 1752).[167] Although still imperfect, the Gregorian calendar was more accurate than the old Julian calendar which had been adopted by Julius Caesar in 46 B.C.[168] Nevertheless, the Gregorian calendar has proven an enduring legacy, as it is still in use today.(4,5)

Historically, this period witnessed two epochal events: The discovery of the New World (1492) by the Genoese navigator, Christopher Columbus (1451-1506), sailing for the Catholic monarchs of Spain, King Ferdinand of Aragon

---

[167] Pope Gregory XIII should not be confused with St. Gregory VII (pope, 1073-1080) of Canossa fame, or St. Gregory I, "the Great" (pope, 590-604), a founder of monasticism.
[168] The calendar was subsequently adjusted by Emperor Augustus to his better liking, by taking a day from February and adding it to the month of August, so that the months of July and August were *a la par* in the number of days contained therein, reflecting both the glory and vanity of their namesakes.

(1452-1516) and Queen Isabella of Castile (1451-1504); and the collapse of the Eastern (Byzantine) Roman Empire with the fall of Constantinople (1453) to the Ottoman Turks – an event still celebrated with great fanfare in Istanbul, Turkey. In fact, some authorities have suggested that following the collapse of the Byzantine Empire, the influx of Greek scholars from Constantinople and other regions of the Empire into northern Italy was at least partially responsible for catalyzing some of the feverish developments associated with the Renaissance.

During this bustling period, new ideas and doctrines challenged the old rules and traditional institutions which had dominated European culture and intellectual life for a millennium. For the first time since classical antiquity, revolutionary discoveries in medicine and astronomy were judged to be within man's grasp. The Renaissance not only witnessed the growth of the humanities but also spurred heated, momentous philosophic and theologic controversies. This era was also associated with the resurgence of old sects (e.g., mysticism) and esoteric cults (e.g., the Cabala) and even the disreputable "sciences" of alchemy and astrology. The formulation of new religious doctrines and the birth of heretic sects, in turn, reactivated the dreaded counterforces of the Inquisition.

THE RULERS AND PATRONS

The Renaissance was an age when autocratic rulers wrestled and vied for power in a world centered in earthly intrigue. Lorenzo the Magnificent (1449-1492) and the de Medici family ruled Florence, the cultural hub of the Italian rebirth. The Church was in turmoil and was led during this time by four of the most enigmatic, flamboyant, powerful, and controversial popes to lead Christendom. They included Rodrigo Borgia (1475-1507), father of the infamous Cesare Borgia (c.1475-1507), who was Nicolo Machiavelli's (1469-1527) model of a ruler and a protagonist in his book *The Prince* (1513), a perennial political science classic. Rodrigo, taking his name from Alexander the Great, ascended to the seat of the papacy as Alexander VI (pope, 1492-1503). Additionally, Florence was well represented in the papacy by the de Medici popes, Giovanni de Medici who became Leo X (pope, 1513-1522) and Giuliano de Medici who became Clement VII (pope, 1523-1534). (6) There was also the "fighting pope," Julius II (pope, 1503-1513) who brought such great artists as Raphael (1483-1520) and Michelangelo Buonarroti (1475-1564) to Rome.

The conflict between Michelangelo and Pope Julius II during the painting of the Sistine Chapel was immortalized in a motion picture based on the Irving Stone novel titled, *The Agony and the Ecstasy*. Pope Julius II not only played a major role in the commission of the painting of the ceiling's frescoes but also participated in the internal decoration of the chapel with beautifully embroidered tapestries (1508-1512).

Although rulers and political theorists did not realize it at the time, many of the attitudes and philosophies formulated in the momentous doctrines relating to the conflict of the state versus the church, and of spiritual versus temporal powers, were being defined and shaped to endure for centuries. Such was the case with the Italian humanist and scholar, Lorenzo Valla (c.1407-1457); the political theorist, Nicolo Machiavelli; and the theologian and Swiss physician, Erastus (16th Century A.D.). Erastus held the political tenet that the power of the state supersedes that of the church, being Erastian philosophy which was later attributed to him went even further, being erroneously interpreted as meaning that the state was omnipotent. This political philosophy carried to its logical conclusion would aptly imply that the clergy were relegated to the status of "the moral police of the state."(3)

This exultant epoch was the age of many other erudite scholars. Desiderius Erasmus (c.1466-1536), the Dutch theologian, translated treatises, commented on Christian writings, and promoted classical scholarship – although he never fully joined the upheaval of the Renaissance reformers.(4) The French moralist, Michel de Montaigne (1533-1592), created the enduring *essay,* a word invented by him specifically for his written personal reflections, *Essais.* Another scholar, the German Renaissance physician Georgius Agricola (1494-1555), compiled a vast amount of knowledge on mining, geology, metals, and smelting, and consequently became "the Father of Mineralogy" – an appropriate accolade – for his efforts led to the development of geology and metallurgy as distinct disciplines of science. The detailed work of this physician was summarized in his book, *De Re Metallica,* which was published posthumously in Basel in 1556, and almost immediately became both a treasured source of reference and a veritable classic.

The storm created by the Reformation surged its gusty winds at the apogee of the Renaissance when the theologian Martin Luther (1483-1546) nailed his 95 Theses to the door of the Castle-Church in Wittenberg in 1517. This momentous event triggered the theologic revolt of the Protestant Reformation whose cascade of events would ultimately lead to a major schism in the Christian faith. Protestantism, in turn, would activate the antithetical forces of the Counter-Reformation.

To the Reformation, the hedonist Leo X (pope, 1513-1522) reacted initially with utter indifference. But just three years later, in 1521, the Pope was forced to respond with the Diet of Worms by which Martin Luther was condemned as a heretic and excommunicated. An extravagant pope, Leo X was an ardent collector of antiquities and to the end continued the policy of the Sale of Indulgences to procure funds for the completion of his dream, St. Peter's Cathedral in Rome – the largest church in the world.(6)

An interesting episode, that deserves mention here because it underscores the great passions elicited during this tempestuous period, concerns the story of a Dominican friar who publicly advocated reformation of the Catholic Church, whilst deeply involved in the perilous political affairs of state. We are referring to the unorthodox Dominican priest, Girolamo Savonarola (1452-1498), friar of the Cathedral of St. Mark in Florence. After the death of Lorenzo de Medici – the true power behind the nobility puppet council of Florence – a temporary power vacuum was left in the prosperous *avant-garde* city; the de Medicis were exiled and driven out of the city. It was in 1494 that the priest Girolamo Savonarola was able to seize control of Florence and unsuccessfully attempted to establish a titularly simple, highly austere, and puritanic Christian state under his rule, based on the rejection of material possessions and the abandonment of worldly enjoyments. In his "fiery sermons," Savonarola condemned what he considered the depravity of the church as well as the corrupting power of the Florentine state. He even claimed divine inspiration for his attacks on the powerful Pope Alexander VI.

But Alexander was not a pope to be taken lightly in political matters or recklessly attacked in fiery theologic sermons. The Borgia pope knew how to wield power in a world of treachery and intrigue that was part of the politics of the Renaissance. This is the same pope that with one mighty stroke of his pen, divided the world between the Catholic rivals, the kingdoms of Spain and Portugal. Alexander forged the Treaty of Tordesillas in 1494 that proposed that all the land to the east of the line would, henceforth, belong to the Portuguese (Africa and most of the still undiscovered Brazil); and any land discovered to the west, would belong to the Spanish Crown.[169]

Eventually, Savonarola was excommunicated by Pope Alexander in 1497 and shortly thereafter fell from power. The old ruling nobility of Florence had him imprisoned, tried for sedition and heresy, tortured, and burnt at the stake as a false prophet.(3,5)

Across the English Channel in England, it was the time of intransigent rulers such as King Henry VIII (1491-1547) who, ironically, had been given the title of *Fidei Defensor*, "Defender of the Faith," by the pope for his opposition to Martin Luther. Yet on the self-serving issue of divorce, Henry would go so far as to splinter the Catholic church in England (beheading his principled minister Sir Thomas More (1478-1535) in the process). For all his faults, Henry VIII yielded to the aspiring barber-surgeons and gave Thomas Vicary the Act of Union Charter in 1540 which consolidated the surgeon's and barber's guilds in London. In 1535, the barber-surgeon Vicary (c.1495-1562), who had been inducted by the Royal Surgeons because of his surgical ability and medical expertise, ascended to the position of "Serjeant-Chirurgeon" to the King. In this capacity, he came to treat the monarch who was afflicted with an indolent leg ulcer. Vicary successfully treated the leg and the ulcer healed. It has been speculated that the professional charter might have been, at least in part, a reward for Vicary's successful treatment of the recalcitrant royal canker. William Clowes (1544-1604) succeeded Vicary, worked and taught at St. Bartholomew's Hospital, and became the greatest surgeon in Elizabethan England. He wrote books on the surgical treatment of gunshot wounds as well as the management of surgical amputations.

As a point of information, we should remember that it was during the Medieval period that professional guilds, provided by local town governments and sanctioned by the authorities, had usually stipulated that barbers were not allowed to practice surgery, nor to bleed patients, but were instead allowed to cut hair, shave, and extract teeth. Conversely, surgeons were not permitted to shave or cut their patients' hair or extract their teeth. This separation between barbers and surgeons held in England for some time (during the Middle Ages) but as the barber-surgeons activities encroached upon these rules, the separation became more hazy, and the restrictions less clear cut.

The medical historian Dr. Richard A. Leonardo points out that it was then (after 1540) that the barber-surgeons of these consolidated professional guilds were permitted to place a blue and white stripped pole in front of their business locations. In France, surgeons of the Long Robes (Master Surgeons) "were permitted to

---

[169] Brazil was claimed formally by Portugal after the Portuguese navigator Pedro Álvarez Cabral (c.1467-c.1570) strayed far west of his course (to India) and landed in Brazil – whether or not he discovered the territory of Brazil remains debatable to this date.(5)

display a galliput and a red pole in addition." [170] In time, the English barber-surgeons and the surgeons were separated by the legal action of Parliament, the College of Surgeons was founded, and a new charter was granted in 1800: "The Barber-Surgeon Company then died a natural death, after an existence of almost four hundred years."(7)

After King Henry VIII's death in 1547, he was followed by the short-lived and ineffective monarchy of his young and chronically infirm son, Edward VI, who reigned from 1547 to 1553. Following Edward, the young Lady Jane Grey ruled briefly for 9 days in 1553. Mary Tudor, "Bloody Mary" (1516-1558), then ascended to the English throne, ruling from 1553 to 1558. Elizabeth I (1533-1603) followed Mary Tudor as queen, ruling from 1558 to 1603. With the long reign of Queen Elizabeth, England reached a pinnacle of glory and relative prosperity.

It was Queen Elizabeth I, along with her accomplished sea captains, Sir John Hawkins (1532-1595), the great navigator and English admiral, and his cousin, the intrepid adventurer Sir Francis Drake (1540-1596), [171] who defeated the Invincible Spanish Armada of King Philip II (1527-1598), sent to subdue and conquer Protestant England. These men in company with other notable buccaneers who comprised in great part the royal Navy with its light but well-armed and highly maneuverable ships, out-performed the large Spanish galleons, and saved Protestant England in 1588.

Elizabeth was succeeded by James I (1556-1625) who came down from Scotland and began the line of Stuart kings. James I was the son of Mary Queen of Scots (1542-1587). Mary Queen of Scots, you will remember, was beheaded by Queen Elizabeth I in 1587 at Fotheringhay Castle.

In France, King Francis I (1494-1547) imported Italian Renaissance works of art, founded the College of France (1530) where medicine was taught amongst other sciences and arts, and repeatedly waged war against the Holy Roman Empire. In 1525, in fact, his royal forces suffered a disastrous defeat at the hands of the imperial forces of Emperor Charles V at the Battle of Pavia. Francis was captured and humiliated in the debacle. But once he had been released and felt safe on French soil, *le enfant terrible* repudiated his treaty with the Emperor and returned to his old belligerent ways.(3) After Francis' death, his son, Henry II (1519-1559) succeeded to the French throne with his queen, Catherine de Medici (1519-1589). In 1559, Henry died from injuries sustained in a fateful joust.(2,8) He would eventually be followed by the outstanding Huguenot leader, Henry of Navarre, later King Henry IV (1553-1610), who sacrificed his Calvinist religion for the good of the nation, becoming one of France's greatest kings. He embraced Catholicism (1595) to heal the wounds of religious strife, and by the Edict of Nantes (1598), granted toleration to as well as political equality for all Protestants. He is also known historically for his publicly expressed sentiment that in France all families deserved, "a chicken in every pot."(3,4)

During this period of cloak and dagger diplomacy, France's main adversary, the King of Spain, was also the greatest of Holy Roman Emperors, the

---

[170] The barbers' rotating blue, red, and white stripped pole is today almost a forgotten lore – a mere vestige of a Medieval and Renaissance legacy.

[171] Sir Francis Drake was the first Englishman to circumnavigate the globe, a task accomplished between 1577-1580. He is also celebrated for his exploits as an English privateer on the Spanish Main, especially his famous attack on *Nombre De Dios* in 1572.(4,5)

Hapsburg monarch Charles V (1500-1558) who, despite being considered overbearing, was a most capable and devout ruler. His empire stretched from its traditional Germanic limits of the Netherlands and the Low Countries to the Mediterranean, as well as most of the known New World at the time. His was the greatest empire in history, except perhaps that of the former Soviet Union. In fact, realizing that his Hapsburg dominion stretched from Vienna to Peru, he once proudly declared, "in my realm, the sun never sets."(9)

In the East, we have some of the ablest rulers to match the Western monarchs – Henry VIII, Francis I, and Charles V – in wit and power: The powerful Sultan Mohammed II, "the Conqueror" (1429-1481), who conquered Constantinople in 1453 (10); Selim I, "the Grim" (1467-1520), who defeated the Persians and assumed the title of Caliph (as well as Sultan) with spiritual as well as temporal powers; and Sulayman the Magnificent (1496-1566), Sultan of the Ottoman Empire, who we met earlier in our saga.

WITCHES, HERETICS, AND THE INQUISITION

During the Renaissance, the persecution of individuals accused of witchcraft reached epidemic proportions, although as we have noted, sporadic persecutions and executions of alleged witches, sorcerers, and magicians had taken place even before the Middle Ages. The persecution of witches started in earnest in the 15th Century and would last well into the 18th Century. During this time, thousands of harmless and dispossessed old women were accused, indicted, convicted, and burned at the stake, or drowned for allegedly collaborating with the devil and practicing satanic rituals.

One must remember that drowning and burning were the favorite methods of execution because the Church abhorred the shedding of blood. These practices were sanctioned by both religious and secular state authorities. The legality of these proceedings was accepted by the legal profession which was armed with unprecedented prosecutorial powers. Witch trials were indeed travesties of history – barbaric and brutal. H.W. Haggard writes: "In solemn courts of law, robed judges listened seriously to fantastic tales mostly of savage and primitive people and condemned harmless old ladies to death."(11)

At the peak of the occurrences of these maleficent acts of unmitigated barbarism in the 16th and 17th Centuries, in which many judges and lawyers participated with the passion and the zeal of sanctimonious fanatics, our own Ambroise Paré was tending to the wounded on the battlefields of Europe, and William Harvey was performing experiments that would lead to the discovery of the circulation of blood. [172]

The Inquisition of the Counter-Reformation became an ecclesiastic tribunal with vested authority to combine the powers of judge and jury, and investigation and prosecution – a powerful entity indeed. The trials were notorious

---

[172] And whilst it is true that the vast majority of ethical physicians were bleeding patients as treatment for a variety of maladies, many others continued to place building blocks of medical information towards the construction of a solid edifice of medical knowledge. All this work would only become self-evident and reach fruition, for the most part, in the mid-19th Century. It is also true that illustrious physicians like Paré and Sir Thomas Browne were compelled to testify in some of the horrible witch trials of the times.

for the harsh and barbarous punishment inflicted upon the accused as well as the gross unfairness of the proceedings.(12,13) The accused had little chance to rebut arguments or refute the charges of his/her accusers and/or prosecutors. Gruesome torture awaited those who denied charges until they confessed; many hapless and innocent victims died from the ordeals of brutal, legal torture. Those who confessed were given a public "verdict," or *auto-da-fé* ("act of faith") judgment. Punishment was execution – agonizing death – by hanging, or by being drawn and quartered, or by burning at the stake.

Ecclesiastic prosecutors participated in earnest in the ghastly inquisitorial trials that would extract the highly-damning infernal confessions, for real or imagined heresies, or the real or fabricated incriminating acts of treason, orchestrated often times to get rid of nagging political opponents rather than genuine traitors. The real purpose of the Inquisition was then both a political and a religious instrument for the establishment of religious conformity and the suppression of political enemies; this was true for both Catholic territories under the Inquisition as well as religious persecutions in Protestant dominions.

At the head of the Inquisition in Spain was the fanatical monk and confessor to Queen Isabella, the Inquisitor-General Tomás de Torquemada (c.1420-1498). Heretics, suspected witches, Jews, and Moslems were all at risk during the Inquisition. In fact, Torquemada was said to have been praised by both Pope Sixtus IV (pope, 1471-1484) and Pope Alexander VI, because these popes considered Jews and Moslems an impediment to the security of the state and the Roman Catholic Church. Nevertheless, although sanctioned by the Church, the Inquisition in Spain, as we have intimated, was under royal control and could be used against political enemies when necessary. It has been estimated that approximately 2000 people were burned at the stake at the height of the Inquisition during its first 20 years of reimplementation in Spain.(14) Countless others died during its entirety. Under these circumstances, it should not be surprising to learn that whenever the Inquisitor-General travelled, he was always escorted by an entourage of armed retainers and horsemen.(15)

In 1492, Torquemada persuaded the Spanish monarchs to extend the Inquisition to the Jews by signing a decree ordering all Spanish Jews to either convert to Catholicism or leave the country within four months.(14) In 1502, all Moslems living in Spain were given the same ultimatum. It is known that "Torquemada particularly distrusted the *Maranos and Moriscos*" – the Jewish and Moorish converts to Catholicism – because the conversions in many instances were thought to be insincere. The Moriscos were ultimately expelled from Spain a century later.

In Spain, the Catholic Church was to be controlled by the monarchy rather than the pope, and as a result of the political and religious unity, and the immense consolidation of power afforded the Inquisition, the Protestant Reformation made no significant headway in Spanish territories. Moreover, it was not until 1560 that the Catholic Church was able to launch its own Counter-Reformation as far as introducing the much needed reforms within the Roman Catholic Church.

History has provided innumerable examples of physicians and health practitioners who have been held unfairly hostage by the ignorance of unruly mobs, the religious fanaticism and intolerance of theologic luminaries, and the political expediency of government leaders and sundry demagogues (as is presently happening). Two examples illustrate this issue of religious and ethnic intolerance that took place in the nation I historically consider the most consistently civilized (perhaps after the Swiss Confederation) – England.

One example, as pointed out by the medical historian, R.S. Roberts, provides a tragic reminder of how easily unwary physicians become the scapegoats of government injustice and the expediency of the moment, and how easily they can become sacrificial lambs to placate the hatred of unruly masses incited via mob psychology by those who wield power. The case of Dr. Lopes – a Jewish Spanish physician (a Marano) who had converted to Catholicism and immigrated to England looking for a better life – illustrates this point. Soon after establishing his medical practice in England, Dr. Lopes was unjustly accused of being the ring leader of a "dastardly plot to kill the Queen while treating her in order to turn England over to the Spaniards and Catholicism." The reality, as Professor Roberts points out, was that "in English eyes he was simply a Catholic Jew and he was executed...."(16) There was never any proof, only the incipient hatred for Maranos, and the perceived threat to the English Protestant political establishment. Dr. Lopes was, as the saying goes, "expendable."

Toward the end of the 17th Century, not only doctors but also midwives, the earliest incarnation of specialized nurse practitioners, were viewed with suspicion (when the need arose by those in power). By the late 1680s, Protestant England had had enough of Catholic King James II (1633-1701), and Protestant leaders were looking for an excuse to oust the oppressive monarch. In 1688, a Catholic midwife was conveniently accused of smuggling a child into the bed-chamber of the queen of the Stuart king. The queen was accused of pretending a pregnancy "in order to obtain a son who would then be brought up as a Catholic and ensure Catholic succession to the English throne."(16) Despite the midwife's testimony as to the legitimacy of the child, it was claimed that an "alleged foundling was brought into the chamber in a warming pan" to accomplish the papist plot.(16) Suffice it to say, the episode led to the so-called Glorious Revolution of 1688 in which Mary II (1661-1694), the Protestant heiress (eldest daughter of James II) and her husband William III, Prince of Orange (1650-1702) and King (1689-1702), ascended to the English throne. England remained Protestant. [173] Queen Anne (1665-1714), the second daughter of James II who was also a Protestant, succeeded after their reign. Anne's death brought to an end the House of Stuart's royal succession in England.

[173] Besides the fact that James II was indecisive and Catholic, there was also the fact that he attempted to disarm Protestant citizens in England and Ireland. The search of homes for the seizure and confiscation of muskets and pistols in private possession was the final straw that broke the camel's back: "...an abominable thing to disarm the nation...." Upon William and Mary ascending to the English throne, they were required to swear to uphold Parliament's Bill of Rights which included "the right to keep and bear arms." [Hardy, David T.: Origins and Development of the Second Amendment. Blacksmith Co., Chino Valley, AZ., 1986, p.33-35].

CHAPTER 30

THE AGE OF EXPLORATION
AND DISCOVERY

The winds and waves are always on the side of the ablest navigator.
Edward Gibbon (1734-1794)

THE AGE OF EXPLORATION

The Renaissance heralded the Age of Discovery, based on explorations of heretofore *terrae incognitae.* As the reader would remember from history, the spices and riches of the Orient were highly prized in Europe, and both the Spanish and the Portuguese lusted for a sea route to exploit those riches. Yes, all of the navigational efforts of the European powers, particularly the Portuguese, had been directed towards the discovery of a sea route to the East – in their search for the riches and the exotic spices of the Orient.

Why the burning desire and need for these products, these spices, for which Europeans with almost religious zeal were willing to spend fortunes, and even risk their lives to go on distant quests around the globe, quests that were fraught with unimaginable hazards, herculean travails, and innumerable dangers? As we have already intimated, spices were more than just food preservatives in those pre-refrigeration days and more than simple condiments used for flavoring food. Most importantly, spices were used as medicinal drugs, and it was for this reason that spices commanded exorbitant prices on the European market. But what were these spices and medicinal herbs that were so highly sought by the explorers?

The exotic spices which triggered the great voyages of discovery in the late 15th and early 16th Centuries indeed deserve mention, at least briefly. First, there was *pepper.* Legend proclaims that one of the ransoms paid in the decadent days of Rome, was paid partly in pepper. The astronomic value of the spices of the East, especially pepper, was one of the main arguments that convinced the Portuguese of the primacy of their decision to seek a sea-route around Africa to the Indies. Land routes were non-existent, having been all but completely blocked by the Moslems. Pepper came primarily from India. Then, there was *ginger,* which in value was rated second only to pepper. Ginger, which had been known since remote antiquity, was cultivated on both the Indian subcontinent and the Island of Sumatra. *Clover,* with its exotic flavor, was used both for flavoring food and preserving meats. It was primarily harvested in the Moluccas, appropriately called the Spice Islands, located between the islands of Celebes (Eastern Indonesia) and New Guinea. *Cinnamon* came from Ceylon (today Sri Lanka) and was used primarily as a flavoring oil. *Nutmeg* and *Mace* came from both Banda and the Moluccas.

Benzoin, a balsamic resin, came from the Island of Sumatra and was used not only as an antiseptic but as a treatment for ulcers. Today, it is still widely used as an adhesive for wound dressings and bandaging. *Musk* and *Camphor* were extracted from plants in China. They were valuable for their medicinal use as liniments, an ingredient that infused strength and permanency to vegetable essences, and as an attar used in compounding perfumes. *Aloes,* which were known in ancient times to both Egyptians and Greeks, were highly valued as purgatives. Exotic varieties of aloes were imported primarily from China. *Rhubarb,* another Chinese herb, was known since 2500 B.C., and was even included in Dioscorides' *De Materia Medica.* Rhubarb was used primarily as a medicament (laxative and astringent) but was also consumed as a vegetable.

In addition to the costly spices available from China, there were silk and porcelain, both treasured in Europe. Prized as these products were in Europe, both the land routes as well as the navigable intervening Red Sea were closed to the Europeans by Mohammedan traders, making these amenities exorbitantly priced commodities. A direct route from Europe had to be found to reach India, China, and the islands of the South China Sea.

Moreover, since the time of Marco Polo (c.1254-1324), who had traveled extensively in China (Cathey) and ventured as far as India and Southeast Asia, the Indies and the entire Far East had dazzled European imagination. Japan (Cipangu), which the Great Khan had tried unsuccessfully to conquer, was also thought to have gold and riches. India and the islands around Indonesia and China were known for their valuable spices. And due to the mesmerizing tales of Marco Polo during the Medieval period, China was already considered the richest empire in the world. After all, it was China that gave birth to paper, gunpowder (used since the late Middle Ages as a powerful siege weapon to blow open the gates of besieged but fortified enemies), silk, and even the compass.

The persistent hurdle was the problem posed by the intervening Moslems who presented a formidable and potential triple threat to the Europeans. Economically, the Moslem traders and middlemen were already an existing threat, since they unabashedly believed in trading and the positive ethics of making profits in legitimate commerce and business transactions. From the religious and military perspective, Islam was a particular threat because of the historic fervor of its tenets, as well as the relatively fresh recollections etched indelibly in the memory of the European Christians that of Moslems as worthy foes (with whom they had previously crossed swords).

Christianity and Islam had known, and kept each other in check, for centuries. Islamic Saracens with their deadly scimitars had been, and continued to be, formidable opponents for the Christian infidels with their halberds and broadswords. The Moors may have been defeated and pushed off the Iberian peninsula, their last major stronghold at Granada taken from them in 1492 (17), but in its stead, Constantinople, the sacred capital of the Byzantine Empire in the East, had been taken by the Turks in 1453.(10) These same Turkish armies and their elite *Janissaries* troops would later be on the march in the Balkans and eastern Europe, even threatening Vienna, led by the intrepid Sultan Sulayman. Whilst on the sea, Moslem privateers and Ottoman allies, such as those commanded by the Turkish Sultan's vassal, Barbarrosa, wreaked havoc on Christian ships and disrupted trade and commerce in the Mediterranean. The point is that the Europeans had to find a viable way to reach the Indies!

But this, of course, did not mean that the Europeans were totally dependent on the East for every amenity, since they had available to them many medicaments within their territories – some of these drugs known to them since the time of Dioscorides in the 1st Century. For instance, there was *opium* from Asia Minor which was used for sedation, for control of pain, and for the treatment of diarrhea. Herbs such as *hepatica* were used for liver ailments, and *foxglove,* whose extract *digitalis* was used for heart problems and other ailments, had been used for centuries according to the old doctrine of signatures. There was also the legendary plant, *mandrake*, with supposedly mythic attributes and from which Belladonna alkaloids were extracted. Mandrake was also known for its toxicity (in higher doses) and thus, had been sometimes conveniently used as a poison.

Be that as it may, the riches and spices of the Orient proved to be a tantalizing lure that Europeans could not ignore. During the Age of Discovery and the epoch of the Renaissance, there would be many men who risked their lives for fame, honor...and the wealth and riches of the Orient. And so, after a series of exploratory voyages, the Portuguese finally succeeded in rounding the Cape of Good Hope.[174] The intrepid seafarer Vasco da Gama (c.1469-1524) reached the seaport of Calicut in the East Indies on May 21, 1498. He had reached India, and with it, he finally established a lucrative spice trade in the Orient. On his second trip in 1502, da Gama returned home with shiploads of spices and exotic riches. In time, although belatedly, da Gama was made Viceroy of India (1524), only to die shortly thereafter, never having had time to enjoy the fruits of his discoveries.

As a point of information, we should cite the tale of a New World miracle drug that, of course, did not become available in Europe until after the Great Discovery. This is the life-saving drug *quinine* which is extracted from the bark of the Cinchona tree of South America (Peru). Quinine, in fact, provides us the first example of an effective drug for a specific illness, a drug that became available only as a result of the Age of Exploration and the discovery of the New World. A product of the late Renaissance, the Cinchona bark was not used until after 1630 when its highly beneficial effects against malaria ("bad air"), then called the *ague*, were discovered. Malaria, known for its periodic attacks of fever and chills, is a debilitating disease caused by the *Plasmodium* protozoan parasite carried by the *Anopheles* mosquito that transmits the disease from the blood of an infected person to that of a healthy individual.

According to a prevalent story of the time, Europeans became acquainted with quinine when it was given to the Countess of Cinchona who had become seriously ill with malaria whilst visiting Lima in 1630. The medicine was given to her by Jesuit priests, and shortly thereafter, miraculously, she was relieved of a severe attack of the disease. The great clinician Thomas Sydenham (1624-1689) was one of the first physicians to introduce and recommend the use of Cinchona bark to treat malaria in England. Later, when the New World was opened to Europe, not only Cinchona bark, but coffee, tea, tobacco, potatoes, as well as gold and silver, were taken to Europe in great quantities in Spanish galleons cruising in their cargo-laden transatlantic voyages. Even these plant and vegetable commodities, including potatoes, were used as medicines.(11,18)

PRE-COLUMBIAN CULTURES AND THE COLUMBIAN LEGACY

If I may digress at this point for the sake and exposition of historic truth to discuss the relevant and still pertinent issue of Christopher Columbus and the

---

[174] The Cape of Good Hope was euphemistically named, as Greenland and perhaps even Tierra del Fuego, to allay the fears of those venturing into their midst. Bartolomeu Dias (c.1450-1500) was the first European to sail around the Cape of Good Hope in the years 1487 and 1488. He assisted Vasco da Gama in planning the latter's expedition a decade later. For his part, Ferdinand Magellan (c.1480-1521) led the first expedition that circumnavigated the globe, proving definitively that the Earth was round and that Columbus had indeed discovered a New World. Magellan was killed by natives in the Philippines.

discovery of the New World as it pertains to today's climate of multiculturalism and historic revisionism. This issue is not only still pertinent but also timely in our discussion, as we have just recently celebrated, as others denigrated, the quincentennial discovery of the New World (1992). With today's liberal zeitgeist – and what Supreme Court Justice, Clarence Thomas called the New Intolerance, and the scholar Thomas Sowell, the New Orthodoxy of political correctness – the American people have been subtly indoctrinated to believe that this epochal event should be scorned and vilified.

The partisan revisionist historians and deconstructionists that regretfully are part of academia and their allies, the liberal media, took great pains to denounce this momentous event by exaggerating facts and creating false imagery to support their revisionists contentions whilst neglecting, suppressing, or ignoring factual events that conflicted with their point of view and their leftist ideologies. The liberal media knowingly placed undue emphasis on the egregious side effects of the European conquest which, as nefarious as they might have been, in many cases were unforeseen and unintentional, whilst at the same time, a conscious effort was made to neglect, reject, or simply cast aside all that was good. Perhaps it would be appropriate for those who seek to misinform and knowingly mislead to remember the Hebrew proverb, "a half-truth is a whole lie."

During the quincentennial, liberal left-wing writers and artists did their utmost to denigrate Columbus at every turn, even if it was necessary to paint or describe a fictitious picture of Pre-Columbian life in Mesoamerica. Thus, the only picture of the New World that was painted by the mass media was one of idyllic or pastoral scenes with beautifully depicted innocent New World natives living in perfect ecologic harmony with their pristine environment in the tradition of the famed Mexican Marxist artist, Diego Rivera (1886-1957), who was ahead of his time with regard to agitprop multiculturalism. In Rivera's paintings, which anyone may still see today in the Palace of Fine Arts and other public buildings throughout Mexico City, his unique style and display of forceful advocacy for liberal social causes is readily evident. The Spanish *conquistadores* are depicted olive-skinned with grotesque and sinister features and always committing perfidious or nefarious acts of social injustice.

The natives, on the other hand, are painted as "noble savages" incapable of evil, or for that matter, incapable of committing any of the cardinal sins of Western lore. Thus, we are led to believe that until the arrival of the European fiends, there was little warfare and no vices, no disease, no greed, no malice, only virtues in the hearts of the natives. In the opposite camp, with a few exceptions, the defenders of Western civilization have recoiled, reluctant to respond to the farce of political correctness and historic revisionism, for fear of being labeled Eurocentrists, racists, or bigots. They are afraid that their defense of Western civilization and its values will be impugned as "racially motivated," or imputed as "insensitive" by the "thought police" patrolling academe because their historic perspectives do not square with prevailing liberal, politically-correct views. Sadly, some scholars, perhaps with justification, feared endangering and even losing their academic positions if they expressed opposition to the chic historic revisionism and deconstructionism.

With this in mind, let us now proceed to elucidate the facts regarding Pre-Columbian history prior to the arrival of *La Pinta, La Niña,* and *La Santa Maria.*

With all due respect to Jean Jacques Rousseau (1712-1778) and his "noble savage" concept, which idealizes primitive man uncorrupted by Western civilization, I would like to relate true historic accounts, some of which have been only recently reconfirmed by scholarly archaeologic and anthropologic research.

Prior to the arrival of the Europeans, the Arawak Indians (*Tainos*) were the relatively peaceful inhabitants of the Caribbean islands whom we associate with idyllic native scenes; but they were not the only native tribe. In fact, the Tainos were preyed upon and suffered as much at the hands of the fierce Carib Indians (*Caribes*) as from the conquering Europeans. Throughout the many islands, the peaceful male Arawaks were hunted, killed, and even cannibalized by the ferocious Caribs who ultimately ended up exterminating the peaceful Arawaks from many of the Caribbean islands in the Lesser Antilles. The female Arawaks were taken as wives or slaves by the male Caribs. Atrocities by the Carib Indians were infamous, and today these atrocities are often discounted or ignored.

As the ferocious Carib warriors invaded northward from the Lesser Antilles to the larger Caribbean islands in the Greater Antilles, they pillaged, plundered, and enslaved their weaker neighbors, raiding island after island. It was the sudden arrival of the Spaniards in the New World that stunted their locust-like invasion in the Antilles.(19)

Never mind all the data we have on the subject, in his book *The Conquest of Paradise*, the zealous environmentalist writer Kirkpatrick Sale, denies that the Carib Indians "were ferocious or engaged in cannibalism."(20) In short, he dismisses their ferocity and cannibalism as a figment of Columbus' and his chroniclers' imagination. Instead, he counters by citing several obscure instances of mob savagery and cannibalism in Europe during the Middle Ages! There is no doubt that Europeans in general and the Spanish and Portuguese in particular perpetrated perfidious and despicable acts during the conquest and colonization of the indigenous peoples of the New World.

One story that remains indelibly in my mind, from happier days as a youth in pre-Castro Cuba, is that of the *Cacique Hatuey*, a brave Taino chief, whose story could be recited by heart by my grammar school classmates. The chieftain Hatuey had waged relentless war against the Spaniards, had refused to surrender, but was finally captured. To his last hour, he remained defiant and unrepentant and was burned at the stake refusing Christian baptism. When he was asked why he did not want to convert to Catholicism and repent so that he could go to heaven, he replied that if heaven was the place where the white colonizers were going after death, that was not the place he wanted to go after he left this existence.

There were indeed many sad and perverse acts perpetrated by the European colonizers during the conquest, but these nefarious and perverse acts were not unique either in European history or in Pre-Columbian annals, as the factual events narrated on the pages that follow will amply testify.

THE MIGHTY AZTECS

In 1978, subway workers in Mexico City discovered archaeologic evidence corroborating previous Aztec and Spanish accounts relating to the dedication of the twin temples of Huitzilopochtli and Tlaloc, the two supreme Aztec gods of war and rain-water, respectively. In 1487, only one generation before the arrival of the Spanish conquistador Hernán Cortes (1485-1547) in Mexico (1519), the *Uey Tlatoani* or "Revered Speaker" of the Aztecs (or Mexica), Ahuitzolt, sacrificed over 20,000 captured prisoners at the dedication of the twin temples (*El Templo Major*). This ceremony went on for four days in which ritualistic killings were performed uninterruptedly, four victims at a time, from dawn to dusk, in a spectacular display of blood, gore, and sacrifice.(21-27) [175]

Hundreds of priests participated in the grisly sacrifices atop the consecrated temples. Chests were ripped open with razor-sharp obsidian knives, and hearts torn out of the briskly bleeding chest cavities. The hearts were often still pulsating and gushing blood and were held up for all in the crowd below to see. The organs were then burned on top of altars named *chacmools,* whilst the corpses were allowed to roll down the descending, steep steps of the infernal temples. Blood was allowed to run down the steps and coagulate at the base of the pyramidal structures. The corpses were then dismembered by spiritually-possessed, frantic butchers located at the base of the pyramid and cannibalized by the frenzied crowds. Blood was also dabbed onto the mouths of the various stone idols in the temples, for they also required satiation with human blood.

In other sacrificial ceremonies, children were solemnly drowned or their throats cut with surgical precision for the Rain God, Tlaloc, and women were ceremoniously decapitated annually for Coatlicue, the proverbial Earth-Mother goddess. In the sacrificial rituals to Xochipilli (the god of flowers) and Xipe-Totec, (the god of youth and Spring), the victims were flayed – whilst still alive. The victims skins were worn as ghastly garments by the bloodied priests whose hair was habitually matted with the coagulated blood of the sacrificial victims.

Vassals, allies, and subjugated peoples alike were coerced or forced to watch, and sometimes participate in, the gruesome ceremonies deliberately to demoralize rivals and terrorize potential adversaries. In this fashion, using terror as a weapon, the Aztecs could extract the desired tribute from their weaker neighbors whilst at the same time, satiating their gods' perpetual thirst for human blood and perennial hunger for human sacrifices.

Contemporary paintings by the native Aztecs themselves, the *Codices,* supplemented by narratives by indigenous as well as European sources (which were later corroborated by archaeologic discoveries) provided evidence of these spectacular sacrificial accounts which until recently were suppressed and attributed to the concoction and imagination of the Spanish colonizers, supposedly as justification for their misdeeds in the New World.

In other words, European historic accounts, indigenous codices, and even pictorial and archaeologic evidence had been suppressed or misinterpreted by liberal-minded scholars because it did not square with their preconceived notions of indigenous peoples. It took relatively recent but fully incontrovertible and irrefutable archaeologic evidence to prove what had been evident and argued by other honest and truth-oriented scholars of Mesoamerican culture for years.(21,24,27,28)

---

[175] Regarding reference #21, the reader may also consult the review of this book that appeared in *The New American*, May 4, 1992; another review was also published in *The Wilson Quarterly*, Spring 1992. Reference #22, *Aztec* by Gary Jennings is an epic historic novel based on over 10 years of research by its author. The adventures of the protagonist, the Aztec, Mixtli "Dark Cloud," are fictitious, but the historic setting and the cultural depictions are based on facts. The book is highly recommended and a must for *aficionados* of Pre-Columbian culture.

THE RESOURCEFUL MAYANS

Farther south, the Mayans of Central America have been considered the "Greeks of the New World." Their civilization arose in the jungles of Mesoamerica to include a vast territory of independent city-states stretching from southern Mexico and the Yucatán peninsula to Honduras and El Salvador in Central America. Yet the glaring fire of this civilization extinguished itself before the arrival of the conquistadors.(28-31) Most of the present theories explaining their decadence in the 10th Century A.D. point toward a poor relationship between the Mayas and their ecosystem.

The Maya reversion to a more primitive level of civilization in the jungles of the Yucatán and Central America have been attributed to soil exhaustion from over-cultivation, topsoil erosion, excessive slash-and-burn agriculture, calamities brought about by plagues, pestilences, and overpopulation (concomitant with poor sanitation and overcrowding), as well as – yes, pollution of their environment. Also entertained as the final cataclysmic event has been the possibility of rebellion of the masses, and annihilation of the planning and ruling theocracy. More recently, evidence has accumulated pointing to rampant internecine warfare amongst the various warring city-states in the 8th and 9th Centuries in Belize, Guatemala, and elsewhere in Central America.(32,33)

Moreover, the Mayans also practiced bloody rites and rituals including human sacrifices, though to a lesser extent than the Aztecs. Royalty participated in complex bleeding ceremonies that included not only sacrifices of captives, but also self-mutilation, and other bleeding ceremonies that brought the participants closer to the gods. These rituals were (and still are) definitely not for the squeamish.(28)

THE INCAS OF PERU

We encounter the Empire of the Sun, the Incas of South America – the road builders and warriors of Peru – in the dense and remote jungles as well as craggy mountain slopes of the Andes. From the onset, it must be stated that the conquest of this empire was not only possible because of the treachery and the technologic advantage (not to mention unfaltering determination) of the Spaniards, but also (and most significantly), because of the intrinsic divisiveness and bellicosity of the Incas.

It is also fair to state that the opulent and ostentatious Atahualpa, King of the Incas, was most responsible for the Inca conquest. Atahualpa claimed descent from the Inca sun-god, but was challenged for this claim by his equally pretentious brothers. Thus, they waged war against each other in a brutal and terrible civil war that ravaged the land and weakened the country – thus making the Inca perhaps easier prey for their soon-to-be adversaries, the men led by Francisco Pizarro (c.1470-1541) and Diego de Almagro (c.1475-1538) during the years of conquest and colonization (c.1524-1538). It was this fratricidal Inca war fought because of greed and naked thirst for power that weakened the Inca empire and made it vulnerable to the iron-willed conquistadors who were there literally, either to die or conquer, regardless of whether their main intentions were for gold, religion, adventure, or for king and country. These were the conquistadors who actually crossed the legendary line drawn in the sand by Pizarro to venture into the unknown and forbidden territory of the Andes.

Once captured, Atahualpa tried to buy his freedom with two and a half rooms filled with the gold and silver extracted from the harrowing travails of his people who struggled laboriously to pay the required ransom demanded for his liberation. The broken Inca population paid the ransom demanded by Pizarro, but Atahualpa's cowardice, notwithstanding, did not save him from the garrote that was used in his execution in 1533.(25,26)

For the sake of intellectual honesty and fairness, it should be said that even though it is true that the Europeans did colonize the New World, and by rules of conquest seized land of the defeated indigenous people, decimation of native populations occurred to the greatest extent as a result of natural cataclysmic and unintentional events. The majority of the casualties in the indigenous population were sustained by disease and pestilences rather than war. It is estimated that nearly 50 million indigenous people died during the 300 year period of colonization as a result of the conquest. An unimaginable calamity, no doubt, but it must be placed in the proper perspective considering the facts and judged by the standards of the age. This depopulation was neither officially sanctioned, anticipated, or even intended by the Spanish or Portuguese authorities.

It should also be ascertained that, although much has been said and written about virulent diseases brought to the New World by the Europeans (such as measles, smallpox, and diphtheria), these calamities were the result of decreased immunity of the indigenous population to the heretofore unknown European maladies. These afflictions had more to do with the mingling of two very different and isolated cultures (which up to this time had not been in contact with each other) than with a deliberate act of genocide. After all, biologic warfare, except for a few isolated instances (i.e., catapulting plague-ridden corpses into besieged cities of the Byzantine Empire), seems to have been for the most part unknown in the 16th Century.

Much less publicized are the diseases that later assailed the Europeans and were likely introduced into Europe from America – a notable example of which is syphilis. It is worth recounting here that this disease was first noted in Europe in the closing decade of the 15th Century. Both medical and epidemiologic evidence suggest that this disease was brought to Europe by Spanish troops returning from the New World, and who were taken to Naples to brake a siege by French troops surrounding the city in 1494. Later, the French army, which was at the time composed largely of mercenaries, was blamed for the disease after the then highly virulent malady spread all over the continent. The dreaded disease was thus called the *morbus gallico*, "the French Disease," and the French conversely, referred to it as the "Neapolitan Sickness." The first two or three generations afflicted by this disease were stricken with fever which was followed by a rapidly debilitating illness that seemingly affected all organ systems and was invariably fatal. As generations passed, the disease lost some of its virulence, became more indolent, and evolved into the disease we know today.(11,34,35)

In short, if Columbus and his legacy were not entirely perfect, it is because the man was human. One thing is for certain and that is that the discovery of the

New World represented a spectacular moment in history. The events it set in motion led to the political documents *par excellence* in the history of man, the American Declaration of Independence and the United States Constitution with its Bill of Rights, documents immersed in a legacy of enlightened European ideas – justice, equality before the law, individual liberty, free enterprise, opportunity for social mobility, the sanctity of private property, and limited government (governance by the consent of the governed).

As has been pointed out by the conservative historian Fr. James Thornton, today we are on a perilous path: "Compromise and conformity to trends are easier than resistance and speaking the truth."(36) This is particularly true in the tacit acceptance of political correctness, historic revisionism, and multiculturalism as ineluctable forces that are easier to conform to than to confront, as if these complaisant qualities were insurmountable, and standing for truth was unimportant and inconsequential. The preservation of America's cultural heritage will depend on the will and resistance of a concerned, vigilant, and well-informed citizenry standing up for truth.

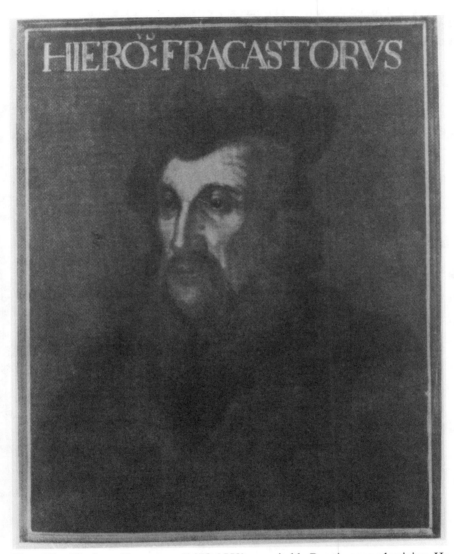

Plate 27 – Girolamo Fracastoro (1478-1553), a veritable Renaissance physician. He wrote a poem about syphilis, supported Copernicus' heliocentric theory of planetary motion, and ahead of his time, was a proponent of the germ theory of disease. Galleria Palatina (Uffizi Gallery), Florence.

CHAPTER 31

RENAISSANCE PHYSICIANS FOR ALL SEASONS

It is very seldom that the same man knows much of science and about the things that were known before science came.

Lord Dunsany (8th Baron, 1878-1957)
Irish writer and poet

PHYSICIANS AND MEDICAL PRACTICE

During the exalted period of the Renaissance, many great medical men dedicated their lives not only to treat the sick and afflicted but also to translate ancient manuscripts and to make critical comments on the newly discovered medical works. Translations of works from Greek into Latin and into the vernacular languages were performed by scholarly physicians. Works of Galen, Hippocrates, Plato, and Dioscorides were re-popularized. Some physicians attempted to reconcile the Humoural doctrines to newly discovered facts and observations. Words such as *institute* and *synopsis* came into vogue during this time, reflecting the accumulation of new learning (34) as well as the revolutionary theory of the specific nature of diseases. The concept of the *contagion* as transmissible material particles was advanced, but the reader must remember that the actual concept of *animalcules,* or living organisms had to wait to the late 17th Century and the invention of the microscope by Anton van Leeuwenhoek (1632-1723). Nevertheless, during the Renaissance, propagation of disease by contact with contagious sources became evident in such widespread diseases as variola, bubonic plague, measles, and syphilis.

Jean Fernel (1497-1588) was just one of the many celebrated Renaissance physicians. He trained in Paris and compiled his great treatise, *A Universal Medicine,* in which he proposed that the study of medicine be divided into three categories: physiology, pathology, and therapeutics. He summarized all of the known medical knowledge of his time. Additionally, his book is credited with planting the seeds of curiosity which later reaped rich harvests of medical information and scientific theories. Fernel, along with Paré and Paracelsus, advanced the idea of the contagious nature of diseases by different causes. In support of this thesis, a unique although unfortunate opportunity presented itself, when in 1494, a new disease made its debut in Europe: *Lues venerae.* Mercurials were first used in ointment form against this devastating disease and were found to be effective. The dreaded malady was later called *syphilis* after the physician-poet Girolamo Fracastoro used the name of a shepherd who was afflicted with the painful and debilitating disease in a poignant poem.(34,37)

The Swiss physician, Paracelsus, on the other hand, has been given the credit for the mercurial therapy that was then widely used against this disease. Contraction of the disease and the required therapy, fraught with undesirable and serious, untoward side effects, has been wittily but aptly described by a contemporary of Paracelsus as: "spending one hour with Venus and the rest of your life with Mercury..." in reference to both the method of transmission and the necessity for long term treatment.(38)

Although Girolamo Fracastoro (1478-1553) has been given credit for coining the term *syphilis* from the aforementioned poem, he was also an established giant in Renaissance medicine. He, along with Jean Fernel, suggested that syphilis was a venereal disease *(Lues venerae)* and concurred in the use of mercurial ointments for treatment. In 1547, Fracastoro wrote a treatise on contagious diseases and adeptly separated the bubonic plague from typhus and meningitis, whilst providing excellent clinical descriptions as well as accurate prognoses for these diseases. He posited transmission by human contact, by contaminated objects, and by air.(37)

Fracastoro was a Renaissance physician in both the modern and historic sense. His treatise on infectious diseases was ahead of its time, and perhaps, if it had been pursued further, could have propelled bacteriology into a true science three centuries earlier. Whilst he followed the physician Theodoric from the Medieval period, he would be the forerunner of such eminent physicians and scientists as Robert Koch, Louis Pasteur, Joseph Lister, and Ignaz Semmelweis – all giants of the scientific era of medicine. Fracastoro, who was interested in a variety of areas of human endeavor besides medicine, was also a proponent of the heliocentric theory proposed by fellow physician, Nicolaus Copernicus.

Quarantining those afflicted was confirmed to be an effective way to control contagious diseases which up to this time had been decimating the populations of Europe and Asia, in both sporadic outbreaks as well as in indolent endemic fashion. Some attention to hygiene, diet, clean water, disinfection with sulfur vapors, and burial of contaminated bodies outside city limits became commonplace during epidemic diseases of the Renaissance. Credit is also due to the French physician, Guillaume De Baillou (1538-1616), court physician to King Henry IV, who separated variola from meningoencephalitis, a pestilence which had severely afflicted the imperial armies of Holy Roman Emperor Maximilian II (reigned, 1564-1576).(34)

The theory of specificity of disease promoted by Paracelsus (of whom we will have more to say shortly) essentially substituted the theory of the "doctrine of signature" which had established that a medicament of nature by its external appearance had been endowed by nature with the proper qualities for the treatment of disease. For example, *digitalis* was discovered and used for heart ailments because of the shape and form of the leaves of the plant from which it was extracted. Botany and chemistry flourished in the search for natural remedies. Many treatises on therapeutics were published encompassing a compilation of all of the known Greek pharmacopoeia, and some even included the new Islamic additions. The old "science" of alchemy, which had been essentially forgotten in Europe during the late Middle Ages, was rediscovered and popularized during this time.

THE NONCONFORMIST: PARACELSUS

The main figure associated with the vivification of alchemy was the controversial Renaissance physician Paracelsus (Theophrastus Bombastus von

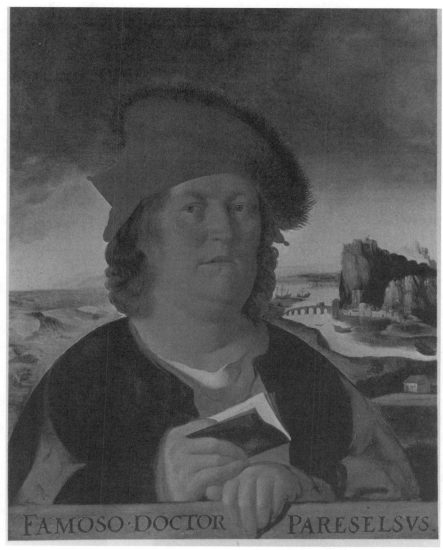

Plate 28 – Paracelsus (1493-1541). Theophrastus Bombastus von Hohenheim, the nonconformist. Musée du Louvre, Paris.

Hohenheim, 1493-1541), the son of a physician from the famed city of Basel, Switzerland, who fashioned himself, Paracelsus, "the equivalent of Celsus," after the celebrated 1st Century Roman physician. This very striking and controversial figure of the Renaissance blended not only magic with mysticism but also alchemy with medicine.

And controversial he was. A recent author writes, "[he came] out of the medieval haze...to leap directly into the bright noon of the Renaissance...." Yet he was said to have been censored for teaching in the vernacular, and even worse, "...he often could be found lecturing, roaring drunk in the lecture halls..." and forever battering the walls of the establishment.(39)

Nevertheless, Paracelsus has been praised for "sowing the seeds of dissatisfaction" in the medical establishment that forced medicine to break with its dogmatic past, and for inciting physicians to discover new theories for the etiology of diseases, and new remedies and surgeries for their treatment. He opposed the medieval reliance on the work of Galen and Avicenna; instead, he emphasized observation, experimentation, and empiricism in medical practice. He has been called the Father of Iatrochemistry for his discoveries of chemical substances, especially minerals, and their application in the practice of medicine. He challenged the traditional theories of the imbalance of the humours and the axiom of *Contraria-Contrariis-Curantur*. He fervently espoused the active intervention of the physician during the crisis of disease. He believed in simple Christianity and in the virtues of herbs and drugs as a product of God's creation, and affirmed that physicians do God's work.(40) Paracelsus was a proponent of the modern examination of the urine as opposed to the old, misleading science of uroscopy.(41)

Perhaps one of his major achievements is that of his regard for – and ultimate establishment that – the practices of surgery and medicine be placed on an equal footing.(2) In fact, in his clinical practice, he performed his own surgery, and thus he described himself as a doctor in medicine and surgery, helping to raise the status of his surgical colleagues as well as others who practiced both. There is no doubt that over the last 400 years his name has been rehabilitated, as most of the more recently written literature about him has emphasized his accomplishments, especially in iatrochemistry: the discovery of vitamins, the description and use of minerals such as arsenic, lead, mercury, iron, as well as tinctures and alcoholic extracts as remedies, etc.(40-42) Paracelsus was also the first physician to recognize the important pharmacologic principle that the dosage of a drug determines its toxicity *(hormesis)*.

Furthermore, his writings and aphorisms are currently very much in vogue. Some examples of his writings are exemplified in his advice to medical students, and as suggested by the writers J.P. Dolan and G.R. Holmes (43,44), may still be applicable today:

> *Prolix writing has no place in medicine; concise writing and great intelligence, brief treatises but great force – that is the standard by which the physician is measured. The longer the book, the less the intelligence; the longer the prescriptions, the poorer their virtue. Therefore, each physician should achieve great things by means of small things. For nature is so excellent in its gifts that...it better benefits a man to know one herb in the meadow without knowing what grows on it.*
>
> *It is better to know and to understand one remedy than to rummage through the great libraries of the monasteries, where of a thousand pages barely one is understood...nature does not call for long recipes.*

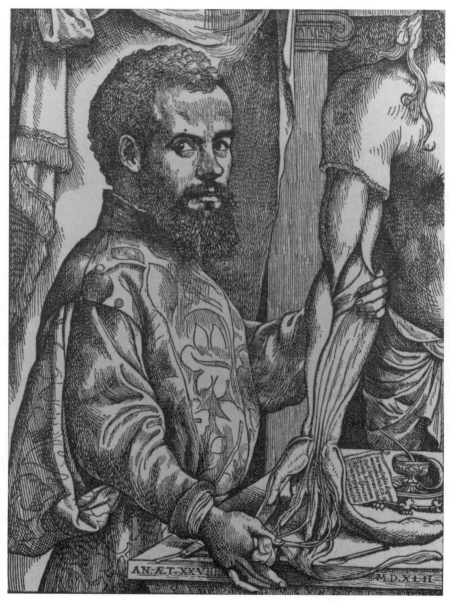

Plate 29 – Vesalius (1514-1564), the genius, at age 28 from his magnum opus, *De Humani Corporis Fabrica* (1543). World Health Organization, Geneva.

THE GENIUS: ANDREAS VESALIUS

If Paracelsus was the most controversial and impetuous proponent of the new learning of the Renaissance, Andreas Vesalius (1514-1564) was the greatest anatomist and medical scientist of his time. He was the beacon of medical genius in an island surrounded by an ocean of darkness (and ignorance). Along with Paré, the greatest surgeon of the Renaissance, the aforementioned physicians exemplified the spirit of the Renaissance at its best. In his *De Humani Corporis Fabrica Libri Septem (On The Fabric of the Human Body*, 1543), Vesalius gave the world one of Western civilization's greatest masterpieces.(45) As professor of anatomy at the University of Padua, he had ample opportunity for human dissection and anatomic studies that led to this monumental work. In *De Fabrica*, he laid the foundation for modern scientific anatomic investigation. The treatise also, for the first time, publicly contradicted and corrected previous anatomic concepts established and accepted as dogma since Galen's time.(1,2)

Though Vesalius revered Galen, he recorded what he observed in his anatomic dissections instead of accepting the inaccuracies and errors contained in the copied and recopied ancient manuscripts. With the publication of *De Fabrica*, Vesalius broke with conventional anatomic misconceptions which had gone uncorrected for 1300 years and thus literally revolutionized the field of anatomy. By actual dissection, Vesalius revealed simple truths that contradicted not only anatomic misconceptions but also philosophic notions. He challenged Aristotle's doctrine that stated that thought and personality were in the heart; Vesalius believed them to be a function of the brain.

Some of the truths that Vesalius revealed through his anatomic works were arrived at by simple observations. For example, he nullified the belief that men have one rib less than women which was assumed by the biblical account of the creation of Eve. Vesalius simply counted the ribs of male and female cadavers in the dissection room to reach that incontrovertible truth. In the same fashion, he also debunked the erroneous idea that men have more teeth than women.(46)

The illustrations in *De Fabrica* were not only precise and accurate but also genuine artistic masterpieces. Moreover, the illustrations were closely integrated with the text, making the book highly effective. Each body system was described with their organs and their interrelation and function. The chambers of the heart were described, and previous errors corrected (i.e., Galen's orifices between the chambers of the heart based on porcine anatomy were not confirmed). Nevertheless, Vesalius has been criticized for not giving proper credit to the artist, his friend John Stephen de Calcar, a student of Titian, who is presumed to have drawn those magnificent human skeletons used to illustrate the book, and for the unusual circumstances surrounding the publication of his work in Basel, Switzerland.(47,48) But in all fairness, Vesalius understood the value of his work as is well exemplified in his letter to Oporinus, his publisher and editor. Vesalius described in minute detail his painstaking work and outlined his instructions on how the woodcuts and text should be carefully handled by the publisher. He wanted the most accomplished publisher of the time to craft his masterpiece.(45)

The publication of Vesalius' monumental book led to a violent academic quarrel between the medical establishment, headed by one of the Renaissance's

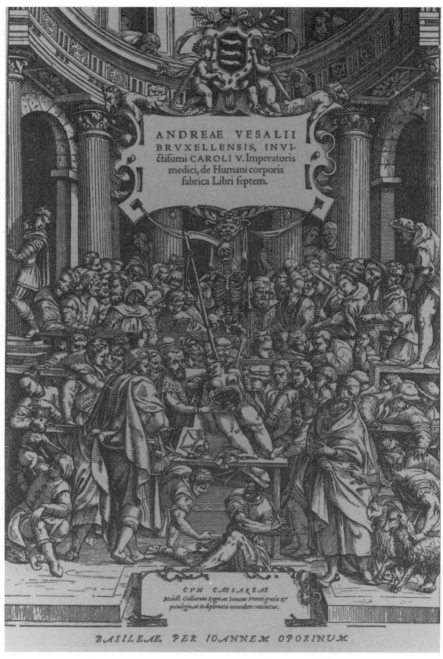

Plate 30 – Title page of Vesalius' 2nd Edition of the *De Humani Corporis Fabrica*, 1555.

great anatomist Jacob Sylvius (Jacob Dubois, 1473-1555), on one side, and the young Vesalius on the other. Sylvius followed Galen's teachings, whose anatomy he accepted without reservation, and could therefore not accept Vesalius's revolutionary findings. Vesalius's revelations were too much for the medical world even during this exalted period. The fuming controversy led Vesalius to relinquish his position as Professor of Anatomy at Padua. These developments were fortunately ameliorated by his temporary good fortune at being installed as personal physician to Holy Roman Emperor Charles V. When the Emperor retired, Vesalius became one of the physicians to his son, Philip II, King of Spain.

Sixtus IV (pope, 1471-1484) was the first prelate to openly approve human dissection. When the pious and immensely religious Emperor Charles V asked the faculty at Salamanca about the position of the Church on human dissection, he was told that an edict of the Church permitted it.(40) We know that anatomic human dissection was common both in Venice in 1552 and in Montpellier in 1556. At Montpellier, human dissections had been performed for years and as a medical student, Francois Rabelais (c.1490-1553) was documented to have dissected there in 1532.(34)

Nevertheless, human corpses for cadaveric dissection were difficult to obtain, and body snatching became a necessity even for conscientious anatomists. In fact, the quest for human corpses for anatomic dissection was such that anatomists were "forced to violate the sanctity of the grave and the threat of excommunication."(46) Vesalius recalled one night when even he remained hidden outside the city walls and then cut from the gallows the corpse of an executed prisoner to use for his cadaveric dissections. A Renaissance account related that Cosimo I de Medici (1519-1574), Grand Duke of Tuscany (1569-1574), offered Dr. Fallopio two condemned criminals for anatomic work. Allegedly, the Grand Duke told the professor, "kill them in any manner you wish and then dissect them."(46)

Vesalius's unhappiness was not to end with the controversy generated by his revolutionary findings but was to culminate with an even greater and more serious calamity. The story goes that he was to dissect the corpse of a Spanish nobleman who had died in his care. It was alleged that when he opened the chest, the heart was still beating! Some authorities deny this occurrence as an abominable calumny perpetrated by his many unforgiving enemies.(49) Nevertheless, following this unfortunate event or despicable fabrication, his life was endangered by the Inquisition. Again, he was saved by royal favor, and his penitence was to make a pilgrimage to Jerusalem where he lived in penance for many years. Vesalius finally decided to return to Padua, where he had again been offered a professorship, but he never made it back. He died on the Greek island of Zakymthos in 1564 during the return trip.(40) Vesalius is now considered the Father of Anatomy, and is warmly remembered for his anatomic masterpieces and scientific legacy.

THE INTREPID BARBER-SURGEON: AMBROISE PARÉ

Considered to be the greatest surgeon of the Renaissance, Ambroise Paré (1510-1590) was born in Laval in northern France. From his humble beginnings, this barber-surgeon elevated himself to a distinguished medical/surgical career at

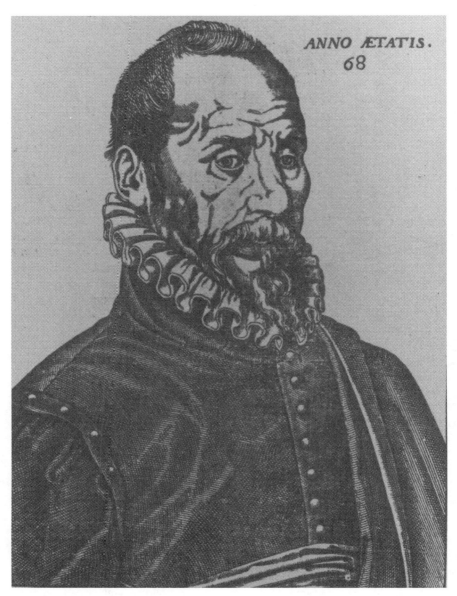

Plate 31 - Ambroise Paré (1510-1590), the greatest of Renaissance surgeons at age 68. Wood engraving (c.1582) unsigned, from the verso of the fourth lead of Paré's *Opera*, Paris, 1582.

the zenith of the Renaissance. Unassuming, compassionate, caring, and always adept at using common sense in medical practice, he came to be revered by royalty, nobility, and peasantry alike, and especially by the countless soldiers whom he treated amidst the wars in which he served as a military surgeon.

In 1533, at age 23, Paré went to Paris and trained as house surgeon at Hôtel Dieu, the first municipal hospital said to have been founded by St. Landry, the Bishop of Paris, in A.D.660.(50) There he performed cadaveric dissections and was taught by Jacob Sylvius, who had taught Vesalius at Padua, and as you will recall, had later become enmeshed in a medical dispute with Vesalius.

After completing his training, Paré was certified for the private practice of surgery, but his plans to commence private medical practice were suddenly interrupted when he was recruited by Colonel de Montejan, commander of the French infantry. Paré left for northern Italy, becoming an active participant in the Cisalpine Wars fought between the Holy Roman Emperor Charles V and the King of France, Francis I. It was subsequently on the battlefields of the various wars between the Habsburg Emperor and the Valois King of France that Paré was to gain most of his surgical experience and expertise for which he became famous. During this time, he not only tended wounds but also drained abscesses and reduced fractures.

It was in the Battle of Chateau de Villane, where the French sustained heavy losses during the siege and storming of the town of Turin, that one of Paré's most celebrated discoveries took place. It was said that he ran out of the boiling oil that was used to neutralize wounds contaminated with gunpowder.[176] That night, Paré improvised in the care of wounds by applying a salve of egg white, rose oil, and turpentine (the latter known today to be a bacteriostatic agent for certain bacteria such as *Escherichia coli* and *Staphylococcus aureus*).(50) The next morning, he got up early to check on his patients. He was worried about those he had not cauterized with the hot oil. But what he found was a different and surprising result. The soldiers who had been treated with his salve spent the night well and experienced less pain and inflammation than those treated with the boiling oil; the latter had experienced fever, swelling, and excruciating pain about their wounds during the night.

From then on, Paré felt that it was "cruel to burn poor people who had suffered shot wounds,"(51) and abandoned the surgical instructions then in vogue by the authoritative Juan de Vigo (c.1460-c.1525), a papal surgeon, who taught the traditional idea that gunshot was poisonous and thus recommended cauterization of gunshot wounds. Paré courageously went against the surgical establishment and practiced surgery guided by the dual principles of always placing the interest of his patient first in medical practice, and enlightened self-interest in his own life. After serving as military surgeon for two years with distinction, Paré was allowed to return to Paris. He bought a comfortable home on the Left Bank near the Mont Saint Michel, was married twice, and fathered several children, none of which survived infancy.

In 1541, Paré joined the College of Barber-Surgeons after passing its entrance examination. He wrote a dissertation on gunshot wounds which, not surprisingly, created an uproar since Paré insisted that gunpowder was not poisonous and that cautery with boiling oil in the treatment of wounds was harmful.(52) Nevertheless, his dissertation would be used by military surgeons as a guide for the

---

[176] Here we must remember that since its introduction from China to the West during the middle of the 13th Century, gunpowder was thought to be poisonous, thus aggressive treatment was deemed necessary for those shot on the battlefield.

treatment of wounds in subsequent wars. In 1549, he wrote a book based on the anatomic dissections of Vesalius, whom he greatly admired. In 1561, *Universal Surgery* followed, describing further refinements in surgical principles and techniques.(40)

Paré's surgical successes led to fame and fortune, but not to peace and tranquility. After King Francis I died in 1547, there were only a few years of peace between Emperor Charles V and the young King Henry II (1519-1559), son of Francis I. Paré was soon summoned for further service to his country. At the siege of Metz, he practiced trephination for head wounds and perfected his technique for amputation. Despite the rigors of war and the muddy and bloody circumstances of the battlefield, he remained committed to the care of his soldiers. He was obsessed with cleanliness, sanitation, and the general well-being of his patients; he even pre-scribed dietary regimes of hyperalimentation for the wounded.(50) On Christmas Eve, 1552, Emperor Charles V finally gave up the siege of Metz, complaining to his aids that "fortune is like the woman, she prefers the young King to the old Emperor."(39) Paré returned to Paris and was handsomely rewarded by the King with 300 gold crowns.

Within months after Metz, Paré found himself in another besieged town, Hesdin, where the situation was so hopeless for the French army that Paré, as an officer, voted with the majority to surrender and was imprisoned. Whilst in prison, he was obliged to treat the leg ulcers of his captor, Lord Vaudeville (1553). After an arduous but successful ordeal, Paré was released by the Knight and rewarded for his treatment with a trumpet-blowing escort to the camp of King Henry II who received the intrepid barber-surgeon with great fanfare.(39)

Paré was subsequently appointed "Surgeon In-Ordinary" to the King, but even with this royal honor, he resented the fact that within professional circles, he was no more than a Master Barber-Surgeon. This situation was corrected in 1554, when he passed a rigorous examination and was granted a license as a member of the Confraternity of St. Côme. We should recollect that in addition to the physicians and the barber-surgeons, there was in France the Confraternity of St. Côme whose members were designated Master Surgeons. This confraternity had been in perpetual conflict with the physicians, who frequently sided with the subservient barber-surgeons to oppose and check the influence of the Master Surgeons.[177] Paré was recruited by the confraternity with the backing of the King and, as previously stated, in 1554, was licensed as Master Surgeon. Though Paré's Latin was inadequate, he was recognized not only because of his popularity amongst royalty, nobility, and the common folk of France, but also because of his truly prodigious surgical knowledge and expertise.(50-54)

In his capacity as royal physician, Paré was invaluable to the reigning kings of France and served five successive French kings. It was Charles IX, King of France (d.1574), who protected Paré by hiding the surgeon in the royal bed dur-ing the infamous Huguenot's massacre that took place on St. Bartholomew's day, August 24, 1572. The massacre was allegedly orchestrated by the Queen Mother, Catherine de Medici (1519-1589), and perpetrated by Paris mobs on the occasion of the celebration and congregation of Huguenot leaders for the wedding of Henry of Navarre, the protestant leader.

Paré was also present at the tournament of St. Quentin on June 30, 1559,

---

[177] Sadly, another historic example of the age-old problem of petty rivalries, professional jealousies and thereof, divi-siveness amongst physicians.

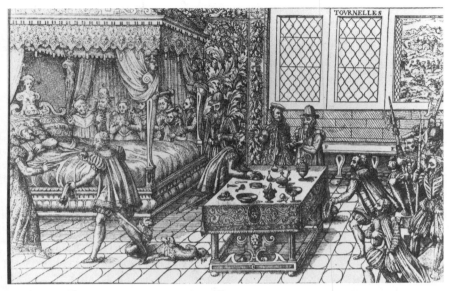

Plate 32 – The Deathbed of King Henry II (1519-1559) of France. Woodcut (c.1560) showing the royal family, and the physicians Vesalius and Paré in attendance. National Library of Medicine, Bethesda.

when King Henry II requested a joust with the dashing Comte of Montgomery, Captain of the Scottish Guard.(8) The King, who had previously been forewarned not to engage in jousts, nor in single combat, impetuously insisted on a second, and then a third joust with the younger opponent. The forewarning had been given in 1558 by the physician-turned-occultist, Michel de Nostradamus (1503-1566), in a famous quatrain:

> *The Lion shall overcome the old*
> *on the field of war in a single combat (duelle);*
> *He will pierce his eyes in a cage of gold*
> *This is the first of two lappings, then he dies a cruel death.(55)*

As prophesied, the King was mortally wounded in the third joust. The wooden lance of the younger opponent pierced the king's headgear, splintering, and blinding him in one eye.(8) Paré was consulted amongst other surgeons including Vesalius who was dispatched from Brussels by King Philip II of Spain, and the illustrious Spanish physician, Dionisio Daza Chacón (1510-1596), who had accompanied the celebrated Spanish general, the Duke of Alba (Fernando Álvarez de Toledo, c.1507-1582) as part of the royal entourage. But destiny had the last word, and Henry died 11 days later.

Henry II's children (by Catherine) also met short, unhappy ends: Francis II, husband of Mary Queen of Scots, died young (d.1560); Charles IX, the young king who hid Paré in his royal bed during the Huguenot's massacre, died at age 24 presumably of tuberculosis (1574); and Henry III, Paré's "fifth king," was stabbed by a demented monk in St. Cloud (1589).

For 30 years, Catherine ruled the affairs of state in France. With the accession of Henry of Navarre as Bourbon King Henry IV (reigned, 1589-1610), civil war intensified, and Catholic Paris rose in full rebellion against the Protestant king. The siege of Paris was led by the obstinate Archbishop of Lyons. At 80 and toward the end of his life, Paré was able to persuade the Archbishop to surrender and end the civil strife that was ravaging France. Henry's triumphant entry into Paris ended the religious wars. The King converted to Catholicism and to pacify the populace is said to have exclaimed, "Paris is worth a mass."(3,4)

As we have seen, like Vesalius, Paré never hesitated to wage war against obsolete methods of treatment even if it meant having to go against the medical establishment. His magnum opus, *Les Oeuvres* (*Collected Works*: first edition, 1575), was published when Paré was 65. In his *Works,* he described techniques for bladder operations, artificial eyes and limbs, the suturing of wounds, and other innovative surgical procedures which were also illustrated in considerable detail.(39,40,51) His *Works* went through several editions. In one of the later editions, he was censured by his dignified colleagues for not asking for their permission to include information from the Parisian medical society.

Paré also offended the establishment for vehemently condemning the use of "unicorn's horn," bezoars stones, and tissue from Egyptian mummies as pharmaceuticals. Even King Charles IX, Paré's "fourth king," was the proud owner of a bezoar stone. Bezoar stones were concretions found in the gastrointestinal tract of cows, goats, and other ruminants which were believed to be endowed with magical and medical power, and therefore were very expensive. When Paré argued with the

King and proved to him that his stone was worthless, the King replied that he must have had a forgery!(40) The sole effect of mummy powder and pulverized "unicorn's horn," Paré claimed, was "vomiting and stinking of the mouth." Moreover, he argued, "the ancient Jews, Egyptians, and Chaldeans never dreamed of embalming their dead to be eaten by Christians."(53)

Paré went on to describe prostatism as a cause of painful urination, and the effects of syphilis on arterial walls including the development of aneurysms. He showed midwives how to stop puerperal hemorrhaging. He advocated prompt caesarean section as soon as the mother died to save the unborn baby, and conversely, urged abortion to remove a dead fetus from a living woman.(56) He popularized the use of truss in the management of hernias.

Paré also showed great insight and common sense when, for example, he requested that a soldier's body be put in the same posture as when he was shot by a musket ball, to assess the trajectory of the projectile's path, and then palpating and removing the bullet. In regard to medicolegal reports, Paré writes:

> DEADLY WOUND. I, Ambroise Paré, have gone today on the order of the court of parliament to the house of X, Rue St. Germain with the ensign of S, and have found him in his bed having a wound on the left part of his head over the temporal bone with fracture. Several parts of this bone have broken through the two membranes and entered the substance of the brain. Therefore, the above-named had lost all consciousness with a convulsion, the pulse is very small, and the sweat cold. He neither drinks nor eats. I, therefore, certify that he will soon die. Testified by my seal, etc.
>
> ABDOMINAL WOUND RESULTING IN ABORTION. I, Ambroise Paré, have come on the order of the great Provost to the Rue St. Houbre, to the house of Mr. M., where I have found a lady called Margaret in bed with a high fever, convulsions, and hemorrhage from her natural parts, as a consequence of a wound that she has received in the lower abdomen situated three fingers below the umbilicus, in the right part, which has penetrated into the cavity, wounded and penetrated the uterus. She has therefore delivered before term a male infant, dead, well formed in all its limbs, which infant has also received a wound in his head, penetrating into the substance of the brain. Therefore, the above-named lady will soon die. Certified this to be true in putting my signature, etc.(46,57)

With this attention to detail, Paré was a forerunner to medical jurisprudence. Yet his greatest single contribution to surgical technique was perhaps the reintroduction of use of ligatures for controlling hemorrhaging during surgery, which was one of the most insoluble surgical problems of his day. Until then, the sole means available to stanch hemorrhage was the cautery iron which had been used extensively by Arabian physicians. Responding to the inquisitorial interrogation of the Parisian medical society, Paré retorted, "You say that tying up the blood vessels after amputation is a new method, and should therefore not be used. That is a bad argument for a doctor."(40)

Allow me, if only for a moment, to make another historic parallel. Despite Paré's unquestionable human compassion and medical charity, he expected and received just compensation and monetary remuneration for the toils of his exemplary career. If sainthood could be bestowed based solely on a person's earthly conduct and good works, then Paré is one person to deserve it – even and in spite of his acceptance of well deserved rewards. Like many of today's devoted physicians, Paré never rested, always gave of himself, and though amassing a small fortune, procuring property, and heading a loving and simple family, he never seemed to have had enough time to enjoy them.

And like Paré, the vast majority of physicians today are hard working, conscientious individuals who are devoted to their beneficent work and to their patients' best interest. Despite their share of altruism, physicians also tend to have an allotment of individualism which, unfortunately, makes them subject to the cardinal sin of professional jealousy. The damage of this truly cardinal sin cannot be overstated, for it greatly diminishes the image of the profession and causes great injury amongst physicians time and again.

Professional jealousy has afflicted the profession throughout the ages, and it is contributing today to the present decline in the image and prestige of the House of Medicine. It is also greatly facilitating, as I write these words, the divide-and-conquer tactic of medicine's adversaries. Sadly, envy and jealousy permeate today's society, even and in spite of the well known Commandment: "Do not covet your neighbor's goods." The corollary to this is, do not covet your peers' success, instead work hard, do your best, and be the best you can be providing for your patients. Paré, our intrepid barber-surgeon, provides a magnificent example of a Renaissance physician who perhaps should be emulated by today's physicians.

Common sensical and witty, many aphorisms are ascribed to Paré. For instance, "I bandaged him but God cured him," and "It is better to prescribe a dubious drug than to leave the patient without help." He also urged physicians to, "always give the patient hope even when death is near."(40)

Because of his advances in the discipline of surgery during the Renaissance, as well as his indomitable moral courage and great technical skills, Paré has been deservedly called "the Father of Modern Surgery."(49) Near death, Paré bequeathed to his family, "his wealth, property, and honor," and to his profession "a burning against mystification and the Ivory Tower."(39)

TOWARDS BLOOD CIRCULATION

Man is but a reed, the weakest thing in nature, but he is a reed that thinks.
Blaise Pascal (1623-1662)
French scientist, mathematician, and philosopher

Other important developments in medicine during the Renaissance include the bougies for strictures of the urethra (1541) and suprapubic cystostomy (1560).(34) The Renaissance also disproved the theory of *ordinary induction* which in essence said that the application of anatomy and physiology from animals to man may be assumed without verification. In fact, the same argument wrapped in different cloth goes on today in a slightly different setting (i.e., the significance of teratogenesis and carcinogenesis produced in laboratory animals following the administration of pharmacologic rather than physiologic doses of drugs, and the

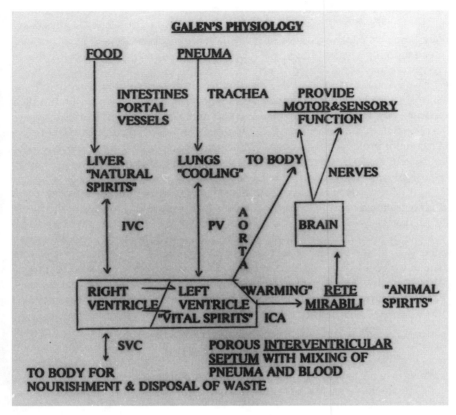

Plate 33 – Author's schematic representation of Galen's ebb and flow theory of the blood, assumed to be true for 14 centuries until Harvey's epochal discovery. IVC stands for Inferior Vena Cava; SCV for Superior Vena Cava; PV for Pulminary Vein; ICA for Internal Carotid Artery. The liver produces the blood from food and adds to it "Natural Spirits"; in the Left Ventricle (LV) blood is mixed with *pneuma* (air) and "Vital Spirits" are added; the rete mirabili at the base of the skull adds "Animal Spirits." The lungs possessed of *pneuma* cool the blood before sending it to the LV. Blood from the Right Ventricle (RV) mixes with the blood charged with *pneuma* in the LV. The latter warms the blood and sends it via the rete mirabili to the brain. The fully energized blood is then distributed throughout the body to provide motor and sensory function via hollow nerves.

induction or extrapolation of this data from animals to humans).[178] Even in this day and age of scientific research and investigation, it has taken us considerable human effort, money, and experimentation to reinvent this wheel – namely, to disprove ordinary induction and reaffirm the fact that the dosage of a drug determines its toxicity, as our predecessors had already demonstrated during the Renaissance.

As we have seen, the work of Andreas Vesalius nullified the erroneous anatomic assumptions based on animal dissections which had gone uncorrected for centuries. Likewise, the work of Miguel de Servetus (1511-1553), a Spanish physician and priest, helped to gather knowledge towards discovering the circulation of the blood. He speculated that blood was transferred from arteries to veins during passage through the lungs and discovered that it changed color during this mystifying passage. Servetus, unfortunately, was burned at the stake in Geneva for his heretical doctrine of the Holy Trinity. On the order of John Calvin, he was tried and sentenced to death, and it was said that the Inquisitors used green wood to prolong his agony and harrowing ordeal.(3) His books were also burned and destroyed with only a few copies remaining, retarding the precious acquisition of knowledge on blood circulation. Nevertheless, it was during this period that major pieces of the puzzle were put in place toward postulating a theory of the general circulation – paving the way for the crowning achievement of William Harvey (1578-1657; *De Motu Cordis*, 1628).

Florence King, a writer for *National Review*, advised in a memorable editorial that when in doubt, one should consult Aristotle. She is correct. From the time of classical Greece and until the time of Galen in the 2nd Century A.D., the authority on the blood vessels remained Aristotle. And it was based on the dissections of the Greek physicians Alcmaeon and Empedocles of Alexandria that Aristotle wrote his treatise, *Historia Animalum*, which not only differentiated arteries from veins, but also indicated the appropriate site of venisection for bloodletting.(58) Galen, of course, refined this knowledge, corrected errors of anatomy and physiology, and came close to discovering the circulation of the blood. His failure to reach a rational explanation for the function of the blood led to the ebb and flow theory of blood motion in the human body, and the abstruse concepts of the infusion of the various "spirits" in the blood as the latter moved to and fro in various organs. And so it was to be 14 centuries later, during the clamor of the late Renaissance, that medicine was fated to give birth to the theory of the circulation of blood.

Miguel de Servetus, Andreas Caesalpinus (1524-1603), and Realdo Colombo (1516-1559) all contributed various pieces to the puzzle, and came close to formulating theories of blood circulation. Both Servetus and Caesalpinus observed that blood was transferred from lung arteries to lung veins. Colombo, who took Vesalius' position at Padua after his resignation, confirmed that blood changed colors in the lungs and that Vesalius' observation regarding the absence of an interventricular orifice in the septum was correct. He also noted that there were no *rete mirabili* at the base of the brain in humans, as had been postulated by Galen and the ancients.

Fabricius de Aquapendente (1537-1619), another professor of anatomy at

---

[178] This argument also brings to the discussion the principle of *hormesis*, which of course dictates that the dosage is the key to whether a drug has beneficial or harmful effects. In other words, toxicity depends on the amount of a drug used during experimentation, so that the dose, in essence, makes the poison. Thereby, today's sensible movement toward the abolition of the obsolete Delaney Clause (1958) that dictates that any amount (even miniscule) of a substance shown to be carcinogenic in animals be banned from the food supply.

Padua, discovered the valves in the veins (1572) and hinted at some knowledge of the general circulation by his observation of unidirectional flow in extremity veins. It was he who inspired his student William Harvey to learn about blood motion.

Harvey went on to describe blood circulation in humans by simple observations, elegant experiments, and the use of mathematical calculations. By the use of simple tourniquets applied to the extremities, he deduced that blood flows toward the heart in veins, and away from it, in the arteries. Blood circulates by the action of the heart that serves as a pump. He calculated that at two ounces per stroke of the heart (one heartbeat), the amount of blood pumped per 24 hours would exceed 16 tons. The blood therefore had to circulate – via two systems, one, pulmonary, and the other, systemic – as it was inconceivable that this huge amount could be produced and dissipated in a 24-hour period.

As the reader will remember, the brilliant Dutch draper, janitor, and naturalist student Anton van Leeuwenhoek (1632-1723) invented the microscope during the late 17th Century at the closing phase of the Renaissance, amidst the "Century of Genius." With the microscope he discovered "animalcules," a living, teeming world of microorganisms including bacteria and protozoa. He dedicated his life to producing better and more complex (higher resolution) microscopes, whilst communicating with the Royal Society of London and the Parisian Academy of Sciences.

The Italian physician Marcello Malpighi (1628-1694) of Pisa, building upon Leeuwenhoek's discovery, used microscopy to observe the actual location of blood transfer from arterioles to venules, the *capillaries,* and along the way, also discovered the air sacs, the alveoli. Nevertheless, in our circulation-puzzle, we have to wait nearly a century for the genius of the aristocratic French chemist, Antoine Laurent Lavoisier (1743-1794), to solve the final conundrum of the circulation of the blood.

Though Harvey had correctly described the blood circulation and Malpighi had discovered the actual site of blood transfer in the capillaries of the lungs, the *raison d'être* for this circulatory system was still debated and remained unknown. It was not until the advent of the numerous discoveries in chemistry and physics of the 18th Century that the way was prepared for the proper placement of the missing piece in the puzzle of the circulation. In particular, gases had to be studied and their properties categorized.

Thus, in 1774 the English physician Joseph Priestley (1733-1804) isolated oxygen and demonstrated that "plants immersed in water give off oxygen." He also discovered that oxygen was essential for animal life.(59) Based on these discoveries, Lavoisier was able to explain the role of oxygen in animal metabolism, the *raison d'être* for the pulmonary circulation: gas exchange, oxygenation, and the release of carbon dioxide – the final act that fitted the last piece of the puzzle of the circulation had been accomplished.(60,61) Another giant step had taken place in medical history.

Unfortunately, the denouement of the drama of the circulation had a tragic ending for the final *dramatis persona*. At the peak of his discoveries and whilst still working on other chemical problems amidst the turbulence of the French Revolution, Lavoisier was accused of being an aristocrat by Jean Paul Marat (1743-1793), the radical Jacobin and the most fanatical physician of the French Revolution. Lavoisier was pronounced an enemy of the revolution and tried by the revolutionaries. Convicted by a radical tribunal, Lavoisier was hurried to the guillotine, complaining that he had not been given enough time to finish a paper on chemistry. He was summarily beheaded. Twenty thousand people were executed during this Reign of Terror in the name of *liberté, egalité*, and *fraternité*.(3) Lavoisier's friend, Joseph Louis Lagrange (1736-1813), a mathematical genius who had verified many of Newton's theorems, was more fortunate; he was admired by the revolutionaries. Lagrange, the man who invented differential calculus, exclaimed at the time of Lavoisier's sentencing with great historic insight, "it only took one moment to get rid of the head which took 100 years to produce."(60)

Let us now return to the period of our narrative, the Renaissance.... There are other Italian physicians and scientists who deserve our citation: Gabriello Fallopio (1523-1562), who also worked at Padua, and Bartolommeo Eustachio (1520-1574), who was in Rome, were two anatomists who were said to have initially ridiculed Vesalius but eventually joined his ranks. Their eponyms for structures that still bear their names (namely the fallopian and eustachian tubes) attest to their stature as Renaissance physicians. Moreover, Dr. Fallopio is credited in his *De Morbus Gallico*, published in 1564, with the first description of a condom. The device was introduced as prophylaxis against syphilis (*Lues venerae*) which was on the rise during the Restoration Period in England (1660) – a time of relative sexual permissiveness and court philandering following the puritanic rule of Lord Protector Oliver Cromwell (1599-1658) and the Interregnum 1649-1660.

The first successful documented case of a Caesarean section on a living woman also took place during the Renaissance. Delivery of a baby through an abdominal and uterine incision was coined a Caesarean or Cesarean (or C-section) from the mistaken belief that the Roman statesman Julius Caesar was delivered from his mother's womb in this fashion. But the fact is that his mother, Aurelia, was still alive and admired as a model of a Roman matriarch when the Roman statesman was 48 years old and at the pinnacle of his career, serving as Roman consul at that time. C-sections were performed then only after the death of the mother in a desperate effort to save the baby. Therefore, it is doubtful that Caesar was delivered by C-section. Centuries later, the Code of Justinian, as we have seen, expressly forbid the burial of a dead pregnant women without the operation being performed by a physician and the fetus removed. This practice was underscored during the Renaissance, when Paré again emphasized the urgency for a C-section as soon as the mother died to save the baby.(56)

The first documented Caesarean section was performed, not by a physician, but by a sow gelder and butcher named Jacob Nufer, who lived in the German village of Sigershufen.(40,42) He controlled the bleeding with hot irons as was commonplace at the time. This first documented successful Caesarean section (c.1500) was an isolated, individual act of desperation that miraculously succeeded. Even in the hands of skilled surgeons, the mortality rate for this operation remained extremely high (86-100%) and therefore out of the reach of most surgeons until the medical advances of the 19th Century.(40,42)

PHYSICIANS: SCHOLARS, POETS... MYSTICS

During this bedazzling period there were an inestimable number of Renaissance physicians who engaged in other activities as well as the practice of medicine. Some excelled in these avocations and achieved even greater fame and notoriety because of their work in those fields. Foremost amongst this group of physicians was Nicolaus Copernicus (1473-1543). A Polish physician, he was also an astronomer who revolutionized the concept of celestial motion. Busy as he was practicing medicine (he even helped combat a plague epidemic in Warmia in 1519)(62), Copernicus found time to make celestial observations and to formulate a revolutionary theory of planetary motions.(63)

In his *Revolutions Of The Heavenly Bodies* (1543), he refuted the theory of Claudius Ptolemy (2nd Century A.D.) which had gone unchallenged for over a millennium. Ptolemy's fixed but complex mechanical world gave way to an old concept which had been forgotten since classical Greece. Copernicus, building on this forgotten theory, proposed his heliocentric theory of the solar system which took Earth from its central position in the universe and in the process revolutionized astronomy.(62,64) Copernicus lived to see a copy of his magnum opus only on the day of his death, May 24, 1543, but confirmation of his theory had to wait until Newton's *Principia* in 1687.(62)

Francois Rabelais (1494-1553), priest and physician, earned his medical degree at Montpellier where he performed cadaveric dissections, and learned medicine, Greek, and Latin. Later, he lectured at Montpellier in anatomy and human dissection, and translated old Greek manuscripts into Latin.(34) Interestingly, the erudite Rabelais also composed bawdy satires and commented on the aphorisms of Hippocrates (Lyons, 1532). He wrote masterful narratives including the tales of *Pantagruel* (1532) and *Gargantua* (1534), in which he lampooned society, mocking the contemporary rules of conduct. He thus anticipated Moliere in the artful derision of ideas and institutions of the times.(3,4,5)

A great mystic and ethicist of this period was the English physician, Sir Thomas Browne (1605-1682). In his celebrated book *Religio Medici*, Browne expressed his innermost feelings and personal reflections whilst exploring the realms of religious mysticism, philosophic paradoxes, and early medical ethics. His style is solemn, whilst at the same time ornate; his yearnings imbued of humanity. At a time of civil strife in England, he wrote his book setting down concepts of religious tolerance, scientific principles, devotion to God and patients, and guidance in moral and ethical principles.

On the duty of imparting knowledge he observed:

> *To this (as calling my self a Scholar) I am obliged by the duty of my condition: I make not therefore my head a grave, but a treasure, of knowledge; I intend no Monopoly, but a community, in learning; I study not for my own sake only, but for theirs that study not for themselves. I envy no man that knows more than my self, but pity them that know less. I instruct no man as an exercise of my knowledge, or with an intent rather to nourish and keep it alive in mine own head then beget and propagate it in his: and in the midst of all my endeavours there is but one thought that dejects me, that my acquired parts must perish with my self, nor can be Legacied among my honoured Friends.(65)*

On the difference of opinions and the settlement of disputes, Browne commented:

> *I cannot fall out or condemn a man for an errour, or conceive why a difference in Opinion should divide an affection; for Controversies, Disputes, and*

argumentations, both in Philosophy and in Divinity, if they meet with discreet and peaceable natures, do not infringe the Laws of Charity. In all disputes, so much as there is of passion, so much there is of nothing to the purpose; for then Reason, like a bad Hound, spends upon a false Scent, and forsakes the question first started. And this is one reason why Controversies are never determined; for, though they be amply proposed, they are scarce at all handled, they do so swell with unnecessary Digressions; and the Parenthesis on the party is often as large as the main discourse upon the subject.(65)

And on the subject of charity and man's intimate knowledge of himself, he thus wrote:

Further, no man can judge another, because no man knows himself: for we censure others but as they disagree from that humour which we fancy laudable in our selves, and commend others but for that wherein they seem to quadrate and consent with us. So that, in conclusion, all is but that we all condemn, Self-love. 'Tis the general complaint of these times, and perhaps of those past, that charity grows cold; which I perceive most verified in those which most do manifest the fires and flames of zeal; for it is a virtue that best agrees with coldest natures, and such as are complexioned for humility. But how shall we expect Charity towards others, when we are uncharitable to our selves? Charity begins at home, is the voice of the World; yet is every man his greatest enemy, and, as it were, his own Executioner.(65)

Lastly, this dissertation would not be complete without expounding on Michel de Nostradamus (1503-1566). A French physician of Jewish descent, Nostradamus was born in the town of St. Remy to a family well versed in science and mathematics. As a young man, he took humanities courses in Avignon and attended medical school at Montpellier, graduating "with great *eclat.*"(55)

Originally intending to practice medicine, Nostradamus' life took a different direction when the plague of 1546 took the lives of his beloved wife and two children. After their deaths, he spent 3 years treating and attending other plague victims. The town of Aix was so grateful to him for his heroic efforts and devotion to his duties that they presented him with a modest pension.

After he remarried and resettled in Salon de Craux, Nostradamus became more secluded and began to have mystic experiences. These experiences culminated in visions of the future. He wrote these prophecies in the form of *Quatrains* which were short four-line verses composed in enigmatic form during periods of solitude. It was his belief that astrology and medicine were inextricably intertwined.

Nostradamus came to be occult consultant to Catherine de Medici (whose personal physician, incidentally, was Jean Fernel), and gained the favor of both the Queen and King Henry II. Amazingly, he was bestowed with great fame and honor after he predicted the death of Henry II (in itself a very dangerous act) in a famous quatrain composed in 1558. The reader will remember that King Henry II of France died in 1559 as a result of the injury that was predicted by Nostradamus in that celebrated quatrain.(55) Nostradamus also predicted the tragic fates of the three royal princes. Ultimately, he presaged his own time and date of death, on July 2, 1566.(55,66)

CHAPTER 32

EPILOGUE

Whosoever, aspiring, struggles on, for him there is salvation.
　　　　　Johann Wolfgang von Goethe (1749-1832), from Faust (1808)
　　　　　German Philosopher

History is a better guide than good intentions.
　　　　　Jeane Kirkpatrick (b. 1926)
　　　　　Former United States Ambassador to the United Nations

　　　　The explosion of ideas during the Renaissance created tidal waves of expanding knowledge that poured over the shores of the world for the next 300 years. These waves of knowledge flowed naturally into the "Century of Genius" in the 17th Century and the "Age of Reason and Enlightenment" in the 18th Century. Then, in the 19th Century, two of the greatest accomplishments in medical history bore fruition: the germ theory of disease and the discovery of general anesthesia. As we look back at the building blocks of medical knowledge, it is easy to recognize that the advances of the Renaissance were essential steps for the completion of these later discoveries, and ultimately, for the forthcoming and even greater achievements of medicine in the 20th Century.

　　　　As we have seen, the Renaissance represented a series of giant steps forward in the acquisition of medical and scientific knowledge in medical history. From the continuum of intuitive medicine of primitive communities to the complex scientific medicine of today's technologic society, the Renaissance represented a truly spectacular period in history.

　　　　Are there any lessons we can learn from the Renaissance that can be applied to the present state of affairs in the field of medicine? Certainly, in view of the seemingly insurmountable obstacles that the medical profession faces today, it is imperative that we look at our past for lessons that might be learned to avoid making old mistakes.

　　　　Perhaps it is to the advantage of today's practicing physicians to be as bold and as resourceful as their medical forefathers to confront successfully the health care problems of our own age. Escalating health care costs; misinterpretation of U.S. perinatal mortality statistics; the inflated numbers of people who are said to be uninsured (whether by choice or by inability to obtain health insurance coverage); the damage inflicted upon the medical profession by the many myths and misconceptions; the devastation wreaked by the litigation juggernaut upon the health care system – are all contributing factors fueling the health care crisis and tarnishing the image of a venerable profession which has served humanity honorably since time immemorial.

　　　　Of these, the adversarial litigious climate wrought by the litigation juggernaut in which physicians are compelled to practice and the looming threat of total government takeover of the health care industry are the two most imminent, mortal dangers presently facing the House of Medicine. The existence of private sector medicine as we know it and academic medicine independent of government are both in peril; both would likely be adversely affected by socialization and government control. Health care would likely deteriorate, that is, unless physicians rise to the occasion and act in concert to face the challenge. Make no mistake about it, these challenges must be confronted *vis-à-vis* with courage, ingenuity, and the perseverance of the Renaissance physicians of yore.

Modern physicians have their job cut out for them. They have the doubly daunting task of fighting to preserve the practice of medicine and the patient-doctor relationship, whilst at the same time educating the public to the fact that individual Americans must take responsibility for their own health. We are, after all, mere mortals prone to disease and destined to death. Detrimental effects to our health and/or disease processes are brought about and/or accelerated by leading unhealthy lifestyles and pursuing self-destructive behaviors. In a brief but now classic article, the medical writer Timothy B. Norbeck has convincingly argued how self-destructive behaviors and abusive, unhealthy lifestyles promote poor health and disease. He writes, "the wise old adage, 'an ounce of prevention is worth a pound of cure,' has gone down the drain," and brings to light the paradoxical situation that despite the punishment that we inflict upon ourselves in lives of self-indulgence and immediate gratification, when the time of serious disease, age-related infirmity, or even a terminal condition is upon us, we then cling tenaciously to life at any price. He cites figures that are astounding: "80% of illnesses can be linked to smoking, alcohol consumption, illicit drugs, poor diet, obesity, or sexual promiscuity. 4% of the people in the United States account for 55% of all hospital costs. 25-35% of Medicare funds are spent on 5-6% of enrollees who will die within a year. 85% of an individual's health care expenses occur in the last two years of life."(67)

Moreover, he bemoans, "even our children are becoming more sedentary...40% of children ages 5-8 already showing risk of heart disease...." Furthermore, on compliance with medical advice, he notes that adults who have been advised to participate in "vigorous 20-minute exercises three times a week" hardly ever comply. He argues, "instead of the expected 60% compliance rate, a paltry 8% is the actual figure." Meanwhile, "Americans are risking their health by eating too much fat, sugar, cholesterol, and salt, and not enough fruit, vegetables, and grain products."(67) Moreover, 1100 people die daily as a result of chronic tobacco use.[179]

Paradoxically these same Americans, says Norbeck, "have a fierce desire to live as long as possible – the cost be damned."(67) Meanwhile, the doctor, hospital, and health care system are blamed for spiraling health care costs. In fact, a whopping one-third of all health care costs is directly attributed to self-abusive and destructive lifestyles beyond the purview of medicine. Increased longevity and improved quality of life could therefore be accomplished by paying attention to dieting, exercising, and no smoking whilst at the same time cutting down health care costs without government rationing.(69)

To accomplish all of these essential objectives, it is imperative that physicians jolt their patients back to reality, and break the seductive spell of the sirens

---

[179] These figures, as we have seen, remain essentially unchanged in the latest statistics.(68) Data from the National Center for Health Statistics (1992) affirm that we have an epidemic of premature low-birth-weight infants (less than 2500 gms) in the context of rising teenage pregnancies (only 50% get the available prenatal care, whilst 20-40% of mothers of all ages continue to smoke despite the warnings of the Surgeon General, etc.). Illicit drug use and alcohol remain rampant in teenage mothers during their pregnancy.

singing the songs of the false security of "free, cradle-to-grave" health care. There is no free lunch. Physicians need to educate the public and their patients about what is really at stake in the battle for health system reform.

First, as leading members of their local communities, physicians must participate in the regional health care discussions to explicate the realities of the health care delivery system. They must also expose myths and misconceptions regarding health care and medical practice. They must also explain the true meaning and intention of such terms as the oxymoronic managed competition (lots of controls and bureaucracy, and little in the way of free market competition), employer mandates, and global budgets (price-fixing). Or the euphemistically styled, National Health Insurance, which is unadulterated single payer (government-run) socialized medicine.

Second, physicians must set aside time to educate their patients about the serious problems brought upon the health care system by the glut of attorney-litigators and the medical liability crisis. Questions should be answered, especially those centered on the true causes of spiraling health care costs (i.e., defensive medicine, the cost of high technology, etc.).

Third, physicians must also explain to their patients the benefits of preventive medicine, for as we have seen, the cost of health care and preventive medicine are two issues which are deeply interrelated. Moreover, physicians must allocate space in their waiting rooms for additional patient information and pabulum material for the consumption, thought, and reflection of their patients.

Studies by the Medical Association of Georgia have determined that there is a real need for patients to obtain information from their physicians about health system reform. And surprisingly, it seems that the majority of physicians are unaware of this. They also seem unaware of the tremendous resources accessible to them: Their own knowledge, the capacity to make available take-home literature for their patients, and the fact that patients want to know what their own doctors think about health system reform. [180] These assets, unfortunately, are not being properly utilized. What a shame! I hear that nothing frightens politicians more than physicians talking with and educating their patients about health care issues. In fact, a recent newspaper editorial described the situation as follows: "If all politics is local, the nation's 653,000 physicians are perfectly placed to influence the course of President Clinton's proposed plan as it winds its way through Congress in the coming months. About 3 million Americans enter doctors' offices daily, and many are likely to get an earful of health reform and an eyeful of American Medical Association brochures.... The White House isn't represented in doctors' offices, where even proponents of health care reform concede the battle could be won or lost."(70)

Physicians need to read and keep abreast of socioeconomic and political developments taking place in America, or they will be swept away by the current. Physicians need to awaken to the reality that there is a social, political, and cultural war that is being fought right now for the heart and soul of America. The battle for the socialization of the American health care delivery system is part of that war and must be seen from that perspective.

The American republic is in mortal danger, in a similar fashion as the Roman Republic was in the 1st Century B.C., and the Roman Empire, was later in

---

[180] According to a survey conducted by an independent firm for the Medical Association of Georgia, 85% of citizens want to know what their own doctors think about health system reform.

the last two and a half centuries of its parlous existence. We should remember the words of the illustrious Supreme Court Justice Louis D. Brandeis (1916-1939) who wisely proclaimed that "the most important office is that of the private citizen." It would be a mistake to underestimate the significance of this battle. The battle for the survival of the practice of medicine represents more than just a struggle between two diametrically opposed, sectarian factions attempting to dictate the mechanism of health care delivery. Even more importantly, philosophically, it symbolizes the titanic conflict between two rival ideologies: one that restores the sacrosanct patient-doctor relationship based on genuine medical ethics, preserves fee-for-service medicine, emanates medical care based on genuine trust and compassion, corroborates the sanctity of voluntarily entered private contracts and free associations, advocates free market incentives, and espouses civil liberties concomitant with individual responsibility.

The opposing view is one that represents the power of an increasingly omnipotent government, dictates medical practice and patient care, mandates coercive compassion, responds not to market forces but to the pressure exerted by special interest groups, and insists on statism and socialism so that our lives are stifled by government regulations and control. Yes, the American republic is in mortal danger. As the moment of reckoning approaches, let us not forget Dante's admonition: "the hottest place in Hell is reserved for those who, in times of great moral crisis, maintain their neutrality."(71)

If we are not successful in our efforts, our fate will be the catastrophic stumble and inevitable plunge down the bottomless pit of socialized medicine with the complete government takeover of the American health care delivery system, representing 14% of the GNP and one-seventh of the U.S. economy. The practice of medicine would then be dictated by the state, health care would inevitably have to be rationed, and in the not-too-distant future of a brave new world, we would likely be treated with government-sponsored, active euthanasia. This conflict thus represents a behemothic struggle that physicians and their patients cannot afford to lose.

If this book points to one salient fact, it is that medicine is a marriage of art and science. The public must recognize that even in the foreseeable future, physicians are not going to obtain 100% perfect results, ameliorate the human condition in every instance, or stop the pain of every soul that knocks on their doors. With compassion, however, ethical physicians can try their best, do their best – as they always have done throughout the ages. Thus, as we face the array of forces arraigned against medicine, physicians must garner all of their resources, energy, and intellect to preserve what is good and to correct the deficiencies. It will take truly Renaissance physicians of the highest order and courage to surmount the titanic hurdles in their path and repel the Vandal hordes massing for the final onslaught, eager to breach the gates, to pillage and plunder the traditional practice of medicine, and sap its substance. Unless physicians act now, the gates will surely fall.

I hope that if anything, this book will be an inspiration for the reader to look within, for his/her own Renaissance consciousness. We need this inspiration to guide us safely through the unchartered troubled waters in which the noble profession of medicine finds itself navigating. Make no mistake about it, all physicians must become involved or the profession as we have known it – independent and dedicated to patients and their well-being – will perish. The profession must not capitulate at this late hour by the sheer and mounting pressure of the lusting barbarian hordes. The gates must not fall, for it would mean the demise of the venerable medical profession and the abject betrayal of their patients' sacred trust.

Physicians and their patients – now educated and transformed into legions of informed and vigilant citizenry – must show the legislators that they will not stand idly by and allow the demoralization, disintegration, and eventual subjugation of Medicine, nor the government takeover of the American health care delivery system.

Physicians, patients...citizens: The world is watching. The future of the American health care delivery system rests in your hands.

We few, we happy few, we band of brothers;
For he to-day that sheds his blood with me
Shall be my brother; be he ne'er so vile
This day shall gentle his condition:
And gentlemen in England, now a-bed
Shall think themselves accursed they were not here,
And hold their manhoods cheap whiles any speaks
That fought with us upon Saint Crispin's Day.

> *Henry V (1387-1422)*
> *Speech to his army on the eve of the Battle of Agincourt in 1415, at the end of the Hundred Years War. The next day, the English army of long-bow men defeated a numerically superior force of heavily armored French knights.*
> *[from Henry V, William Shakespeare (1564-1616)]*

BIBLIOGRAPHY

PART ONE

1. Haggard, Howard W.: *The Doctor in History*. Reprinted in New York by Dorset Press, 1989.

2. *The Columbia Encyclopedia*. Columbia University Press (1989). Franklin Electronic Publishers, Inc., Mt. Holly, N.Y. 08060, 1991.

3. Tylor, Edward B.: *Primitive Culture*. New York, Henry Holt and Co., 1874.

4. Frazer, James G.: *The Golden Bough* (1890). Reproduced in New York by Avenel Books, Crown Publishers, Inc., 1981.

5. Cavendish, Richard (Ed.): *Man, Myth and Magic*. New York, Vol. I., M. Cavendish Co., 1970.

6. Mathews, Holly F.: "Rootwork: Description of an Ethnomedical System in the American South." *South Med J* 1987;80:885-390.

7. McWhorter, John H. and Ward, Steven D.: "American Indian Medicine." *South Med J* 1992;85: 625-638.

8. Accardo, Pasquale: "Dante and the Circle of Malpractice." *South Med J* 1989;82:624-628.

9. Sayers, D.L.: *The Comedy of Dante Alighieri, the Florentine. Cantica I Hell*. Penguin Books, Hardmondsworth, 1951.

10. Campbell, Joseph: *Transformation of Myth Through Time*. Public Media Video, Williams Free Productions and Mythology Ltd., Vol. I, Tape 2, 1989.

11. Leonardo, Richard A.: *History of Surgery*. New York, Froben Press, 1943.

12. Rifkinsn-Mann, Stephanie R.: "Cranial Surgery in Ancient Peru." *Neurosurgery* 1988;23(4):411-416.

13. Walker, A. Earl: *A History of Neurological Surgery*. New York, Hafner Publishing Co., 1967.

14. Stone, James L.: "Paul Broca and the First Craniotomy Based on Cerebral Localization." *J Neurosurg* 1991;75:154-159.

15. Budge, Sir Ernest A. Wallis (Trans.): *Tutankhamen: Amenism, Atenism and Egyptian Monotheism* (1900). Reprinted by Bell Publishing Co., New York.

16. Bloch, Harry: "Solartheology, Heliotherapy, Phototherapy, and Biologic Effects: A Historical Overview." *J Nat Med Assoc* 82(7):517-521.

17. *Ancient Secrets of the Bible*. TV Documentary produced by P. Klein and C.E. Sellier. SUN-PKO Productions, Inc., 1992.

18. Bucaille, Maurice: *Mummies of the Pharaohs: Modern Medical Investigations*. New York, St. Martin Press, 1990.

19. Lyons, Albert S. and Petrucelli, R. Joseph: *Medicine: An Illustrated History*. New York, Harry N. Abrams, Inc. Publishers, 1978.

20. *Plutarch's Lives*. The Dryden Translation. Random House, New York, 1984.

21. Tavallali, Morad: "Origins of the Rx Symbol: The Medical Legacy of the Egyptian God Horus." *Surgical Rounds* 1988;11(12):57-60.

22. Budge, Sir Ernest A. Wallis (Ed. and Trans.): *The Book of the Dead*. New York, Dover Publications, Inc., 1967.

23. Woodward, Theodore E.: "Religion and Medicine: An Ancient Relationship." *Maryland Medical Journal* 1989;38(7):568-572.

24. Goodrich, Norma L.: *Priestesses*. New York, Franklin Watts, 1989.

25. Metzer, W. Steven: "The Caduceus and the Aesculapian Staff: Ancient Eastern Origins, Evolution, and Western Parallels." *South Med J* 1989;82(6):743-748.

26. Goldfarb, Bruce: "Learning from Ancient Medical History." *Am Med News* 1986;(5):32-36.

27. Neuberg, M.: *History of Medicine*. London, 1910, 2 Vols. Trans. by Ernest Playfair. Cited by Leonardo, R.A.: *History of Surgery*, op.cit.

28. Adams, Francis (Trans.): *The Genuine Works of Hippocrates*. London, Sydenham Society, 1849.

29. Dolan, John P. and Holmes, George R.: "Some Important Epochs in Medicine." *South Med J* 1984;77(8):1022-1026.

30. Cumston, Charles G.: *The History of Medicine* (1926). New York, Dorset Press, 1987.

31. Brinton, C., Christopher, J.B., and Wolff, R.L.: *A History of Civilization*. 3rd edition, Vols. I & II. Englewood Cliff, New Jersey, Prentice-Hall, Inc., 1967.

32. Faria, Miguel A., Jr.: "Enemies of Private Medicine Bide Their Time." *Private Practice* 1992;24(9):33-34.

33. Wooley, Sir Leonard: *UR: The First Phases*. The King Penguin Books, London, 1946.

34. Cooke, J., Kramer, A., and Rowland-Entwistle, T.: *History's Timeline*. F. Franklin (Ed.). New York, Crescent Books, 1981.

35. Severy, Merle: "Iraq the Crucible of Civilization." *National Geographic* 1991;179(5):102-115.

36. Smith, U.: *Daniel and the Revelation*. Review and Herald Publishing Assn., Washington, D.C., 1905.

37. Clayton, Peter and Price, Martin (Eds.): *The Seven Wonders of the World*. Routledge, 1988. Reprinted in New York by Dorset Press, 1989.

38. Halford, John A. and Stump, Keith: *Babylon – Past, Present and Future* (1990). Pasadena, California. © 1991 Worldwide Church of God.

39. Creasy, Edward S.: *Fifteen Decisive Battles of the World* (1851). Reprinted in New York by Dorset Press, 1987.

40. Garrison, F.H.: *History of Medicine*. W.B. Saunders, Philadelphia, 1913, 4th edition, 1929. Cited by Leonardo, R.A.: *History of Surgery*, op.cit.

41. Hart, Michael H.: *The 100 – A Ranking of the Most Influential Persons in History*. Citadel Press Books, Carol Publishing Group Edition, 1989.

42. Topping, Audrey and Yang, Hsien-Min: "The First Emperor's Army – China's Incredible Find." *National Geographic* 1977;(3):293-311.

43. Fitzhenry, Robert I. (Ed.): *Barnes and Nobles – Book of Quotations*. New York, Harper and Row Publishers, 1987.

44. *Parade Magazine*: "Our Best Books." December 29, 1991, p.20.

45. Parrinder, Geoffrey (Ed.): *World Religions – From Ancient History to the Present* (1971). Reprinted by Facts on File Publications, New York, 1984.

46. *The World Almanac and Book of Facts*. 114th Year Special Edition. Newspaper Enterprise Association, Inc., New York, 1982.

47. Jaggard, Robert S.: "Which Moral Code Do You Choose." *Iatrofon,* Vol. 7, No.2, December 1987.

PART TWO

1. *The Columbia Encyclopedia*. Columbia University Press (1989). Franklin Electronic Publishers, Inc., Mt. Holly, N.Y. 08060, 1991.

2. Brinton, C., Christopher, J.B., and Wolff, R.L.: *A History of Civilization*. 3rd edition, Vols. I & II. Englewood Cliff, New Jersey, Prentice-Hall, Inc., 1967.

3. Woodward, Theodore E.: "Religion and Medicine: An Ancient Relationship." *Maryland Medical Journal* 1989;38(7):568-572.

4. Metzer, W. Steven: "The Caduceus and the Aesculapian Staff: Ancient Eastern Origins, Evolution, and Western Parallels." *South Med J* 1989;82(6):743-748.

5. Carver, Lou: "The True Symbol of Medicine: One Snake or Two?" *J Med Assoc Ga* 1989;76: 809-810.

6. Friedlander, Walter J.: *The Golden Wand of Medicine: A History of the Caduceus Symbol in Medicine.* Westpoint, Connecticut, Greenwood Press, 1992.

7. Geelhoed, Glenn W.: "The Caduceus as a Medical Emblem: Heritage or Heresy?" *South Med J* 1988;81(9):1155-1162.

8. Meade, James W.: "Letter to the Editor – the Symbol of Medicine." *JAMA* 1989;262(13):1771.

9. Michael, Ronald: "Letter to the Editor – the Symbol of Medicine." *JAMA* 1989;262(13):1771.

10. Smith, Dennis M.: "Letter to the Editor – the Symbol of Medicine." *JAMA* 1989;262(13):1771.

11. Vincent, L.M.: "Letter to the Editor – The Caduceus." *South Med J* 1989;82(11):1454-1455.

12. Eich, W. Foster: "Letter to the Editor – The Caduceus." *South Med J* 1989;82(11):1455.

13. Parrish, D.O.: "The Symbol of Medicine: One Snake, Not Two." *JAMA* 1989;261:3412.

14. Hæger, Knut: *The Illustrated History of Surgery.* New York, Bell Publishing Co., 1988.

15. Faria, Miguel A., Jr.: "The Litigation Juggernaut – Part I: The Dimensions of the Devastation." *J Med Assoc Ga* 1993;82(8):393-398.

16. Faria, Miguel A., Jr.: "The Litigation Juggernaut – Part II: Strategies and Tactics for Victory." *J Med Assoc Ga* 1993;82(9):447-451.

17. Schiller, Francis: "The Inveterate Paradox of Dreaming." *Archives of Neurology* 1985;42:903-908.

18. Aristotle: *De Insomniis* in D. Ross (Ed.): *Parva Naturalia.* Oxford, England, Clarendon Press, 1955, p. 266-280.

19. Hippocrates: On Dreams in W.H.S. James (Trans.): *Hippocrates.* Cambridge, Mass., Harvard University Press 1959;4:422-427.

20. Galenus, Claudius (Galen): *De Dignitione ex Insomniis* in C.G. Kühn (Ed.) *Opera Omni,* Leipzig, Germany, Knobloch, 6:832-835, 16:219-223 and 19:32, 1824.

21. Freud, Sigmund: *The Interpretation of Dreams.* New York, Avon Books, 1953.

22. Cooke, J., Kramer, A., and Rowland-Entwistle, T.: *History's Timeline.* F. Franklin (Ed.). New York, Crescent Books, 1981.

23. Clayton, Peter and Price, Martin (Eds.): *The Seven Wonders of the World.* Routledge 1988. Reprinted in New York by Dorset Press, 1989.

24. Harvey, Douglas and Fehrenbacher, Don E. (Eds.): *The Illustrated Biographical Dictionary.* New York, Dorset Press (3rd edition), 1990.

25. Welch, Robert: "Republics and Democracies." *The New American,* June 30, 1986.

26. Brownell, D. and Conkle, N: *Great Lawyers.* Bellerophon Books, Santa Barbara, CA., 1988.

27. Sagan, Carl: *Cosmos.* New York, Random House, 1980.

28. Herodotus: *The Histories.* A. De Selincourt (Trans.), Penguin Books. Cited by Brinton, Christopher and Wolff: *A History of Civilization,* op.cit.

29. Thucydides: *History of the Peloponnesian War.* T. Hobbs (Trans.) and R. Schlatter (Ed.). New Brunswick, Rutgers University Press, 1975.

30. Haggard, Howard W.: *The Doctor in History.* Reprinted in New York by Dorset Press, 1989.

31. Cumston, Charles G.: *The History of Medicine* (1926). New York, Dorset Press, 1987.

32. Dolan, John P. and Holmes, George R.: "Some Important Epochs in Medicine." *South Med J* 1984;77(8):1022-1026.

33. Hart, Michael H.: *The 100 – A Ranking of the Most Influential Persons in History.* Citadel Press Books, Carol Publishing Group Edition, 1989.

34. Plato: *Five Great Dialogues*. B. Jowett (Trans.) and L.R. Loomis (Ed.). Roslyn, New York, Walter J. Block, Inc., 1941.

35. Benatar, S.R.: "Traditional and Evolving Concepts in Medical Ethics." *Medicine and Law* 1989;7:423-426.

36. Aristotle: *On Man in the Universe*. L.R. Loomis (Ed.). Roslyn, New York, Walter J. Block, Inc., 1943.

37. Prindle, Robert F.: "Disinfection – Yesterday and Today." *Resident and Staff Physician* 1977;100:1s-11s.

38. Faria, Miguel A., Jr.: *The Forging of the Renaissance Physician*: "The Philosophic Basis for Pre-Renaissance Medical Knowledge." *J Med Assoc Ga* 1992;81(3):124-126.

39. Robinson, V.: *The Story of Medicine*, New York, 1931. Cited by Leonardo, R.A.: *History of Surgery*, op.cit.

40. Osler, William: "The Evolution of Modern Medicine – Galen's Written Works." Silliman Foundation. Yale University, New Haven Connecticut, April 1913. Reproduced in *JAMA* 1988;260:318.

41. Celsus, Aulus C: *De Medicina*. W.G. Spencer (Trans.) 3 Vols., London, W. Heinemann, 1935-38.

42. Norman, Jeremy M. (Ed.): *Morton's Medical Bibliography* (5th edition). Garrison and Morton, Scolar Press. Gower Publishing Co. Printed in Great Britain at the University Press, Cambridge, 1983.

43. Leonardo, Richard A.: *History of Surgery*. New York, Froben Press, 1943.

PART THREE

1. Brinton, C., Christopher, J.B., and Wolff, R.L.: *A History of Civilization*. 3rd edition, Vols. I & II. Englewood Cliff, New Jersey, Prentice-Hall, Inc., 1967.

2. Virgil: *The Aeneid*. Washington Square Press, Inc., New York, 1965.

3. Goodrich, Norma L.: *Priestesses*. New York, Franklin Watts, 1989.

4. Cavendish, Richard (Ed.): *Man, Myth and Magic*. New York, Vol. I., M. Cavendish Co., 1970.

5. Altman, Alexander: *Studies in Religious Philosophy and Mysticism*. Ithaca, 1969. Cited by N.L. Goodrich in *Priestesses, op.cit.*

6. Metzer, W. Steven: "The Caduceus and the Aesculapian Staff: Ancient Eastern Origins, Evolution, and Western Parallels." *South Med J* 1989;82(6):743-748.

7. *The Columbia Encyclopedia*. Columbia University Press (1989). Franklin Electronic Publishers, Inc., Mt. Holly, N.Y. 08060, 1991.

8. Strabo: *Geographia*. 8 Vols. Germaine Aujac (Trans.), Introduction by G. Aujac and Francois Laserne, Paris, 1969. Cited by N.L. Goodrich in *Priestesses, op.cit.*

9. Welch, Robert: "Republics and Democracies." *The New American*, June 30, 1986.

10. Grant, Michael: *The Roman Emperors, A Biographical Guide to the Rulers of Imperial Rome 31BC-AD476*. New York, Charles Scribners Sons, 1985.

11. Fitzhenry, Robert I. (Ed.): *Barnes and Nobles – Book of Quotations*. Harper and Row Publishers, New York, 1987.

12. Harvey, Douglas and Fehrenbacher, Don E. (Eds.). *The Illustrated Biographical Dictionary*. New York, Dorset Press (3rd edition), 1990.

13. Dirckx, John H.: "Virgil and Medicine," *JAMA* 1981;246(12):1326-1329.

14. Livy quoted by William Norman Grigg in "Trial by the Mob," *The New American*, May 31, 1993.

15. Suetonius: *The Twelve Caesars*. Robert Graves (Trans.) and Michael Grant (Ed.). Penguin Books, London, 1979.

16. Cicero, Marcus T.: *Oratory and Orators*. Guthrie (Trans.). London, England, Wright Printer, 1808.

17. Cicero, Marcus T.: *General Letters*. W. Melmoth (Trans.). S. Hamilton, London, Weybridge, Surrey Printers, 1814.

18. Norman, Jeremy M. (Ed.): *Morton's Medical Bibliography* (5th edition). Garrison and Morton, Scolar Press. Gower Publishing Co. Printed in Great Britain at the University Press, Cambridge, 1983.

19. Spivack, Betty S.: "A.C. Celsus: Roman Medicus." *J Hist Med Allied Sci*, 1991, p. 143-157.

20. Jones, W.H.S.: Introduction in Celsus *De Medicina*. 3 Vols. W.G. Spencer (Ed. and Trans.). Cambridge, Massachusetts: Loeb Classical Library, Harvard University Press, 1935. Cited in Spivack, B.S.: "A.C. Celsus: Roman Medicus," op.cit.

21. Pliny: *Natural History*. 10 Vols. H. Rockham, W.H.S. Jones, D.E. Eichholz (Eds. and Trans.). Cambridge, Massachusetts: Loeb Classical Library, Harvard University Press, 1938-1963. Cited in Spivack, B.S.: "A.C. Celsus: Roman Medicus," op.cit.

22. Hart, Michael H.: *The 100 – A Ranking of the Most Influential Persons in History*. Citadel Press Books, Carol Publishing Group Edition, 1989.

23. Grant, Michael: *The Twelve Caesars*. New York, Charles Scribners Sons, 1975.

24. Gibbon, Edward: *The Decline and Fall of the Roman Empire*. New York, The Heritage Press, 1946.

25. Rice, Charles E.: "Gifts from God – Basic Rights Transcend the State!" *The New American* 1993;(5):21-26.

26. Creasy, Edward S.: *Fifteen Decisive Battles of the World* (1851). Reprinted in New York by Dorset Press, 1987.

27. Cartwright, Frederick F. and Biddiss, Michael D.: *Disease and History* (1972). Reprinted in New York by Dorset Press, 1991.

28. Ferrill, Arthur: *The Fall of the Roman Empire: The Military Explanation*. Thames and Hudson, London, 1986.

29. MacMullen, Ramsey: *Corruption and the Decline of Rome*. New Haven, Connecticut, Yale University Press, 1988.

30. Thornton, Fr. James: "Crumbling from Within." *The New American* 1991;7(24):23-29.

31. Beedham, Brian: "A Better Way to Chose." *The Economist* (150 Economists Years Special Edition), 11th Sept.1993, p.5-7.

32. Putnam, John J.: "Switzerland – the Clockwork Country." *National Geographic* 1986;169(1): 96-127.

33. Bastiat, Frederic: *The Law* (1850). The Foundation for Economic Education, Inc., Irvington-on-Hudson, New York, 1990.

34. The Tax Foundation: "Taxes Based on the Proposed Fiscal 1993 Federal Budget."

35. McManus, John F.: "Examining the Rule of Law." *The New American*, June, 1991.

36. Dye, T.R. and Zeigler, L.H.: *The Irony of Democracy – An Uncommon Introduction to American Politics*. Duxbury Press, Wadsworth Publishing Co., Inc., Belmont, CA., 1971.

37. Lee, Robert W.: "Collectivist Clichés." *The New American*, July 13, 1992.

38. Fowler, W. Warde: *Julius Caescr and the Foundation of the Roman Imperial System*. G.P. Putnam and Sons, New York, The Knickerbocker Press, 1902.

39. Balsdon, J.P.V.D.: *Julius Caesar – A Political Biography*. Atheneum, New York, 1967.

40. Eidsmore, J.: "The Bill of Rights – Securing that which is God-Given." *The New American* 1991;26(7):21-28.

41. Pomeroy, Susan B.: *Goddesses, Whores, Wives and Slaves – Women in Classical Antiquity*. New York, Schocken Books, 1975.

42. Davis, Philip G.: "The Goddess and the Academy." *Academic Questions* 1993;6(4):49-66.

43. deBeer, Sir Gavin: *Hannibal – Challenging Rome's Supremacy*. New York, Viking Press, 1969.

44. Cooke, J., Kramer, A., and Rowland-Entwistle, T.: *History's Timeline*. F. Franklin (Ed.). New York, Crescent Books, 1981.

45. Wells, H.G.: *The Outline of History*. Vol.1. Garden City Books, New York, 1949.

46. Churchill, Winston S.: *A History of the English Speaking Peoples*, Vol.1: The Birth of Britain, 1956. Reprinted in New York by Dorset Press, 1990.

47. Stump, Keith W.: *Europe and the Church*. Worldwide Church of God, Pasadena, CA., 1983.

48. Halford, John A.: *Introduction to Prophecy*. Worldwide Church of God, 1989.

49. Sade, Robert M.: "The Clinton Health Care Plan – Implications for Medicine in the Future." *J Med Assoc Ga* 1993;82(12):667-671.

50. Moffit, Robert: "Comparable Worth for Doctors – A Severe Case of Government Malpractice." The Heritage Foundation, Washington, D.C., 1991.

51. Orient, Jane: *AAPS News*, June, 1991.

52. Goodgame, Dan: "Ready to Operate." *Time,* September 20, 1993, p.54-58.

53. "American Survey – Kill or Cure?", *The Economist,* September 25, 1993, p.31-32.

54. Congressman Fortney "Pete" Stark quoted in *The Macon Telegraph*, September 23, 1993.

55. Faria, Miguel A., Jr.: "On the True Numbers of the Uninsured." *J Med Assoc G*a 1993;82(5): 203-204.

56. Faria, Miguel A., Jr.: "The Litigation Juggernaut – Part I: The Dimensions of the Devastation." *J Med Assoc Ga* 1993;82(8):393-398.

57. Faria, Miguel A., Jr.: "The Litigation Juggernaut – Part II: Strategies and Tactics for Victory." *J Med Assoc Ga* 1993;82(9):447-451.

58. Faria, Miguel A., Jr.: "Crisis in Health Care Delivery – Rescuing Medicine From the Clutches of Government." *J Med Assoc Ga* 1992;81(11):615-620.

59. The Health Security Act of 1993.

60. Goodman, William E.: "Health Care in Canada: Face to Face with Reality." *J Med Assoc Ga* 1993;82(12):647-649.

61. O'Rourke, P.J.: "Health Reform: A License to Kill." *Wall Street Journal*, September 23, 1993.

62. Olson, Walter K.: *The Litigation Explosion – What Happened When America Unleashed the Lawsuit*. Truman-Talley Books, Dutton, New York, 1991.

63. McManus, John F.: "America's Vanishing Liberty – Onerous Federal Regulations are Turning our Republic into a Dictatorship." *The New American* 1993;9(10):5-8.

64. Lee, Robert W.: "Regulatory Attack – It's Killing Our Economy and Enslaving Our Nation." *The New American* 1992;8(9):21-28.

65. Faria, Miguel A., Jr.: "Enemies of Private Medicine Bide Their Time." *Private Practice* 1992;24(9):33-34.

66. Lee, Robert W.: "A Law Unto Itself." *The New American* 1993;9(10):65-66.

67. Faria, Miguel A., Jr.: "On the Liability Crisis and the Glut of Litigators." *J Med Assoc Ga* 1993;82(4):155-157.

68. Hoar, William P.: *Our Corrupt Congress*. Soundview Publications, Dunwoody, Ga., 1992. Cited in *The New American*, November 2, 1992.

69. Rusher, William A.: *The Coming Battle for the Media: Curbing the Power of the Media Elite*. William Morrow and Co., Inc., New York, 1988.

70. Irvine, Reed and Kincaid, Cliff: *Profiles of Deception – How the News Media are Deceiving the American People.* Book Distributors, Inc., New York, 1990.

71. Harvard Medical Practice Study Group: "Patients, Doctors and Lawyers: Medical Injury, Malpractice Litigation, and Patient Compensation in New York." Report to the State of New York, 1990.

72. Norbeck, Timothy B.: "Telling the Truth about Rising Health Care Costs." *Private Practice,* February 1990.

73. Burckhardt, Jacob: *The Age of Constantine the Great.* Moses Hadas (Trans.). Pantheon Books, 1949. Reprinted in New York by Dorset Press, 1989.

74. Friedlander, Walter J.: "On the Obligation to Treat AIDS: Is There a Historical Basis?" *Review of Infectious Disease* 1990;12(2):191-203.

75. Bettenson, H.(Ed.): *Documents of the Christian Church.* New York, 1947, p. 140. Cited by Brinton, Christopher, and Wolff: *A History of Civilization,* op.cit.

76. Sagan, Carl: *Cosmos.* Random House, Inc., New York, 1980.

77. Roberts, Wess: *Leadership Secrets of Attila the Hun.* Warner Books, New York, 1987.

78. Brownell, D. and Conkle, N.: *Great Lawyers.* Bellerophon Books, Santa Barbara, CA., 1988.

79. Thornton, Fr. James: "The Barbarians are Back." *The New American,* July 16, 1990, p.41-42.

80. Panati, Charles: *Extraordinary Endings of Practically Everything and Everybody.* New York, Harper and Row Publishers, 1989.

81. Downey, Glanville: *Constantinople in the Age of Justinian.* University of Oklahoma Press (1960). Reprinted in New York by Dorset Press, 1991.

82. Payne, Robert: *The History of Islam* (1959). New York, Dorset Press, 1990.

83. Craig, Charles F. and Faust, Ernest C.: *Clinical Parasitology.* Lea and Febiger, Philadelphia, 1941, pp.621-628.

84. Kirkland, Larry R.: The Black Death – A Primer and a Critique. *Emory Univ J Med* 1991;5(3): 169-175.

85. Haggard, Howard W.: *The Doctor in History.* Reprinted in New York by Dorset Press, 1989.

86. Cumston, Charles G.: *The History of Medicine* (1926). New York, Dorset Press, 1987.

PART FOUR

1. Faria, Miguel A., Jr.: *The Forging of the Renaissance Physician*: "The Influence of Hippocrates, Galen and the Islamic Physicians" and "The Philosophic Basis for Pre-Renaissance Medical Knowledge." *J Med Assoc Ga* 1992;81(3):119-126.

2. Adams, Francis (Trans.): *The Genuine Works of Hippocrates.* London, Sydenham Society, 1849.

3. Cumston, Charles G.: *The History of Medicine* (1926) New York, Dorset Press, 1987.

4. Richardson, Daniel D., Gray, Stephen W., and Skandalakis, John E.: "The History of the Small Bowel." *J Med Assoc Ga* 1991;80(8):439-443.

5. Bloch, Harry: "Solartheology, Heliotherapy, Phototherapy, and Biologic Effects: A Historical Overview." *J Nat Med Assoc* 82(7):517-521.

6. Edelstein, Ludwig: *The Hippocratic Oath – Text, Translation and Interpretation.* The Johns Hopkins Press, Baltimore, 1943.

7. Veith, Ilza: "Medical Ethics Throughout the Ages." *Quarterly Bulletin Northwestern University Medical School* 1957;31:351-358.

8. Faria, Miguel A., Jr.: "Crisis in Health Care Delivery – Rescuing Medicine from the Clutches of Government." *J Med Assoc Ga* 1992;81(11):615-620.

9. Tanner, Michael: *Getting Off the Critical List – A Prescription for Health Care Reform in Georgia.* Georgia Public Policy Foundation, Inc., Atlanta, GA., 1992.

10. Goodman, John C. and Musgrave, Gerald L.: *Patient Power – Solving America's Health Care Crisis.* Cato Institute, Washington, D.C., 1992.

11. Haggard, Howard W.: *The Doctor in History.* Reprinted in New York by Dorset Press, 1989.

12. Walsh, Joseph: "Refutation of the Charges of Cowardice Made Against Galen." *Annals Medical History* 1931;3:195-208.

13. Hæger, Knut: *The Illustrated History of Surgery,* Bell Publishing Co., New York, 1988.

14. Bunting, Bruce W. and Stanfield, James L.: "Bhutan: Kingdom in the Clouds." *National Geographic* 1991;179(5): 79-101.

15. Newman, Art: *The Illustrated Treasury of Medical Curiosa.* New York, McGraw Hill Book Co., 1988.

16. Lyons, Albert S. and Petrucelli, R. Joseph: *Medicine: An Illustrated History.* New York, Harry N. Abrams, Inc. Publishers, 1978.

17. Osler, William: "The Evolution of Modern Medicine – Galen's Written Works." Silliman Foundation. Yale University, New Haven Connecticut, April 1913. Reproduced in *JAMA* 1988;260:318.

18. Faria, Miguel A., Jr.: "To Treat or Not – Can a Physician Choose?" *The Pharos* 1992;55(1):39-40.

19. Fox, Daniel M.: "The Politics of Physicians' Responsibility in Epidemics: A note on History." *Hastings Center Report,* April-May, 1988.

20. Friedlander, Walter J.: "On the Obligation to Treat AIDS: Is There a Historical Basis?" *Review of Infectious Disease* 1990;12(2):191-203.

21. Thucydides: *History of the Peloponnesian War.* T. Hobbs (Trans.) and R. Schlatter (Ed.). New Brunswick, Rutgers University Press, 1975.

22. O'Flaherty, Jennifer: "The AIDS Patient: A Historical Perspective in the Physician's Obligation to Treat." *The Pharos* 1991;54(3):13-16.

23. Panati, Charles: *Extraordinary Endings of Practically Everything and Everybody.* New York, Harper and Row Publishers, 1989.

24. Aurelius, Marcus: *Meditations.* G. Long (Ed.). Roslyn, New York, Walter J. Block, Inc., 1945.

25. Hart, Michael H.: *The 100 – A Ranking of the Most Influential Persons in History.* Citadel Press Books, Carol Publishing Group Edition, 1989.

26. *The Columbia Encyclopedia.* Columbia University Press (1989). Franklin Electronic Publishers, Inc., Mt. Holly, N.Y. 08060, 1991.

27. Harvey, Douglas and Fehrenbacher, Don E. (Eds.): *The Illustrated Biographical Dictionary.* New York, Dorset Press (3rd edition), 1990.

28. Riddle, John M.: *Dioscorides on Pharmacy and Medicine.* Austin, Texas, University of Texas Press, 1985.

29. Augustine, St.: *The City of God.* M. Dods (Trans.). New York, The Modern Library, 1950.

30. Fitzhenry, Robert I. (Ed.): *Barnes and Nobles – Book of Quotations.* Harper and Row Publishers, New York, 1987.

31. Augustine, St.: *The Confessions of St. Augustine.* J.G. Pilkington (Trans.). New York, The Heritage Press, 1963.

32. Carré, Meyrick H.: *Realists and Nominalists.* Oxford University Press, London, 1946.

33. Aquinas, St. Thomas: *Philosophical Tests.* T. Gibby (Ed. and Trans.). New York, Oxford University Press, 1960.

34. Aquinas, St. Thomas: *The Summa Theologica and Summa Contra Gentales.* A.C. Pegis (Ed.). The Modern Library, New York, Random House, Inc., 1948.

35. Brinton, C., Christopher, J.B., and Wolff, R.L.: *A History of Civilization*. 3rd edition, Vols. I & II. Englewood Cliff, New Jersey, Prentice-Hall, Inc., 1967.

36. Cartwright, Frederick F. and Biddiss, Michael D: *Disease and History* (1972). Reprinted in New York by Dorset Press, 1991.

PART FIVE

1. Osler, William: "The Evolution of Modern Medicine – Galen's Written Works." Silliman Foundation. Yale University, New Haven Connecticut, April 1913. Reproduced in *JAMA* 1988;260:318.

2. Cumston, Charles G.: *The History of Medicine* (1926). New York, Dorset Press, 1987.

3. Cartwright, Frederick F. and Biddiss, Michael D: *Disease and History* (1972). Reprinted in New York by Dorset Press, 1991.

4. Herodotus: *The Histories*. A. De Selincourt (Trans.), Penguin Books. Cited by Brinton, Christopher and Wolff: *A History of Civilization*, op.cit.

5. Thucydides: *History of the Peloponnesian War.* T. Hobbs (Trans.) and R. Schlatter (Ed.). New Brunswick, Rutgers University Press, 1975.

6. Friedlander, Walter J.: "On the Obligation of Physicians to Treat AIDS: Is There a Historical Basis?" *Review of Infectious Disea*se 1990;12(2):191-203.

7. Faria, Miguel A., Jr.: "To Treat or Not – Can a Physician Choose?" *The Pharos* 1992;55(1):39-40.

8. Fox, Daniel M.: "The Politics of Physicians' Responsibilities in Epidemics: A Note on History." *Hastings Center Report*. April-May 1988.

9. Council on Ethical and Judicial Affairs: "Ethical Issues Involved in the Growing AIDS Crisis." *JAMA* 1988;259: 1360-1361.

10. American Medical Association: Principles of Medical Ethics – as adopted by the House of Delegates, July 22, 1980.

11. American Association of Neurological Surgeons Code of Ethics, approved May 1987.

12. Edelstein, Ludwig: "The Professional Ethics of the Greek Physician." *Bull Hist Med* 1956;30:391-419.

13. American Medical Association: "U.S. Health Care System Facts on How U.S. Health Care Dollars are Spent." *Advocacy Brief*s, October 1991.

14. "American Survey – Kill or Cure?," *The Economist,* September 25, 1993, p.31-32.

15. Goodgame, Dan: "The Clinton Health Care Plan." *Time* 1993;142(12):54-63.

16. The Health Security Act of 1993.

17. Faria, Miguel A., Jr.: "On Clinton's Health Care Reform Proposal, Further Reflections." *J Med Assoc Ga* 1994;83(1):11-14.

18. Stang, Alan: Quotation cited by R.W. Lee: "A New OSHA Assault," *The New American* 1992;8(26):19-26.

19. Edelstein, Ludwig: "William Osler's Philosophy." *Bull Hist Med* 1946;(20).

20. Osler, William: *The Principles and Practice of Medicine*. 1905.

21. Orient, Jane: "Health Care Crisis: Made in Washington." *AAPS News* 1992;48(8).

22. Bohmfalk, George: "Medical Practice Has Lost Its Glamour." *Am Med New*s, May 12, 1990.

23. Krieger, Gary F.: "How can we stop the Exodus? Physicians giving up and getting out." *Am Med News*, September 1991.

24. Gibbs, Nancy: "Sick and Tired – Doctors and Patients, Image vs. Reality." *Time,* July 31, 1989.

25. Faria, Miguel A., Jr.: "Crisis in Health Care Delivery – Rescuing Medicine from the Clutches of Government."*J Med Assoc Ga* 1992;81(11):615-620.

26. "In Brief, New Survey Shows Lawyers More Dissatisfied," *The New York Times*. Reported by *The Macon Telegraph*, August 17, 1990.

27. Benson, Sam: "My Turn: Why I Quit Practicing Law." *Newsweek,* November 4, 1991.

28. Faria, Miguel A., Jr.: "Enemies of Private Medicine Bide Their Time." *Private Practice* 1992;24(9):33-34.

29. Faria, Miguel A., Jr.: "Doctor Unity Needed to Save Profession." *Am Med News* 1990;33(37).

30. "Nationalized Medicine Worries." *Am Med News*, February 20, 1992.

31. Edelstein, Ludwig: "The Relation of Ancient Philosophy to Medicine." *Bull Hist Med* 1952;26.

32. Aristotle: *On Man in the Universe*. L.R. Loomis (Ed.). Roslyn, New York, Walter J. Block, Inc., 1943.

33. Plato: *Five Great Dialogues*. B. Jowett (Trans.) and L.R. Loomis (Ed.). Roslyn, New York, Walter J. Block, Inc., 1941.

34. Fitzhenry, Robert I. (Ed.): *Barnes and Nobles – Book of Quotations*. Harper and Row Publishers, New York, 1987.

35. Berg, Robert N.: "The Ethical Practice of Medicine." *J Med Assoc Ga* 1990;79(11):863-864.

36. Merriam Webster – Language Master. Franklin Electronic Publishers, Inc., 1991.

37. Helmreich, G.: *Compositiones*. Leipzig, Teubner, 1887. Cited in Edelstein, L: "The Professional Ethics of the Greek Physician," op cit.

38. Galdston, I.: "Humanism and Public Health." *Bull Hist Med* 1940;8:1032.

39. Pellegrino, Edmund D. and Pellegrino, Alice A.: "Humanism and Ethics in Roman Medicine – Translation and Commentary on a Text of Scribonius Largus," in *Literature and Medicine*. D.Heyward Brock and Richard M. Ratzan (Eds.) *Literature and Bioethics* 1988;7:22-38.

40. Suetonius: *The Twelve Caesars*. Robert Graves (Trans.) and Michael Grant (Ed.). Penguin Books, London, 1979.

41. Cicero, Marcus T.: "On Moral Obligations." A New Translation of Cicero's *De Officiis* with Introduction and Notes by John Higginbotham. Berkeley, University of California Press, 1967. Cited by Pellegrino E.D. and Pellegrino A.A.: "Humanism and Ethics in Roman Medicine," op. cit.

42. Amundsen, Darrel W. and Ferngren, Gary B.: "Evolution of the Physician Patient Relationship, Antiquity Through the Renaissance." *The Clinical Encounter*. E. Shelp (Ed.). Dordrecht, Holland: Reidel, 1983.

43. Pellegrino, Edmund D.: "Agape and Ethics: Some Reflections on Medical Morals from a Catholic Christian Perspective." *Catholic Perspective in Medical Morals: Foundational Issues, Philosophy, and Medicine Series*. Dordrecht, Holland: Reidel in press. Quoted by Pellegrino E.D. and Pellegrino A.A. in "Humanism and Ethics in Roman Medicine," op. cit.

44. Hanlon, C. Rollins: "Surgery and the Humanities." *Emory Univ J* 1990;4(4)276-280.

45. Harvey, Douglas and Fehrenbacher, Don E. (Eds.): *The Illustrated Biographical Dictionary*. New York, Dorset Press (3rd edition), 1990.

46. Pellegrino, Edmund D.: *Humanism and the Physician*. University of Tennessee Press, 1979. Cited in C.R. Hanlon: "Surgery and the Humanities," op.cit.

47. Page, Leigh: "Association of American Medical Colleges 14-Year Application Decline May Have Bottomed Out." *Am Med News*, November 17, 1989.

48. Page, Leigh: "Record Number of Medical Students Failing Boards." *Am Med News*, October 26, 1990.

49. Mitgang, L.: "Applications to Medical School Jump Following a Near-Decade of Decline." *The Associated Press*. Reported by *The Macon Telegraph*, March 2, 1991.

50. Kirk, Russell: "Civilization Without Religion?" *Modern Age*, Summer 1990, p.151-156.

51. Muggeridge, Malcolm: "The Great Liberal Death Wish." Quoted by Russell Kirk, op.cit.

52. McGinnis, J. Michael and Foege, William H.: "Actual Causes of Death in the United States." *JAMA* 1993;270(18):2207-2212.

53. Dawson, Christopher: *Religion and Culture* (1949). Cited by Russell Kirk, op.cit.

54. Burke, Edmund: *First Letter on a Regicide Peace* (1796). Cited by Russell Kirk, op.cit.

55. Dickey, L.E.: "Whose Bread I Eat – His Song I Must Sing." *HCA Coliseum Medical Center Newsletter,* Macon, GA., August 9, 1990.

56. Lichter, S. Robert and Rothman, Stanley: "Survey of the Media." *Public Opinion.* American Enterprise Institute for Public Policy Research, October-November 1981. Cited by William A. Rusher in *The Coming Battle for the Media: Curbing the Power of the Media Elite,* op.cit.

57. Irvine, R., Goulden, J. and Kincaid, C.: *The News Manipulators.* Accuracy In Media, Washington, D.C., 1994.

58. Rusher, William A.: *The Coming Battle for the Media: Curbing the Power of the Media Elite.* William Morrow and Company, Inc. New York, 1988.

59. Wilkinson, John D.: "Smoke and Mirrors." *J Med Assoc Ga* 1993;82(11):568.

60. *Physicians Prescription for Georgia – Building A Better State of Health.* Medical Association of Georgia, July 1993.

61. Watt, Clark: "Americans With Disabilities Act: Implications for the Practice of Neurosurgery." *AANS Bulletin,* Fall 1993, p.16-17.

62. Tanner, Michael: *Getting Off the Critical List – A Prescription for Health Care Reform in Georgia.* Georgia Public Policy Foundation, Inc., Atlanta, GA., 1992.

63. Breo, Dennis L.: "Sidney Wolfe, M.D. – Healing the System or Just Raising Hell?" *JAMA* 1991;266(8):1131-1133.

64. Faria, Miguel A., Jr.: "The Data Bank: Why It Should be Abolished." *J Med Assoc Ga* 1991;80(9):477-478.

65. Jaffe, B.M.: "Big Brother is Looking Askance at You." *Surgical Rounds* 1991;183-185.

66. Page, Leigh: "Rocky Start-Up for Fledgling Federal Data Bank." *Am Med News,* December 12, 1991, p.1.

67. Page, Leigh: "Which Malpractice Payouts Need To Be Reported?" *Am Med News,* December 16, 1991, p.9.

68. McCormick, Brian: "House Wants Data Bank Dismantled – Delegates See Bank as Example of Government's Betrayed Trust." *Am Med News,* December 23-30, 1991.

69. Oberman, Linda: "Data Bank Access Debate." *Am Med News,* May 24-31, 1993.

70. Faria, Miguel A., Jr.: "Data Bank Violates Due-Process Rights." *Am Med News,* January 27, 1992.

71. O'Brien, Richard P.: "Data Bank Should Die." *Am Med News,* January 27, 1992.

72. Kravitz, Richard L., Rolph, John E., and McGuigan, Kimberly: "Malpractice Claims Data As a Quality Improvement Tool." *JAMA* 1991;266(15):2087-2098.

73. Gianelli, Diane M.: "Bad Guy Kusserow Will Keep Health Care Focus." *Am Med News,* June 22, 1992.

74. Fishman, Howard: "Will HHS Call Off the Dogs? Or Will Feds Continue to Harass Physicians?" *Private Practice* 1992;24(8):9-14.

75. Schwartz, Harry: "Physicians Have Little Chance Against Anti-Medical Propaganda." *Am Med News,* September 9, 1988.

76. Schwartz, Harry: "Where are M.D.'s who Make $600,000 a Year?" *Am Med News,* February 17, 1989.

77. Schwartz, Harry: "Media's Final Word: Doctors Make Too Much Money." *Am Med News,* June 3, 1991.

78. AAPS News: "AAPS Sues to Open Secret Task-Force Meeting." 49(4): April 1993.

79. Schwartz, Harry: "Is the AMA Headed in the Right Direction?" *Private Practice* 1992;(1):17-21.

80. Oberman, Linda: "AMA Has Record Membership: Looks to Market Share Gains." *Am Med News*, February 22, 1993.

81. AAPS News: "Do Physicians Have Civil Rights?" 42(11): November 1990.

82. AAPS News: "AAPS Challenges Ex Post Facto Law." 46(12): December 1990, *ibid.*

83. AAPS News: "Civil Rights Act Annulled" and "On Euthanasia" 47(11): November 1991, *ibid.*

84. AAPS News: "Are Doctors Like Drug Dealers?" 48(6): June 1992, *ibid.*

85. Oberman, Linda: "Data Bank Access Debate: Any Middle Ground?" *Am Med News*, January 3, 1994.

86. McManus, John F.: "America's Vanishing Liberty – Onerous Federal Regulations are Turning Our Republic into a Dictatorship." *The New American* 1993;9(10):5-8.

87. Perna, John: "Government on the Take – Private Property Falls Victim to Forfeiture Laws." *The New American* 1993;9(11):23-27.

88. Roberts, Paul Craig: Scripps Howard News Service (11/1/93) Reported by AAPS News: "Asset Forfeiture Exceed Losses from Burglary." 1993;49(12):3.

89. AAPS News: May 1992, *ibid.*

90. Schwartz, Harry: "Up Against the Wall – Are Doctors Running Out of Options." *Private Practice* 1993;25(3):13-16.

91. Public Opinion Survey. Commissioned by the Medical Association of Georgia, conducted by Market Fact, Inc.,Chicago, Ill. July 19-26, 1993, and made public in Atlanta, August 24, 1993.

92. Bell, Reuben P.: "Who will Call the Shots in American Medicine's Future?" *Private Practice* 1992;(6):45-57.

93. Kozlov, A.M.: "From the History of the Soviet Medical Oath." *La Sante Publique* 1984;27(2): 141-146.

94. Mises, Ludwig Von: *Socialism: An Economic and Sociological Analysis*. J. Kahone (Trans.). Liberty Classics, Indianapolis, 1981.

95. Jasper, William F.: *Global Tyranny...Step by Step – The United Nations and the Emerging New World Order*. Western Islands Publishers, Appleton, WI., December, 1992.

96. Dennis, Kimberly O.: "Philanthropy and the Free Society." *Imprimis* 1993;22(5), Hillsdale College, Hillsdale, MI.

97. Lifton, Robert J.: *The Nazi Doctors – Medical Killing and the Psychology of Genocide*. Basic Books, Inc., New York, 1986.

98. Scherzer, Anna: "The Holocaust Museum – Lessons for American Medicine." *AAPS*, pamphlet No.1027, January, 1994.

99. Scherzer, Joseph M.: "The Holocaust Memorial, Ayn Rand, and Politics in Pre-Revolutionary New York – Lessons for Today." *AAPS*, pamphlet No.1027, January, 1994.

100. Goodman, John C. and Musgrave Gerald L.: *Patient Power – Solving America's Health Care Crisis*, Cato Institute, Washington, D.C., 1992.

101. Glavin, Matthew J.: "Health Care and a Free Society." *Imprimus* 1993;22(11). Hillsdale College, Hillsdale, MI.

102. Goodman, John C.: "An Agenda for Solving America's Health Care Crisis." National Center for Policy Analysis, Dallas, TX., 1991.

103. Friedman, Milton: "Health Care and Gammon's Law." *Private Practice* 1992;24(2).

104. Moffitt, Robert: "Consumer Choice in Health: Learning From the Federal Employee Health Benefits Program." The Heritage Foundation, Washington, D.C., 1992.

105. Royal, C. Ashley and Alexander, Thomas C: *A Handbook on Georgia Medical Malpractice Law.* The Harrison Company, Norcross, GA., 1991.

106. Olson, Walter K.: *The Litigation Explosion – What Happened When America Unleashed the Lawsuit.* Truman Talley Books, Dutton, New York, 1991.

107. Benatar, S.R.: "Traditional and Evolving Concepts in Medical Ethics." *Medicine and Law* 1989;7:423-426.

108. Moore, Roy E.: "Insurance, Lawyers, and Government have Ruined our Health-Care System." *The Atlanta Constitution*, January 5, 1992.

109. Wills, Robert V.: "Rx for Physicians: Fight Back Before It's Too Late." *Surgical Rounds* 1987;(10):119-125.

110. AAPS News: April, 1991, *ibid.*

111. Letters to the Editor: *Am Med News*, June 29, 1992; July 6 and 13, 1992; and August 17, 1992.

112. Orient, Jane: "Hippocrates, the Constitution, and the Samaritan." *AAPS News*, Banquet Address 43rd Annual Meeting, Bermuda, October 24, 1986.

113. Sade, Robert M.: "The Political Fallacy that Medical Care is a Right." *N Engl J Med*, December 2, 1971, Reprinted by AAPS, 1990.

114. Scott, Otto: "The Gelded." The Chalcedon Report, No.303, October 1990. Reprinted by AAPS, 1990.

115. Durante, Salvatore J.: "The Fallacy and Danger of Public Service." *AAPS,* April 1990.

116. Jaggard, Robert S.: "Which Moral Code Do You Choose." *Iatrofon,* Vol. 7, No. 2., December 1987.

117. Wilson, E.J.: "Deceptive Legislation Produces Involuntary Servitude." *Private Practice*, June 1992.

118. *The Columbia Encyclopedia.* Columbia University Press (1989). Franklin Electronic Publishers, Inc., Mt. Holly, N.Y. 08060, 1991.

119. Thornton, Fr. James: "Lysenkoism is Alive and Well." *The New American* 1993;9(3):31-33.

120. Zirkle, Conway: *Death of a Science* (1949). Cited by Fr. James Thornton in "Lysenkoism in Alive and Well," op. cit.

121. Conquest, Robert: *The Great Terror: A Reassessment.* Oxford University Press, 1992.

122. Dorman, Thomas A.: "It's Called Protection." *Practice Newsletter.* Cited in AAPS News 48(6), June 1992, *ibid.*

123. *The Associated Press*: "Former Soviet dissident testifies Against Party that Persecuted Him." Reported in *The Macon Telegraph*, August 1, 1992.

124. Altman, Lawrence K.: "Experts Ponder Cuban Epidemic." *The New York Times,* May 25, 1993.

125. McGeary, Johanna and Booth, Cathy: "Cuba Alone." *Time* 1993;142(24):42-54.

126. Benoit, Gary: "Castro's Cuba – Correction Please." *The New American* 1993;9(26):42.

127. Faria, Miguel A., Jr.: "Paraguay is a Paradise Compared to Castro's Cuba." *The Macon Telegraph*, February 22, 1989.

128. Valladares, Armando: *Against All Hope: The Prison Memoirs of Armando Valladares.* H. Andrew (Trans.). Ballantine Books, New York, 1986.

129. Faria, Miguel A., Jr.: "Latin Communists – No Idle Threat." *The Macon Telegraph*, August 23, 1987.

130. Lazo, Mario: *American Policy Failures in Cuba – Dagger In The Heart.* Twin Circle Publishing Co. Inc., New York, 1968.

131. U.S. Department of Commerce: "Investment in Cuba, 1956" and "Statistical Abstract of the United States, 1962." Washington, DC., Government Printing Office. Cited in Mario Lazo's *American Policy Failures in Cuba*, op.cit.

132. Draper, Theodore: *Castroism – Theory and Practice.* New York, Frederik A. Praeger, 1965.

133. Hoar, William P.: "The Right Answers." *The New America*n, October 5, 1992.

134. White, Peter T.: "Cuba at a Crossroad." *National Geographic* 1991;180(2):90-121.

135. O'Connor, Anne-Marie: "Cuba Fed Up, Not Taking it Anymore." *Atlanta Constitution,* August 8, 1993.

136. Roberts, Paul Craig: "The Coming Cuban Collapse." *National Review*, June 21, 1993.

137. de Cordoba, Jose: "Survival Tactics – Its Economy Dying, Cuba Seeks Salvation in Dollars – and Exiles." *The Wall Street Jour*nal 1993;222(12):July 19.

138. Makhov, Alexander: "Insights from Moscow." *Moscow News*, Fall 1990. Quoted by *AAPS News*, January 1991.

139. Coffey, Robert J.: "International Perspective: Neurological Surgery in Nicaragua." *Surgical Neurology* 1990;33:356-61.

140. Faria, Miguel A., Jr.: "Rebuttal to Neurosurgery in Nicaragua." *Surgical Neurology* 1990;34:352.

141. "Sandinistas Sufren Pérdida de Popularidad." *El Nuevo Herald* 5A. 16 de Agosto de 1993.

142. Evans-Pritchard, Ambrose: "Nicaragua's Killing Fields." *National Review* 1991;43(7):38-44.

143. "Freedom Fighters." *National Review* 1993;45(4):19-20.

144. Gray, Michael: "3 British Physicians Found Guilty for Roles in Paid Kidney Donations." *Am Med News*, April 29, 1990.

145. Butler, Eamonn: "The National Health Service in the United Kingdom: Model for the United States." *J Med Assoc Ga* 1993;82(12):643-645.

146. "Insurance for Blood Centers Cancelled after AIDS Scandal." *Associated Press*. Reported in *The Macon Telegraph*, August 12, 1992.

147. *The Associated Press*: "Officials to Stand Trial in French AIDS Scandal." Reported in *The Macon Telegraph*, December 20, 1992.

148. "Dr. Gallo says HIV Isolate came from Pasteur Institute Sample." *Am Med News*, June 17, 1991.

149. Munro, Ian R.: "How Not to Improve Health Care." *Reader's Digest*, September 1992.

150. Goodman, William E.: "Health Care in Canada – Face-to-Face with Reality." *J Med Assoc Ga* 1993;82(12):647-649.

151. Spivack, Betty S.: "A.C. Celsus: Roman Medicus." *J Hist Med Allied Sci*, 1991, p.143-157.

152. Pellegrino, Edmund D.: "The Metamorphosis of Medical Ethics" – 30 year Retrospective." *JAMA* 1993;269(9):1158-1162.

153. Emanuel, Ezekiel J. and Emanuel, Linda L.: "Four Models of the Physician-Patient Relationship." *JAMA* 1992;267(16):2221-2226.

154. Hamilton, E. and Cairns, H. (Eds.), Emanuel, Ezekiel J. (Trans.): *Plato – The Collected Dialogues.* Princeton University Press, 1961. Cited in E. J. Emanuel and L. L. Emanuel, "Four Models of the Physician-Patient Relationship," op.cit.

155. Thompson, Ian E.: "The Implications of Medical Ethics." *J Med Ethics* 1976;2:74-82.

156. Senator Jay Rockefeller quoted by AAPS News: "Universal Means Compulsory." 1993;49(12):2.

157. Faria, Miguel A., Jr.: "The Litigation Juggernaut – Part I: The Dimensions of the Devastation." *J Med Assoc Ga* 1993;82(8):393-398.

158. Faria, Miguel A., Jr.: "The Litigation Juggernaut – Part II: Strategies and Tactics for Victory." *J Med Assoc Ga* 1993;82(9):447-451.

PART SIX

1. Duckett, Eleanor S.: *The Gateway to the Middle Ages: Monasticism* (1938). Reprinted in New York by Dorset Press, 1990.

2. *The Columbia Encyclopedia.* Columbia University Press (1989). Franklin Electronic Publishers, Inc., Mt. Holly, N.Y. 08060, 1991.

3. Johnson, Peter C.: "Guy de Chauliac and the Grand Surgery." *Surg Gynecol Obstet* 1989;169(8): 172-176.

4. Ackernecht, E.H.: *A Short History of Medicine.* New York, The Ronald Press Co., 1968. Cited in P.C. Johnson: "Guy de Chauliac and the Grand Surgery," op.cit.

5. Haggard, Howard W.: T*he Doctor in History.* Reprinted in New York by Dorset Press, 1989.

6. Suetonius: *De Vita Caesarum: Julius Caesar – Domitian.* Cited by H.W. Haggard: *The Doctor in History,* op.cit.

7. Hæger, Knut: *The Illustrated History of Surgery.* New York, Bell Publishing Co., 1988.

8. Beeching, Jack: *The Galleys at Lepanto.* Charles Scribner's Sons, New York, 1983.

9. Leonardo, Richard A.: *History of Surgery.* New York, Froben Press, 1943.

10. Cartwright, Frederick F. and Biddiss, Michael D.: *Disease and History* (1972). Reprinted in New York by Dorset Press, 1991.

11. Castiglioni, Arturo: *A History of Medicine.* E.B. Krumbhaar (Trans. and Ed.), New York, 1941.

12. Brinton, C., Christopher, J.B., and Wolff, R.L.: *A History of Civilization.* 3rd edition, Vols. I & II. Englewood Cliff, New Jersey, Prentice-Hall, Inc., 1967.

13. Haggard, Howard W.: *Mystery, Magic and Medicine.* Garden City, New Jersey, Doubleday, 1938.

14. Harvey, Douglas and Fehrenbacher, Don E. (Eds.): *The Illustrated Biographical Dictionary.* New York, Dorset Press (3rd edition), 1990.

15. Bagwell, Charles E.: "Ambroise Paré and the Renaissance of Surgery." *Surg Gynecol Obstet* 1981;152:350-354.

16. Nicaise, E.: *La Grande Chirurgie de Guy de Chauliac.* Paris, 1890. In E. Grant (Ed.): *A Source Book in Medieval Science.* Harvard University Press, 1974. Cited in P.C. Johnson: "Guy de Chauliac and the Grand Surgery," op.cit.

17. Bishop, W.J.: *The Early History of Surgery.* London, Oldbourne, 1962. Cited in P.C. Johnson: "Guy de Chauliac and the Grand Surgery," op.cit.

18. Anson, Berry J.: "The Ear and The Eye in the Collected Works of Ambroise Paré, Renaissance Surgeon to Four Kings of France." *Treatise of the American Academy of Ophthalmology and Otology,* 1970;74:249-277.

19. Whipple, A.O.: "Wound Healing and Wound Repair." Springfield, Illinois, Charles C. Thomas, 1983. Cited in P.C. Johnson: "Guy de Chauliac and the Grand Surgery," op.cit.

20. Cumston, Charles G.: *The History of Medicine* (1926) New York, Dorset Press, 1987.

21. Ferngren, Gary B.: "Early Christianity as a Religion of Healing." *Bull Hist Med* 1992;66(1):1-15.

22. Sigerist, Henry: *Civilization and Disease.* The University of Chicago Press, Chicago, 1943.

23. Amundsen, Darrel W.: "Medicine and Faith in Early Christianity." *Bull Hist Med* 1982;56:326-350.

24. Newman, Art: *The Illustrated Treasury of Medical Curiosa.* New York, McGraw Hill Book Co., 1988.

25. Richardson, Andrea: "Compassion and Cures – A Historical Look at Catholicism and Medicine." *JAMA* 1991;266(21):3063.

26. Jones, C.: "Sisters of Charity and the Ailing Poor." *Soc Hist Med* 1989:339-348.

27. O'Boyle, Cornelius: "Medicine, God, and Aristotle in the Early Universities: Prefatory Prayers in Late Medieval Medical Commentaries." *Bull Hist Med* 1992;66(2):185-209.

28. Amundsen, Darrel W.: "Casuistry and Professional Obligations – The Regulation of Physicians by the Court of Conscience in the Late Middle Ages." *Trans Studies Coll Physician Philadelphia* 1986;3(2):93-112.

29. Amundsen, Darrel W.: "Medical Deontology and Pestilential Disease in the Late Middle Ages." *J Hist Med* 1977;(10):403-421.

30. Campbell, Anna M.: *The Black Death and Men of Learning* (1931). Cited in Darrel W. Amundsen: "Medical Deontology and Pestilential Disease in the Late Middle Ages," op.cit.

31. Lyons, Albert S. and Petrucelli, R. Joseph: *Medicine: An Illustrated History*. New York, Harry N. Abrams, Inc. Publishers, 1978.

32. Quétel, Claude: *History of Syphilis*. J. Braddock and B. Pike (Trans.). The Johns Hopkins University Press, Baltimore, Maryland, 1990.

33. Sigerist, Henry E.: "Bedside Manner in the Middle Ages." *Quarterly Bulletin Northwestern University Medical School* 1946;20:1-8.

34. Veith, Ilza: "Medical Ethics Throughout the Ages." *Quarterly Bulletin Northwestern University Medical School* 1957;31:351-358.

35. Tenery, Robert M., Jr.: "Answer to Question: Do Doctors Really Make Too Much Money?" *Am Med News*, December 13, 1993.

36. Schwartz, Harry: "Physicians Have Little Chance Against Anti-Medical Propaganda." *Am Med News*, September 9, 1988.

37. Schwartz, Harry: "Where are M.D.'s who Make $600,000 a Year?" *Am Med News*, February 17, 1989.

38. Schwartz, Harry: "Media's Final Word: Doctors Make Too Much Money." *Am Med News*, June 3, 1991.

39. Buckley, Jerry and Creighton, Linda L.: "How Doctors Decide Who Shall Live and Who Shall Die." *U.S. News and World Report,* January 22, 1990.

40. Gibbs, Nancy: "Sick and Tired – Doctors and Patients, Image vs. Reality." *Time,* July 31, 1989.

41. Cook, Robin: Quoted by Somerville, Janice: "Greedy Lawyers, Dedicated Doctors, Macabre Medicine." *Am Med News,* March 2, 1990.

42. Wills, Robert V.: "Rx for Physicians: Fight Back Before Its too Late." *Surgical Rounds* 1987;(10):119-125.

43. Olson, Walter K.: *The Litigation Explosion – What Happened When America Unleashed the Lawsuit*. Truman Talley Books, Dutton, New York, 1991.

44. Benson, Sam: "My Turn: Why I Quit Practicing Law." *Newsweek,* November 4, 1991.

45. "In Brief, New Survey Shows Lawyers More Dissatisfied," *The New York Times*. Reported by The Macon Telegraph, August 17, 1990.

46. "Less Litigation, More Justice." *Wall Street Journal*, August 14, 1991.

47. "ABA Won't Open Discipline Records." *The Associated Press*. Reported in *The Macon Telegraph*, February 5, 1992.

48. McCormick, Brian: "Doctors Fighting Back, Taking Lawyers to Court." *Am Med News*, May 11, 1992.

49. "Litigation Abuse is Crippling American Business." *The Macon Telegraph*, July 28, 1992.

50. De Marco, Edward: "Atlanta's Ide Takes on Nation's Legal Woes." *Atlanta Business Chronicle,* October 1-7, 1993.

51. AAPS News: "On Euthanasia." 1991;47(11):4.

52. National Public Radio: "Morning Edition – Dutch Ethicists Comment on Euthanasia in the Netherlands," December 14, 1993.

53. Payne, Robert: *The History of Islam* (1959). Reprinted in New York by Dorset Press, 1990.

54. Severy, Merle: "Iraq the Crucible of Civilization." *National Geographic* 1991;179(5):102-115.

55. Torao, Mozai: "The Lost Fleet of Kublai Khan." *National Geographic* 1982;162(5):634-649.

56. Accardo, Pasquale: "Dante and the Circle of Malpractice." *South Med J* 1989;82:624-628.

57. Spector, Benjamin: *One Hour of Medical History – Selected Excerpts.* Reprinted in *Surgical Neurology* 1990;33:64-73.

58. Faria, Miguel A., Jr.: *The Forging of the Renaissance Physician*: "The Influence of Hippocrates, Galen and the Islamic Physicians" and "The Philosophic Basis for Pre-Renaissance Medical Knowledge." *J Med Assoc Ga* 1992;81(3):119-126.

59. Faria, Miguel A., Jr.: *The Forging of the Renaissance Physician*: "The Physicians and the Period of Rebirth" and "Physicians For All Seasons." *J Med Assoc Ga* 1992;81(4):165-176.

60. Riddle, John M.: *Dioscorides on Pharmacy and Medicine.* Austin, Texas, University of Texas Press, 1985.

61. Bacon, Francis: *Novum Organum.* J. Devey (Ed.). New York, American Home Library, 1902.

62. Bloch, Harry: "Francois Magendie, Claude Bernard and the Interrelation of Science, History, and Philosophy." *South Med J* 1989;82:1259-1261.

PART SEVEN

1. Faria, Miguel A., Jr.: *The Forging of the Renaissance Physician:* "The Influence of Hippocrates, Galen and the Islamic Physicians" and "The Philosophic Basis for Pre-Renaissance Medical Knowledge." *J Med Assoc Ga* 1992;81(3):119-126.

2. Faria, Miguel A., Jr.: *The Forging of the Renaissance Physician*: "The Physician and the Period of Rebirth" and "Physicians for All Seasons." *J Med Assoc Ga* 1992;81(4):165-176.

3. Brinton, C., Christopher, J.B., and Wolff, R.L.: *A History of Civilization.* 3rd edition, Vols. I & II. Englewood Cliff, New Jersey, Prentice-Hall, Inc., 1967.

4. Harvey, Douglas and Fehrenbacher, Don E. (Eds.): *The Illustrated Biographical Dictionary.* New York, Dorset Press (3rd edition), 1990.

5. *The Columbia Encyclopedia.* Columbia University Press (1989). Franklin Electronic Publishers, Inc., Mt. Holly, N.Y. 08060, 1991.

6. Chamberlin, E.R.: *The Bad Popes* (1969). Reprinted in New York by Dorset Press, 1986.

7. Leonardo, Richard A.: *History of Surgery.* New York, Froben Press, 1943.

8. Faria, Miguel A., Jr.: "The Death of Henry II of France." *J Neurosurg* 1992;77:964-969.

9. Stump, Keith W.: *Europe and the Church.* Worldwide Church of God, Pasadena, CA., 1983.

10. Severy, Merle and Stanfield James L.: "The Byzantine Empire – Rome of the East." *National Geographic* 1983;164 (6):708-737.

11. Haggard, Howard W.: *The Doctor in History.* Reprinted in New York by Dorset Press, 1989.

12. Roth, Cecil: *The Spanish Inquisition* (1937). W.W. Norton and Co., New York, 1964.

13. Hroch, Miroslav and Skýbová, Anna: *Ecclesia Militans – The Inquisition.* Janet Fraser (Trans.). New York, Dorset Press, 1988.

14. Hart, Michael H.: *The 100 – A Ranking of the Most Influential Persons in History.* Citadel Press Books, Carol Publishing Group Edition, 1989.

15. Hendrickson, Robert: *The Henry Holt Encyclopedia of Word and Phrase Origins.* Henry Holt and Co., New York, 1987.

16. Roberts, R. S.: "Historical Aspects of Medical Ethics." *Central African Journal of Medicine* 1978;24(10):214-216.

17. Abercrombie, T.J.: "When The Moors Ruled Spain." *National Geographic* 1988;174(1):86-119.

18. Haggard, Howard W.: *Mystery, Magic and Medicine.* Garden City, New Jersey, Doubleday, 1938.

19. Barquin Lopez, Ramón M. and Valdes Jimenez, Roberto: *Cuba – Ayer, Hoy, y Mañana.* Vol. I. Editorial Barval, Puerto Rico, 1968.

20. Sale, Kirkpatrick: *The Conquest of Paradise – Christopher Columbus and the Columbian Legacy*. Penguin Books, Inc., New York, 1991.

21. Clendinnen, Inga: *Aztecs: An Interpretation*. Cambridge, England, Cambridge University Press, 1991. See also the review of this book by Fr. James Thornton: "Aztec Atrocities." *The New American*, May 4, 1992.

22. Jennings, Gary: *Aztec*. Avon Books, The Hearst Corporation, New York, 1980.

23. Diaz del Castillo, Bernal: *The Discovery And Conquest Of Mexico*. Farrar, Straus, and Cudahy Publishers, New York, 1956.

24. Matos-Moctezuma, Edwardo: *The Great Temple Of The Aztecs*. Thames and Hudson Ltd, London, England, 1988.

25. Blacker, Irwin R.: *Prescott's Histories: The Rise and Decline Of The Spanish Empire*. New York, Dorset Press, 1990.

26. Innes, Hammond: *The Conquistadors*. Alfred A. Knopf, Inc., New York, 1969.

27. McDowell, Bart: "The Aztecs." *National Geographic* 1980;158(6):714-752.

28. Schele, Linda and Miller, Mary E.: *The Blood of Kings*. George Braziller, Inc., New York, 1986.

29. De Landa, Fr. Diego: *Yucatan Before And After The Conquest*. Dover Publications, Inc., New York, 1978.

30. LaFay, Howard: "The Maya Children of Time." *National Geographic* 1975;148(6):729-767.

31. Stuart, George E.: "The Maya Riddle of the Glyphs." *National Geographic* 1975;148(6):768-791.

32. Demarest, Arthur A.: "The Violent Saga of a Maya Kingdom." *National Geographic* 1993;183(2):94-111.

33. Lemonick, Michael D.: "Secrets of the Maya." *Time* 1993;142(6):44-50.

34. Cumston, Charles G.: *The History of Medicine* (1926). New York, Dorset Press, 1987.

35. Quétel, Claude: *History of Syphilis*. J. Braddock and B. Pike (Trans.). The Johns Hopkins University Press, Baltimore, Maryland, 1990.

36. Thornton, Fr. James: "Crumbling From Within." *The New American* 1991;7(24):23-29.

37. Prindle, Robert F.: "Disinfection – Yesterday and Today." *Resident and Staff Physicians* 1977;100:1s-11s.

38. Graham, Harvey: Story of Surgery. Cited by A. Singer: "Letter to the Editor." *J Med Assoc Ga* 1991;80:333.

39. Bendiner, Elmer: "From Barbershop to Battlefield – Paré and the Renaissance of Surgery." *Hospital Practice* 1983;(8):193-225.

40. Hæger, Knut: *The Illustrated History of Surgery*. New York, Bell Publishing Co., 1988.

41. Bloch, Harry: "Paracelsus Resolute Renaissance Pioneer." *South Med J* 1986;79:1564-1566.

42. Lyons, Albert S. and Petrucelli, R. Joseph: *Medicine: An Illustrated History*. New York, Harry N. Abrams, Inc. Publishers, 1978.

43. Dolan, John P. and Holmes, George R.: "Some Important Epochs in Medicine." *South Med J* 1984;77(8):1022-1026.

44. Jacobi, J. (Ed.) and Gutterman, N. (Trans.): *Paracelsus: Selected Writings*. New York, Pantheon Books, 1951. Cited by J.P.Dolan and G.R. Holmes: "Some Important Epochs in Medicine," op.cit.

45. Vesalius, Andreas: *De Humani Corporis Fabrica Libri Septem*. Basel, Oporinus, 1543. Reprinted by Saunders, J.B. de C.M. and O'Malley, Charles D.: *The Illustrations From The Works of Andreas Vesalius*. The World Publishing, Co., Cleveland, OH, 1950.

46. Newman, Art: *The Illustrated Treasury of Medical Curiosa*. New York, McGraw Hill Book Co., 1988.

47. Bendiner, Elmer: "Andreas Vesalius: Man of Mystery in Life and Death." *Hospital Practice* 1986;(2):199-234.

48. Silverman, Mark E.: "Andreas Vesalius and De Humani Corporis Fabrica." *Clinical Cardiology* 1991;14:276-279.

49. Spector, Benjamin: *One Hour of Medical History – Selected Excerpts.* Reprinted in *Surgical Neurology* 1990;33:64-73.

50. Bagwell, Charles E.: "Ambroise Paré and the Renaissance of Surgery." *Surg Gynecol Obstet* 1981;152:350-354.

51. Paré, Ambroise: *A Method of Curing Wounds by Gunshot.* W. Hammond (Trans.). London, 1617.

52. Paré, Ambroise: *The Apologie and Treatise.* Geoffrey Keynes (Ed.). The University of Chicago Press, Chicago, 1952.

53. Bloch, Harry: "Ambroise Paré and His Times (1510-1590), Father of Surgery as Art and Science." *South Med J* 1991;84:763-765.

54. Paget, S.: *Ambroise Paré and His Times* (1510-1590). New York, Putnam, 1897. Cited by H. Bloch: "Ambroise Paré and His Times (1510-1590), Father of Surgery as Art and Science," op.cit.

55. Nostradamus, Michel de: *Prophecies.* Basel, 1558. Reproduced in New York by Avenel Books, Crown Publishers, Inc., 1980.

56. Houtzager, H.L.: "Cesarean Section Till the End of the 16th Century." *European Journal of Obstetrics and Gynecology and Reproductive Biology* 1982;13:57-58.

57. Ackerknecht, E.H.: *CIBA Symposia.* CIBA-Geiga Corporation, 1950. Cited by A. Newman: *The Illustrated Treasury of Medical Curiosa,* op.cit.

58. Osler, William: "The Evolution of Modern Medicine – Galen's Written Works." Silliman Foundation. Yale University, New Haven Connecticut, April 1913. Reproduced in *JAMA* 1988;260:318.

59. Norman, Jeremy M. (Ed.): *Morton's Medical Bibliography* (5th edition). Garrison and Morton, Scolar Press. Gower Publishing Co. Printed in Great Britain at the University Press, Cambridge, 1983.

60. Gordon, Everet J.: "William Harvey and the Circulation of the Blood." *South Med J* 1991;84(12):1493-1498.

61. Silverman, Mark E.: "William Harvey and the Discovery of the Circulation of Blood." *Clinical Cardiology* 1985;8:244-246.

62. Miller, Joseph M.: "Copernicus, Medicine, and the Heliocentric Concept." *South Med J* 1983;76:1167-1168.

63. Copernicus, Nicolai: *De Revolutionibus Orbitum Coelestium.* 1543.

64. Sliwinski, M.: "Doctor Copernicus." *World Health* 1973:12-15.

65. Browne, Thomas: *Religio Medici.* MacMillan and Co., London, 1936.

66. Cohen, Daniel: *The Encyclopedia of the Strange.* New York, Dorset Press, 1985.

67. Norbeck, Timothy B.: "Telling the Truth About Rising Health Care Costs." *Private Practice,* February 1990.

68. McGinnis, J. Michael and Foege, William H.: "Actual Cases of Death in the United States." *JAMA* 1993;270(18):2207-2212.

69. Faria, Miguel A., Jr.: "Crisis in Health Care Delivery – Rescuing Medicine from the Clutches of Government." *J Med Assoc Ga* 1992;81(11):615-620.

70. Feinsilber, M.: "Untouchables Are Fair Game For Legislators – Tobacco, Doctors, Guns Are No Longer Safe." *The Associated Press.* Reported in *The Macon Telegraph,* April 3, 1994.

71. Fitzhenry, Robert I. (Ed.): *Barnes and Nobles – Book of Quotations.* Harper and Row Publishers, New York, 1987.

INDEX

SPECIAL RECOGNITION

I would like to take this opportunity to recognize my family, friends, and professional colleagues who through the years have provided me with much support and encouragement in my professional pursuits.

My mother, Clara, my sister, Mercedes Bland, and my cousin, Clara Gómez – for their support and understanding; my love to my son, Miguelito, and my daughter, Elenita – who were so patient and understanding despite the countless hours that research, writing, and preparation of my book took away from them.

My ever-vigilant friends, Rick (and Debbie) Stappenbeck, M.D., and Mrs. Billie Harris, R.N. – for being my eternal comrades-in-arms through the best and the worst of times. Their strong beliefs in conservative principles have never wavered.

My mentors, Ludwig Kempe, M.D. and Russell Blaylock, M.D., for their philosophic influence and for teaching me the value of convictions as well as introducing me to the beautiful art of neurosurgery; Isabel Lockard, Ph.D., for teaching me neuroanatomy.

My high school 20th Century history teacher, Mrs. Gloria Henderson, for instilling in me a love of history; my friends, Don Crone, Ronnie Amick (and Carmen), and the memory of our friend, David Price; Jim (and Linda) Bethea, M.D., John (and Toni) Paylor, M.D., McCrea (and Jan) Ewart, M.D., and my medical school classmates....

My special appreciation to – George T. Tindall, M.D., Professor and Chairman of the Department of Neurosurgery, for teaching me to use the surgical knife and the mighty (purple-editing) pen; and my other great mentors, Roy Bakay, M.D., Alan S. Fleischer, M.D., William (Bill) Moore, M.D., and Mark S. O'Brien, M.D.

My unforgettable friends: Charles Bearden, P.A., Linda Lane, R.N., Sharon Neal, R.N., Olga Duffey, Carol Caughman, R.N., Dan Barrow, M.D., Steve Stranges, M.D., and Mark Artusio, M.D.

My gratitude also goes to my friend, W. Douglas Skelton, M.D., Dean, Mercer University School of Medicine, for providing me a sanctuary when it was most needed, where I could perform my classic research and write undisturbed. To my colleagues at Mercer University School of Medicine, especially Drs. Charles Hockman, David Innes, and Paul D'Amato who made me feel welcomed from the start; and Joe Sam Robinson, Jr., M.D. and Martin L. Dalton, M.D. for their faculty and academic support; and my colleagues and friends at large – Carl Schuessler, M.D., Larry Grant, M.D., John Dean, M.D., Charles Kellum, M.D., Richard Lennington, M.D., Rex Tidwell, M.D., Susan Raybourne, M.D., Peter Holliday, M.D., Harvey Roddenberry, M.D., Charles May, M.D., Rodney Browne, M.D., Maria Bartlett, M.D., Bill Acton, M.D., Cash Stanley, M.D., Kent Kyzar, M.D., Chip Ridley, M.D., Alex Mitchell, M.D., Norman Smith, M.D., Bob Lane, M.D., Gary Prim, M.D., Edwin Slappey, M.D., Sam Shaker, M.D., Steve Noller, M.D., David Plaxico, M.D., Winston Wilfong, M.D., William Birdsong, M.D., Louis Wexler, M.D., Fernando (and Renee) Hernandez, M.D., and many other fellow physicians still in the trenches – I can not name them all.

My gratitude goes to the best hospital administrators that I have ever known, Mr. Charles Neal, and his successor at HCA Coliseum Medical Centers, Mr. Michael Boggs; and the Officers of the Bibb County Medical Society; and Milton Johnson, M.D. (for his unwavering moral support).

My thanks also go to two friends who also happen to be two of the most ethical attorneys I have ever known, C. Ashley Royal and John Draughon – who have always been there to give me legal advice.

And my thanks also go to my friend and advisor, James O. Taylor, for his wise perspective and advice.

My gratitude is also extended to my friends at Accuracy In Media (AIM), Mr. Reed Irvine and Mr. Joseph Goulden, for an enlightening trip to El Salvador which, I am now certain, contributed to the final peaceful resolution of a longstanding conflict by bringing forth the truth – and for fighting pervasive liberal media bias and leftist disinformation.

My thanks to the leadership of the Medical Association of Georgia (MAG) for appointing me editor of the *Journal* – a job I cherish; and to the membership and staff, particularly Mr. Paul Shanor, Executive Director, for their overwhelming support.

My thanks are also extended to the new wave of medical warriors: Billie L. Jackson, M.D., John D. Wilkinson, M.D., and the members of the Editorial Board of the *Journal,* who along with others (too many to mention), have contributed in their own special way – to fight and repel the onslaught of the hordes of modern-day Vandals battering at the gates of the House of Medicine.

COLOPHON

This edition of *Vandals at the Gates of Medicine*
is produced solely by Hacienda Publishing, Inc., Macon, Georgia, USA.

The design and production coordination of the book is
by Hank Richardson, Chameleon, Inc., Atlanta, Georgia, USA.
Special design assistance is by Corinne Cox, Chameleon, Inc., Atlanta, Georgia, USA.

Special editorial assistance of the book is by
Susan T. Johnson, Managing Editor, *Journal of the Medical Association of Georgia*
Atlanta, Georgia, USA.

Typography by Graphic Center, Atlanta, Georgia, USA.

The type face is Adobe Systems, Inc., Times New Roman.
The design and production were done on Apple™ Macintosh.

The printing is done by offset lithography on Georgia Pacific offset
by Ovid-Bell Press, Fulton, Missouri, USA.